PRECIS

AN UPDATE IN OBSTETRICS AND GYNECOLOGY

Gynecology

Fourth Edition

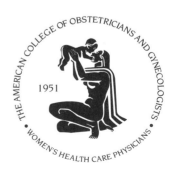

Precis: An Update in Obstetrics and Gynecology represents the knowledge and experience of experts in the field and does not necessarily reflect policy of the American College of Obstetricians and Gynecologists (the College). This publication describes methods and techniques of clinical practice that are accepted and used by recognized authorities. The recommendations do not dictate an exclusive course of treatment or of practice. Variations taking into account the needs of the individual patient, resources, and limitations unique to the institution or type of practice may be appropriate.

Medicine is an ever-changing field. As new research and clinical experience emerge, changes in treatment and drug therapy are required. Every effort has been made to ensure that the drug dosage schedules contained herein are accurate and in accordance with standards accepted at the time of publication. Readers are advised, however, to check the product information literature of each drug they plan to administer to be certain that there have been no changes in the dosage recommended or in the contraindications for administration. This recommendation is of particular importance for new or infrequently used drugs.

Lists of web sites provided in this volume were prepared by the College Resource Center librarians and are provided for information only. Referral to these web sites does not imply College endorsement. The lists are not meant to be comprehensive; the exclusion of a web site does not reflect the quality of that site. Please note that web sites and URLs are subject to change. Web sites were verified on December 7, 2010.

Library of Congress Cataloging-in-Publication Data

Precis : an update in obstetrics and gynecology. Gynecology. -- 4th ed.
    p. ; cm.
  Precis. Gynecology
  Gynecology
  Includes bibliographical references and index.
  ISBN 978-1-934984-05-5
  1. Gynecology--Outlines, syllabi, etc. 2. Obstetrics--Outlines, syllabi, etc. I. American College of Obstetricians and Gynecologists. II. Title: Precis. Gynecology. III. Title: Gynecology.
  [DNLM: 1. Genital Diseases, Female. WP 140]
  RG112.P74 2011
  618.1--dc22
2010046938

The American College of Obstetricians and Gynecologists
409 12th Street, SW
PO Box 96920
Washington, DC 20090-6920
www.acog.org

CONTENTS

CONTRIBUTORS   v

PREFACE   vii

Introduction   1

Hysteroscopy and Other Transcervical Procedures   3
Howard T. Sharp

Laparoscopy   8
Anthony A. Luciano, Rachel LaMonica, and Danielle E. Luciano

Gynecologic Imaging   17
Daniel M. Breitkopf

Cervical Cytology and Cervical Intraepithelial Neoplasia   26
Mark Spitzer

Perioperative Care   39
Thomas E. Snyder

Benign Disorders of the Vulva   55
Colleen K. Stockdale and Lori A. Boardman

Vulvovaginitis   67
Rudolph P. Galask and Diane Elas

Pelvic Support Defects   78
Amy J. Park and Peter L. Rosenblatt

Surgical Management of Incontinence   97
Cheryl B. Iglesia

Management of Uterine Leiomyomas   104
Deborah S. Lyon

First-Trimester Management of Nonviable Pregnancy   108
Charles Ascher-Walsh and Terri-Ann Samuels

Management of Ovarian Cysts and Adnexal Masses   117
Richard G. Moore and Shannon MacLaughlan

Recognition and Management of Surgical Injuries   124
Fidel A. Valea

Postoperative Complications   132
Daniel L. Clarke-Pearson

Surgical Site Infections   140
David A. Eschenbach

Sterilization   147
Amy J. Voedisch and Paul D. Blumenthal

Pregnancy Termination   157
Anitra Beasley, Ana Cepin, and Carolyn Westhoff

Chronic Pelvic Pain   164
Roger P. Smith

Benign Breast Disease   171
Catherine Takacs Witkop

Pediatric Gynecology   178
Samantha Schon and Diane F. Merritt

APPENDIX. INFORMATION RESOURCES   183

INDEX   187

CONTRIBUTORS

EDITORIAL TASK FORCE

Thomas E. Snyder, MD, Chair

John F. Greene Jr, MD, Chair

Deborah S. Lyon, MD

Christine Ann LaSala, MD

Joseph M. Montella, MD

Martin Larry Gimovsky, MD

Abbey Belina Berenson, MD

ADVISORY COMMITTEE

Donald R. Coustan, MD, Chair

Jonathan Berek, MD

Roger P. Smith, MD

AUTHORS

Charles Ascher-Walsh, MD, MS

Anitra Beasley, MD

Paul D. Blumenthal, MD, MPH

Lori A. Boardman, MD, ScM

Daniel M. Breitkopf, MD

Ana Cepin, MD

Daniel L. Clarke-Pearson, MD

Diane Elas, ARNP

David A. Eschenbach, MD

Rudolph P. Galask, MD

Cheryl B. Iglesia, MD

Rachel LaMonica, MD

Anthony A. Luciano, MD

Danielle E. Luciano, MD

Deborah S. Lyon, MD

Shannon MacLaughlan, MD

Diane F. Merritt, MD

Richard G. Moore, MD

Amy J. Park, MD

Peter L. Rosenblatt, MD

Terri-Ann Samuels, MD, MS

Samantha Schon, MD

Howard T. Sharp, MD

Roger P. Smith, MD

Thomas E. Snyder, MD

Mark Spitzer, MD

Colleen K. Stockdale, MD, MS

Fidel A. Valea, MD

Amy J. Voedisch, MD

Carolyn Westhoff, MD, MSc

Catherine Takacs Witkop, MD, MPH

STAFF

Sterling Williams, MD, MS
Vice President for Education

Thomas Dineen
Senior Director of Publications

Deirdre Allen, MPS
Editorial Director

Nikoleta Dineen, MA
Senior Editor

Mark D. Grazette
Senior Graphic Designer

PREFACE

Education is a lifelong process. In no field is this process more important than in medicine. As scientific advances unfold, new techniques and technologies emerge, knowledge expands, and the art and science of medicine undergo dynamic change. Progress in medicine is ongoing, and so too must be the continuing medical education of those who practice it.

Precis: An Update in Obstetrics and Gynecology is intended to meet the continuing education needs of obstetricians and gynecologists. It is a broad, yet concise, overview of information relevant to the specialty. As in earlier editions, the emphasis is on innovations in clinical practice, presented within the context of traditional approaches that retain their applicability to patient care.

Precis is an educational resource to be used in preparation for the cognitive assessment of clinical knowledge, regardless of the form of the assessment—formal or informal, structured or independent. It is one of the recognized vehicles useful in preparing for certification and accreditation processes, and it is designed to complement those evaluations while serving as a general review of the field.

Each year, one volume of this five-volume set is revised. This process provides continual updates that are critical to the practice of obstetrics and gynecology, and it echoes the dynamic nature of the field. The focus is on new and emerging techniques, presented from a balanced perspective of clinical value and cost-effectiveness in practice. Hence, discussion of traditional medical practice is limited. The information has been organized to unify coverage of topics into a single volume so that each volume can stand on its own merit.

This fourth edition of *Precis: Gynecology* reflects current thinking on optimal practice. The information is intended to be a useful tool to assist practicing obstetrician–gynecologists in maintaining current knowledge in a rapidly changing field and to prepare them better for the role of women's health care physicians.

Some information from the previous edition continues to be of value and, thus, has been retained and woven into the new structure. The efforts of authors contributing to previous editions, as well as the work of those authors providing new material, must be recognized with gratitude. Collectively, they represent the expertise of the specialty. With such a breadth of representation, differences of opinion are inevitable and have been respected.

Other *Precis* volumes are *Obstetrics*, Fourth Edition; *Primary and Preventive Care*, Fourth Edition; *Oncology*, Third Edition; and *Reproductive Endocrinology*, Third Edition. Each is an educational tool for review, reference, and evaluation. Precis establishes a broad scientific basis for the delivery of quality health care for women. Rather than being a statement of the American College of Obstetricians and Gynecologists (the College) policy, Precis serves as an intellectual approach to education. An effort has been made, however, to achieve consistency within Precis and with other College recommendations. Variations in patient care, based on individual needs and resources, are encouraged as an integral part of the practice of medicine.

—THE EDITORS

PRECIS

AN UPDATE IN OBSTETRICS AND GYNECOLOGY

Gynecology

Fourth Edition

Introduction

The editors of *Precis: Gynecology*, Fourth Edition, are excited to present an up-to-date review of a variety of topics in gynecology. Our goal is to provide a succinct presentation of the most recent developments in gynecology for the practicing obstetrician–gynecologist. We have solicited the input of authors with significant expertise in their topic areas and used the most current publications as references.

Highlights of the new edition include discussions of technologic advances in areas, such as robotic surgery and hysteroscopy. The section on cervical cytology and cervical intraepithelial neoplasia has been completely revised to provide the clinician with the latest recommendations for management of cytologic abnormalities and cervical intraepithelial neoplasia, especially in the adolescent patient. The section on perioperative care has been updated with the latest information on the use of β-blocker therapy, bowel preparation, and prophylaxis of deep vein thrombosis. Other areas where new guidelines have emerged also have been updated, such as the sections on recognition and management of surgical injuries and antibiotic prophylaxis. The resulting text is comprehensive and easy to read. In addition, algorithms and illustrations have been included where relevant.

The members of the Editorial Task Force and Advisory Committee as well as other selected individuals have reviewed the content to ensure that the information is accurate, complete, and current. During this review, every effort was made to ensure consistency with guidelines of the American College of Obstetricians and Gynecologists and to identify emerging areas of gynecology. As further advances unfold, physicians are urged to consult current recommendations.

—THOMAS E. SNYDER, MD
Chair, Editorial Task Force

—JOHN F. GREENE JR, MD
Chair, Editorial Task Force

Hysteroscopy and Other Transcervical Procedures

Howard T. Sharp

Visual examination of the uterine cavity can be performed with an endoscope by distending the uterine cavity with either a liquid or carbon dioxide gas. Whereas hysterosalpingography and ultrasonography allow indirect evaluation of the uterine cavity's contour, endoscopy offers the ability to diagnose and treat intrauterine abnormalities directly. In addition, new transcervical therapies are being introduced as alternatives to hysteroscopic procedures.

Hysteroscopy

Equipment

Hysteroscopes are available in a variety of designs, with sheaths of various outer diameters. Hysteroscopes with small-caliber sheaths generally are used for diagnostic evaluation, whereas hysteroscopes with sheaths of larger outer diameters are used for therapeutic purposes.

Rigid, diagnostic hysteroscopes consist of two components: 1) an outer sheath, generally between 2.7 mm and 5 mm in diameter with a single port for instillation of a distending medium, and 2) a central telescope with varying view angles (0, 12, 15, 30, and 70 degrees). Continuous-flow hysteroscopes consist of three elements: 1) fluid inflow sheath, 2) outer fluid return sheath, and 3) telescope. These typically have a 4–6-mm outer diameter and also can be used in the office setting for diagnosis and performance of minor therapeutic procedures. A small operating channel may allow for biopsy and other minor surgical procedures.

Operative hysteroscopes are larger (outer diameter of 7–10 mm) and include a 4-mm scope as well as a retractable handle or working element. The working element can be fitted with electrosurgical tips (eg, loops, vaporizing tips, and rollerballs), lasers, or scissors. Flexible hysteroscopes range in diameter from 2.7 mm to 5 mm and have a bendable tip (up to 160 degrees). Most hysteroscopes contain an operating channel for biopsy or fallopian tube catheterization.

Role in Gynecologic Practice

A number of tests are available for the evaluation of the uterine lining, including transvaginal ultrasonography, hysterosalpingography, sonohysterography, and hysteroscopy. As a diagnostic tool, hysteroscopy is considered the standard procedure in the evaluation of structural abnormalities, such as endometrial polyps and submucosal leiomyomas. The benefits of diagnostic hysteroscopy compared with other diagnostic procedures should be weighed against the small risk of complications.

Studies have shown sonohysterography to have a similar diagnostic accuracy for diagnosing submucosal leiomyomas compared with hysteroscopy, whereas transvaginal ultrasonography may be less sensitive (60–77%) and specific (69%) (1). In the evaluation of congenital anomalies, sonohysterography has been shown to be superior to hysteroscopy (2). Before surgical resection of endometrial polyps or submucosal leiomyomas, office diagnostic hysteroscopy or hysterosalpingography should be considered.

Hysteroscopy permits a systematic exploration of the cervical canal and uterine cavity. It provides the opportunity to detect most pathologic conditions of these areas, including the uterotubal junctions. Indications for diagnostic use of this technique are as follows:

- Endocervical canal lesions
- Suspected endometrial polyps
- Suspected submucosal leiomyomas
- Intrauterine foreign bodies
- Uterine anomalies
- Intrauterine adhesions
- Evaluation of the endometrium
- Evaluation of the tubal ostia

Office Hysteroscopy

The use of small-caliber hysteroscopes (less than 5 mm in outer diameter) facilitates office hysteroscopy. Because cervical dilation usually is not necessary, the procedure can be performed in the office setting under local or no anesthesia for a relatively quick, easy, and safe hysteroscopic evaluation.

The main use for hysteroscopy in the office is the evaluation of abnormal uterine bleeding to rule out intracavitary pathology. Two different methods can be used to distend the uterine cavity. The first is carbon dioxide gas insufflation using hysteroflators that calibrate the flow of the gas. Carbon dioxide (CO_2) gas flow should be limited to 100 mL/min with intrauterine pressures less than 100 mm Hg. This method is used particularly with rigid endoscopes that have a single unidirectional channel for introduction of the gas. The second method of uterine distention uses low-viscosity fluids with a continuous-flow hysteroscope, now available in a small-caliber design. This method permits the washing of the uterine cavity should any debris, blood, or blood clots be present. Additionally, it permits minor manipulations of the hysteroscope within the uterine cavity, such as for removal of misplaced intrauterine devices (IUDs) and small (less than 1-cm) polyps or pedunculated leiomyomas. To facilitate the performance of minor procedures in the office, vaporizing electrodes have been introduced that involve less cumbersome manipulation.

Hysteroscopy is useful in the selective evaluation of infertile patients with abnormal hysterosalpingography results, but its routine use in infertile patients is not warranted. Hysterosalpingography remains the best screening method for evaluating both the uterine cavity and the fallopian tubes in these patients.

Surgical Procedures

Although hysteroscopy originally was developed for diagnosis, it has evolved into a tool for treatment. Lesions that are abnormal or suspected of being abnormal can be biopsied, and pathologic conditions can be treated. The therapeutic applications of operative hysteroscopy include the following conditions and procedures:

- Endometrial polyps
- Submucosal leiomyomas
- Uterine septa
- Intrauterine foreign bodies (including misplaced IUDs)
- Intrauterine adhesions
- Menorrhagia (endometrial ablation)
- Treatment of tubal occlusion
- Tubal occlusion for sterilization

The operative hysteroscope or resectoscope is useful in the systematic resection of submucosal leiomyomas, particularly sessile submucosal leiomyomas with an intramural component but also pedunculated submucosal leiomyomas. Selective ultrasound mapping of sessile submucosal leiomyomas that penetrate the uterine wall is useful to determine both the extent of uterine wall penetration and the configuration of the leiomyomas. In this way, the feasibility of complete removal can be evaluated and uterine perforation avoided. Sonohysterography may be required to allow appropriate mapping of these leiomyomas (3).

Endometrial ablation was initially performed by way of a resectoscopic technique, which involved the use of a monopolar electrode in the form of a loop or rollerball to resect or ablate the endometrium respectively, or by using a bare laser fiber threaded through the operative channel (4). When rollerball endometrial abla-

tion is chosen, it is important to thin the endometrium preoperatively using a hormone, such as a gonadotropin-releasing hormone agonist or danazol, or by performing a suction curettage at the time of surgery (5). Preoperative thinning of the endometrium not only permits complete destruction of the endometrium by coagulation but also allows the coagulating energy to penetrate the superficial portion of the myometrium (6).

Some hysteroscopic procedures, such as uterine septum resection and lysis of intrauterine synechiae, often are performed with the concomitant use of laparoscopy; however, ultrasonography by an experienced practitioner can be considered an alternative to laparoscopy.

Currently, two devices have been approved by the U.S. Food and Drug Administration (FDA) for hysteroscopic sterilization. The first system (Essure) gained approval in 2002. This system uses a nickel titanium outer coil and a stainless steel inner coil wrapped around polyethylene terephthalate fibers as a "microinsert" to be placed into the proximal fallopian tube under hysteroscopic visualization. The other system (Adiana) was approved by the FDA in 2009. This system initially applies bipolar radiofrequency within the proximal fallopian tube and subsequently, a silicone "matrix" is placed within the treated proximal tube. Both systems rely on tissue in-growth to ultimately achieve fallopian tube occlusion. The procedure requires a confirmatory hysterosalpingography result 3 months after the placement to document bilateral occlusion. The phase III trial of the microinsert documented that 8% of women had persistent patency at 3 months (7). The matrix was shown to have similar patency rates at 3 months (8). These tubal sterilization methods should not be used in conjunction with endometrial ablation because intrauterine scarring may significantly interfere with the ability of hysterosalpingography to assess fallopian tube patency. For more details on hysteroscopic sterilization, see the section on "Sterilization."

Contraindications

Hysteroscopy should not be performed in the presence of certain conditions. It should not be performed in patients with pelvic inflammatory disease, endomyometritis, known early pregnancy, or known carcinoma of the endometrium.

Nonresectoscopic Methods of Global Endometrial Ablation

Several new methods of endometrial ablation have been developed that do not require direct visualization or the use of a resectoscope. These methods systematically destroy the endometrium using nonhysteroscopic, computerized energy delivery systems to avoid fluid overload syndrome and the subjective variables involved in performing these procedures manually. Currently, the FDA has approved five global ablation procedures: 1) balloon thermal ablation, 2) cryoablation, 3) thermal fluid ablation, 4) radiofrequency ablation, and 5) microwave ablation (9).

Balloon thermal ablation involves the use of a balloon that is inserted in the uterine cavity and inflated with fluid heated to 87°C to accomplish endometrial destruction in 8 minutes. The approved balloon thermal ablation system was designed to be used in uterine cavities between 6 cm and 10 cm in length. Safety features include monitoring of intraballoon pressure and volume as well as a temperature cutoff.

Cryoablation is performed by placing a 6-mm cryoprobe into the endometrial cavity to create a temperature of –120°C at the tip, creating an ice ball. The method requires two applications (each cornu) with the cryoprobe with a treatment time of 10–12 minutes. It is designed for use on endometrial cavities up to 10 cm in length. Ultrasound guidance is used to verify placement of the cryoprobe into the endometrial cavity and subsequent ice ball formation.

Thermal fluid ablation is a global ablation method that uses diagnostic hysteroscopy for visualization of the endometrial cavity while heated saline (90°C) is instilled into the endometrial cavity through a 7-mm sheath for a treatment time of 10 minutes. It is designed for use in uterine cavities between 6 cm and 10.5 cm in length with submucosal leiomyomas up to 4 cm. As a precaution heated fluid is circulated into the endometrium at a low pressure (less than 55 mm Hg) to avoid fluid loss through the fallopian tubes. Other safety features include the use of concomitant diagnostic hysteroscopy for direct visualization of the endometrium and an automatic fluid shut off system if more than 10 mL of fluid loss occurs. Initially, nonheated saline is circulated to test for leakage.

Radiofrequency ablation involves the use of an 8-mm bipolar device that is inserted into the endometrial cavity for coagulation and desiccation of the endometrium and superficial myometrium. As tissue destruction proceeds, tissue impedance increases. When the impedance at the tissue interface reaches 50 ohms, or if the procedure lasts 2 minutes, the procedure is terminated. The average treatment time is 90 seconds. The device is designed to treat uterine cavities between 4 cm and 6.5 cm (this measurement excludes the length of the cervix).

Microwave ablation uses microwave energy to ablate the endometrium. With this technique, microwave power at a frequency of 9.2 GHz is applied to the lining of the uterus to achieve a layer of tissue destruction to 3 mm at temperatures usually between 70°C and 80°C. A treatment time of 3–4 minutes is typical. Patients whose uterine cavities have lengths of 6–14 cm and those with leiomyomas of 3 cm or less and polyps may

be treated. Temperature and power indications are displayed graphically in real time on a monitor. Safety features, such as warnings and cutoff devices, are incorporated into the system.

Satisfaction rates are uniformly high, ranging from 85% to 92%. However, on an intention-to-treat basis, amenorrhea rates from randomized clinical trials vary significantly from 13% to 55%.

Appropriate selection and preparation of patients are critical factors in predicting success. Patients with dysfunctional uterine bleeding not amenable to hormonal or pharmacologic treatment are the best candidates, and others with organic pathologies should be evaluated carefully and counseled for alternative methods of treatment.

Complications

Uterine Perforation

Perforation occurs most often when uterine sounding is used to determine the depth of the uterine cavity or during cervical dilation. Because these procedures are not necessary during diagnostic hysteroscopy, perforation is rare. When operative hysteroscopy is performed, cervical dilation usually is necessary; however, uterine perforation can be avoided by advancing the dilators carefully through only the internal cervical os, without touching the uterine wall. Uterine perforation with a hysteroscope may occur, but it can be avoided by the introduction of the endoscope under direct vision. When there is no panoramic view in front of the hysteroscope, the instrument should not be advanced, particularly when resistance is encountered and the view becomes blurred.

Uterine perforation also can occur during resection of leiomyomas, and care should be taken to discontinue the resection when the surface is level with the uterine wall. The procedure should be terminated if the natural uterine contractions do not force the remaining portion of the leiomyoma to protrude. Preoperative ultrasound mapping of the leiomyoma may warn the physician of its proximity to the serosal surface.

When dividing a uterine septum, the uterine fundal configuration should not be concave but rather should be somewhat convex, which is the normal anatomy of the uterine cavity. Laparoscopy, with a decreased or dimmed light, may be used in conjunction with a hysteroscopic procedure to help avoid perforation. The uniform translucency through the uterine wall produced by the lighted hysteroscope helps the operator determine the limit of resection.

When intrauterine adhesions are extensive and thick, laparoscopy is useful in detecting early damage to the uterine wall during dissection. When endometrial resection with the cutting loop is performed, extreme care should be exercised in shaving only the superficial portion of the myometrium and avoiding the cornual regions, where the uterine wall is thinnest. The cornual areas should be treated by coagulation with a rollerball rather than by resection. When the rollerball electrode is used for endometrial ablation, care should be taken to activate the electrode only while it is moving to prevent extensive transmural necrosis and perforation.

Because of the scatter of fiberoptic lasers and the small diameter of the fibers used, care should be taken to prevent deep uterine penetration and perforation. The energy source should not be activated when neither an electrode nor laser fiber is in full view of the operator.

Bleeding

Bleeding can occur after operative hysteroscopy, particularly if the myometrial wall is entered. Bleeding from a diagnostic hysteroscopy is unusual, and although spotting may occur, it is usually brief and self-limited. When bleeding occurs after operative hysteroscopy, it may be due to division of a uterine septum too close to the uterine wall near the vascular arches; this bleeding may be controlled by selective coagulation. Bleeding also can occur if a submucosal leiomyoma is not completely removed. Occasionally, bleeding may ensue if an endometrial resection is performed too deep in the myometrium. When bleeding cannot be controlled by selective coagulation or when it occurs after the patient has left the operating suite, an intrauterine Foley catheter may be useful for temporary tamponade of the bleeding. A pediatric Foley catheter (no. 8) with a trimmed tip is introduced into the uterus and inflated with 3–4 mL of saline. Tamponade of 12–24 hours usually is sufficient to control the bleeding, and the catheter may then be removed.

Fluid Management

Contemporary operative hysteroscopy usually involves the use of a low-viscosity distending medium; however, high-viscosity fluids also may be used. The high-viscosity fluid used is a high-molecular-weight dextran, which provides good visualization because of its transparency and high refractory index. Because of its viscosity, the fluid does not mix easily with blood, which permits visualization even if a small amount of bleeding occurs during the procedure. However, because it is a hyperosmotic substance, it attracts fluids and can cause fluid overload and noncardiac pulmonary edema if a significant amount enters the intravascular compartment. Additionally, it may cause an anaphylactic reaction and alter clotting factors, producing secondary bleeding (10).

Because a highly viscous solution cannot be easily retrieved once injected through the hysteroscope, there is danger of intravasation with either increased volume or pressure. Therefore, the total volume of the fluid used in hysteroscopy should not exceed 500 mL, and the patient should be observed carefully for signs of decompensation if more than 300 mL is absorbed.

Low-viscosity fluids used for hysteroscopy may contain electrolytes (particularly sodium) or be devoid of electrolytes. With mechanical instruments or laser energy, only fluids containing electrolytes, such as normal saline, 5% dextrose in half-normal saline, or lactated Ringer's solution, should be used. All these fluids offer similar visual properties. Normal plasma osmolality is maintained with sodium, even if considerable absorption occurs. Pulmonary edema can occur, but it is much less common than with the use of high-viscosity fluids. If a deficit of 2,500 mL has occurred with a low-viscosity electrolytic fluid, the procedure should be concluded promptly. Electrolytes should be assessed and use of diuretics considered.

Electrolyte-free solutions, such as 1.5% glycine, 3% sorbitol, and 5% mannitol, are required when electrosurgery is used in the uterus. It is important to measure carefully the fluid inflow and outflow to determine the deficit of fluid not recovered. Guidelines for fluid monitoring have been published (11) and adopted by the American College of Obstetricians and Gynecologists (12). It is recommended that a 750 mL deficit implies excessive intravasation, and the fluid deficit should be monitored at an extremely close interval. In older patients and patients with comorbid medical conditions, consideration should be given to immediate termination of the procedure. Depending on the size of the patient and other factors, a fluid deficit of 1,000–1,500 mL, should warrant prompt conclusion of the surgery. The patient should be assessed for fluid overload syndrome.

One of the difficulties in estimating fluid input and output is that 3 L bags may be overfilled by up to 5–10%. Thus, if 10 L of fluid are used, it could be possible to have a balanced input and output on paper but actually have 1,000 mL of intravasation. Newer methods of fluid collection based on fluid weight have made the estimation of fluid balance easier; however, these systems may not be available in all settings. An alternative method of evaluating the patient's serum sodium level is to obtain a venous blood sample for blood gas analysis at frequent intervals. This is available at most hospitals and can be analyzed within minutes. These complications of operative hysteroscopy are most common during prolonged removal of submucosal leiomyomas or extensive destruction of tissue during endometrial resection or ablation (13).

Embolism

A gas embolization may occur when gas is used to distend the uterine cavity (14). The conscious patient may report chest pain or dyspnea. In the anesthetized patient, cardiopulmonary status may show sudden hypotension, a decrease in oxygenation and end tidal CO_2, or both. A "mill wheel" type of cardiac murmur may be detected and other signs of cardiopulmonary collapse may be present. If a gas embolism is suspected, immediate resuscitative measures are necessary. The patient should be placed on her left side, oxygen should be administered, and direct percutaneous cardiac aspiration of gas should be performed. Air embolization can occur through open uterine venous channels and sinuses. Thus, excessive use of the Trendelenburg position should be avoided, and hysteroscopic or resectoscopic cannulas should not be left in the uterus while obturators, electrodes, or telescopes are removed. Treatment measures for room air embolism are similar to those for CO_2 embolism.

References

1. Farquhar C, Ekeroma A, Furness S, Arroll B. A systematic review of transvaginal ultrasonography, sonohysterography and hysteroscopy for the investigation of abnormal uterine bleeding in premenopausal women. Acta Obstet Gynecol Scand 2003;82:493–504.

2. Soares SR, Barbosa dos Reis MM, Camargos AF. Diagnostic accuracy of sonohysterography, transvaginal sonography, and hysterosalpingography in patients with uterine cavity diseases. Fertil Steril 2000;73:406–11.

3. Cohen LS, Valle RF. Role of vaginal sonography and hysterosonography in the endoscopic treatment of uterine myomas. Fertil Steril 2000;73:197–204.

4. O'Connor H, Magos A. Endometrial resection for the treatment of menorrhagia. N Engl J Med 1996;335:151–6.

5. Romer T, Schmidt T, Foth D. Pre- and postoperative hormonal treatment in patients with hysteroscopic surgery. Contrib Gynecol Obstet 2000;20:1–12.

6. Valle RF. Endometrial ablation for dysfunctional uterine bleeding: role of GNRH agonists. Int J Gynaecol Obstet 1993;41:3–15.

7. Cooper JM, Carnigan CS, Cher D, Kerin JF. Microinsert nonincisional hysteroscopic sterilization. Selective Tubal Occlusion Procedure 2000 Investigators Group. Obstet Gynecol 2003;102:59–67.

8. Vancaille TG, Anderson TL, Johns DA. A 12-month prospective evaluation of transcervical sterilization using implantable polymer matrices. Obstet Gynecol 2008;112:1270-7.

9. Sharp HT. Assessment of new technology in the treatment of idiopathic menorrhagia and uterine leiomyomata. Obstet Gynecol 2006;108:990–1003.

10. Witz CA, Silverberg KM, Burns WN, Shenken RS, Olive DL. Complications associated with the absorption of hysteroscopic fluid media. Fertil Steril 1993;60:745–56.

11. Loffer FD, Bradley LD, Brill AI, Brooks PG, Cooper JM. Hysteroscopic fluid monitoring guidelines. The ad hoc committee on hysteroscopic training guidelines of the American Association of Gynecologic Laparoscopists. J Am Assoc Gynecol Laparosc 2000;7:167–8.

12. Hysteroscopy. ACOG Technology Assessment No. 4. American College of Obstetricians and Gynecologists. Obstet Gynecol 2005;106:439–42.

13. Istre O, Bjoennes J, Naess R, Hornbaek K, Forman A. Postoperative cerebral oedema after transcervical endometrial resection and uterine irrigation with 1.5% glycine. Lancet 1994;344:1187–9.

14. Stoloff DR, Isenberg RA, Brill AI. Venous air and gas emboli in operative hysteroscopy. J Am Assoc Gynecol Laparosc 2001;8:181–92.

Laparoscopy

Anthony A. Luciano, Rachel LaMonica, Danielle E. Luciano

Compared with laparotomy, laparoscopy is associated with smaller incisions, reduced tissue trauma, shorter hospitalization, less postoperative pain, and shorter recuperation time. Although laparoscopic surgery is considered a minimally invasive procedure, it can be associated with serious and occasionally fatal complications when proper safeguards are not respected. Important perioperative steps lead to safer and more effective laparoscopic surgery and may help to avoid or manage some of the more common complications.

Preparation of Patient for Surgery

Proper evaluation of the patient before surgery can potentially decrease morbidity by preventing intraoperative and postoperative complications. During gynecologic laparoscopy, patients often are placed in a steep Trendelenburg position, which may make ventilation difficult in obese patients, smokers, or those with cardiopulmonary disease. For such cases, consultation with ananesthesiologist prepares the patient, the anesthesiologists, and the entire operative team to anticipate and take necessary steps to prevent intraoperative complications or adverse events. Examination of previous surgical scars on the abdomen may help

the surgeon plan a safer entry point and avoid access injuries as described later. Proper informed consent for the procedure should be obtained, and all risks and potential complications, including the possibility of laparotomy if the procedure cannot be completed safely by laparoscopy, should be explained.

Intraoperative Considerations

The American College of Obstetricians and Gynecologists' guidelines recommend that prophylactic antibiotics not be used for diagnostic laparoscopy; however, for extensive operative procedures, a first generation cephalosporin should be used (1). If the patient is allergic to cephalosporins, metronidazole can be used.

Proper patient positioning, as illustrated in Figure 1, can avoid neurologic injuries and facilitate the surgeon's manipulation of laparoscopic instruments. Tucking the patients' arms along her sides, using boot stirrups, and avoiding excessive abduction at the patients' hips can avoid brachial plexus, sciatic, and femoral nerve injuries. The patient's position should be rechecked periodically throughout the procedure to ensure there has been no movement, especially when the patient is placed in a steep Trendelenburg position

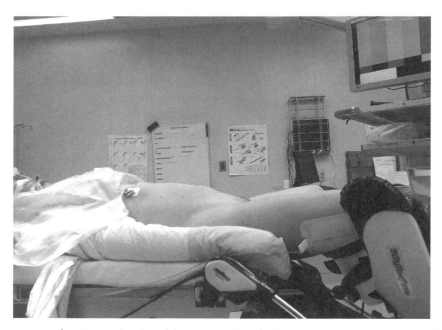

Figure 1. Proper positioning of patient in the dorsolithotomy position for laparoscopic surgery. Trunk-to-thigh angle should be less than 180 degrees to facilitate manipulations of instruments through the lower trocar ports and to prevent excessive stretching of the sciatic, femoral, and iliopsoas nerves. Knee flexion should be between 90 degrees and 120 degrees to support calves and promote circulation and to avoid prolonged compression of the calves. Arms should be tucked along the side of the patient.

(2). A patient with previous back or leg injuries can be placed in dorsolithotomy position before anesthesia induction so that she can assume a comfortable position on the operating table. Checking all instruments before making an incision, especially ensuring that any hemostatic instruments are working properly, can avoid excess bleeding and delays during the operation.

Measures to prevent adhesion, such as gentle handling of tissue, use of minimally invasive technique, and hemostasis, are as important in laparoscopy as in open surgery. Adhesion barriers approved for laparotomy have not been approved for laparoscopy and may not be useful, with the exception of 4% icodextrin solution, which has been shown to decrease postoperative adhesion formation at laparoscopy by 40% (3).

Laparoscopic Entry

Most common and severe complications occur during peritoneal access and include bowel and vessel injuries as well as extraperitoneal insufflation and procedure failure. A surgeon should adopt a laparoscopic access technique that is safe, effective, and reproducible in most patients, taking into account their weight, body habitus, and previous abdominal or pelvic surgery. Several approaches have been described in an effort to reduce complications and include the following:

- The classic approach of closed Veress–pneumoperitoneum–trocar method
- The Hasson or open technique
- Direct trocar insertion without prior pneumoperitoneum
- Optical Veress trocar method
- Visual access cannula method
- Optical trocar method
- Shielded trocar method
- Radially expanding trocar method

A Cochrane meta-analysis reviewed 17 randomized controlled studies comparing open versus closed entry methods, Veress-needle entry versus direct trocar entry, radially expanding trocars versus sharp trocar or direct vision entry methods. The review found no evidence of benefit in terms of safety of one technique or specialized instrument over all others in gaining access to the peritoneal cavity for laparoscopic surgery. Consequently, the authors concluded that it is difficult to recommend one method over the other (4).

Placement of Veress Needle

Intraabdominal placement of the Veress needle has been traditionally used to establish pneumoperitoneum. Because the Veress needle is inserted blindly, the needle may enter other spaces or puncture other organs and cause injury. The factors that increase the risk of injury include previous surgery, body weight (obese or very thin), and a large uterus or distended bladder or stomach, or the presence of a large abdominal mass. Complications from the placement of the Veress needle include preperitoneal insufflation, injury to bowel or mesentery, perforation of major blood vessels (inferior vena cava, aorta, and common iliac vessels) and injury to the stomach or urinary bladder. The latter may be avoided by the routine preoperative placement of a nasogastric tube and Foley catheter to decompress and keep these organs out of harm's way. The risk of other complications may be significantly reduced by using the safest and least vascular point of entry, which is the base of the umbilicus. As shown in Figure 2, the skin, fascia, and parietal peritoneum converge at the base of the umbilicus without any intervening subcutaneous fat, muscle, or large blood vessels. All abdominal wall structures converge forming an avascular fulcrum at the base of the umbilicus where the shortest distance between the skin and the peritoneal cavity occurs, regardless of the patient's body mass index (BMI). Moreover, because the umbilicus serves as a fulcrum for the abdominal wall, as demonstrated in Figure 3, the distance between the parietal peritoneum and retroperitoneal major vessels is maximally increased (5). If the patient has bowel adhesions to the abdominal wall from previous abdominal surgery, especially when the incision extends above the umbilicus, the risk of bowel or mesenteric injury is high and other ports, such as the left upper quadrant or Palmer's point (approximately 1–3 cm below the left subcostal border of the midclavicular line) should be used instead. Even for patients with a previous vertical incision, if the incision does not extend above the umbilicus, the intraumbilical entry is safe because adhesions to the anterior abdominal wall rarely involve the umbilical parietal peritoneum. However, the needle or trocar must be inserted through the base of the umbilicus perpendicularly, as shown in the Figure 3, to avoid bowel and mesenteric attachment to the anterior abdominal wall that in most cases occurs below and not directly under the umbilicus.

The amount of subcutaneous tissue at the Palmer's point correlates with the patient's BMI; thus, in severely obese women longer Veress needles may be required. The stomach may be distended by the ventilation before intubation and may be at risk of perforation by the needle or the trocar. Therefore, it is important that the stomach be aspirated with a nasogastric tube before introducing the needle or the trocar at the Palmer's point. Entry at the Palmer's point is contraindicated in patients with prior gastric or splenic surgery and in patients with hepatosplenomegaly. The correct placement of the Veress needle is confirmed by the opening

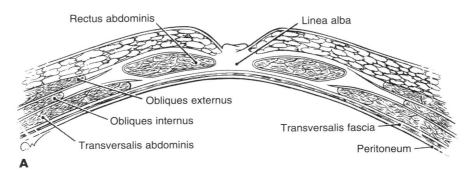

The level of the umbilicus

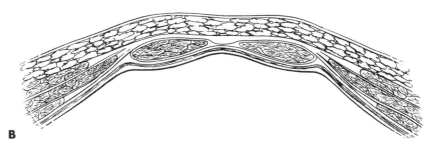

Below the arcuate line

Figure 2. A cross-section of the abdominal wall showing convergence of all layers of the abdominal wall into a single aponeurosis at the umbilicus **(A).** A cross-section of the abdominal wall below and above the umbilicus **(B).** (Nezhat C, Nezhat C, Nezhat F, Ferland R. Laparoscopic access: principles of laparoscopy. In: Nezhat C, Nezhat F, Nezhat C, editors. Nezhat's operative gynecologic laparoscopy and hysteroscopy. 3rd ed. New York (NY): Cambridge University Press; 2008. p. 40–56. Reprinted with the permission of Cambridge University Press.)

pressure of less than 6 mm Hg, suggesting intraperitoneal placement regardless of patient's BMI or parity. Adequate insufflation usually is reached at intraperitoneal pressure of 15 mm Hg, which is considered safe and does not compromise venous return, ventilation, or cardiopulmonary function. In some cases, especially in very thin or very obese patients, to maximize the space between the peritoneum and underlying viscera, the insufflating pressure should be increased to 20–25 mm Hg only during the trocar insertion, after which the insufflating pressure is immediately restored to 15 mm Hg.

Laparoscopic Trocar

The entry of the trocar into the peritoneal cavity is the most critical point in the procedure and has been associated with catastrophic complications. Although the adequate pneumoperitoneum affords a measure of safe distance between the anterior abdominal wall and the pelvic viscera or retroperitoneal vessels, injuries from the trocar still may occur. The reasons for such injuries may include bowel immobilization by peritoneal adhesions or excessive force required to advance the trocar when the umbilical incision is too small, the skin and fascia may be fibrotic and hard, or the trocar is dull. Other potential reasons include inadequate elevation

of the abdominal wall, improper insufflation, lateral displacement of the trocar during insertion, laceration of vessels within the abdominal wall, perforation of the stomach if insufflated during preintubation ventilation, or injury to the liver and spleen, if they are enlarged. Methods of avoiding trocar injuries logically follow from the predisposing conditions associated with an increased risk of the injury. Aspiration of the stomach and the establishment of a large pneumoperitoneum before trocar insertion have been suggested as ways of decreasing the chance of bowel and vascular injuries. The best safeguard is the slow and controlled advancement of the trocar through an adequate skin incision while maximally elevating the abdominal wall at the umbilicus, as shown in Figure 3. The distance created by such elevation of the abdominal wall exceeds the length of the trocar.

The trocar should be inserted with the patient in a completely horizontal position. Premature Trendelenburg positioning does not avoid bowel injuries, particularly if bowel adhesions are present, and may significantly alter important landmarks, such as the sacral promontory and sacral hollow (6). Many surgeons insert and advance the trocar at a 45-degree angle toward the hollow of the sacrum to provide the greatest distance between the point of the trocar and the dor-

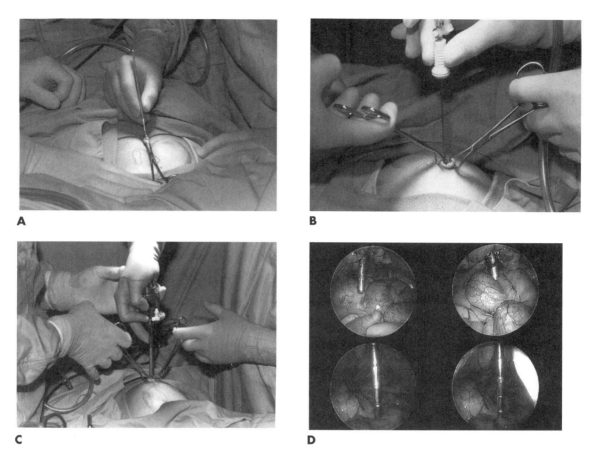

Figure 3. The intraumbilical incision involves everting the umbilicus with Allis clamps and making a 5-mm vertical incision at the center of the umbilicus **(A).** The edges of the incision are grasped with towel clips and maximally elevated while introducing either the Veress needle **(B)** or the 5 mm trocar **(C).** Lifting of the abdominal wall manually **(D—upper panels)** creates a space of less than 2.5 cm between the umbilicus and the viscera below. When the abdominal wall is lifted with towel clips placed at the edges of the intraumbilical incision **(D—lower panels)** it creates a space of greater than 6.5 cm, reducing the risk of visceral injury and essentially eliminating the risk of injury to the retroperitoneal vessels (aorta and vena cava).

sal spine. In obese patients, whose abdominal wall is thick, the intraumbilical, perpendicular entry is useful.

When adhesions are present, the bowel cannot slide out of the way, and because they usually occur on the abdominal wall from just below the umbilicus toward the pelvis, the bowel is in harm's way when the trocar is directed toward the hollow of the sacrum. Therefore, the umbilical trocar should be inserted in a perpendicular direction through the base of the umbilicus taking advantage of the shortest distance through the abdominal wall into the peritoneal cavity, which is usually less than 4 cm. This technique may not completely avoid adherent bowel under the abdominal wall.

Direct Trocar Insertion

Trocar insertion without creating a pneumoperitoneum reduces the number of preliminary procedures and saves operative time. Several studies have compared the ease and safety of creating a pneumoperitoneum with the Veress needle versus direct trocar insertion,

and the results have been similar. However, most authors recommend Veress needle insufflation in patients who have had multiple laparotomies. Whether direct trocar insertion or Veress needle insufflation is used, the intraumbilical port is safest for accessing the peritoneal cavity at laparoscopy (6).

Open Laparoscopy

Open laparoscopy eliminates the risk associated with the blind insertion of the Veress needle and trocar. This technique involves making a small (approximately 2 cm) skin incision at the level of the umbilicus and extending the incision through the abdominal wall into the peritoneal cavity. A special cannula and cone-shaped sleeve are placed through the small abdominal incision and are secured with a suture to the fascia and peritoneum. At the end of the procedure, the same suture is used to close the puncture wound of the abdominal wall. Although this technique does not significantly reduce abdominal wall bleeding or bowel injury (0.1%), it significantly reduces the incidence of failed procedures, inappropriate gas insufflation, or punctures to major retroperitoneal blood vessels. The major criticism of open laparoscopy is that it takes longer than a closed technique and is cumbersome. A higher complication rate with an open entry than with a closed entry technique has been reported (7). However, this report was not a randomized study, and the results may have reflected the surgeon's bias of choosing the open entry for the complicated cases and the high-risk patients.

Alternative Techniques and Equipment

Single Port Access Laparoscopy

Single port access laparoscopy is a technique involving only one incision placed infraumbilically where the scar is hidden, hence the name "scarless surgery." A 2-cm umbilical incision is made using the Hasson technique into which a single flexible donut-shaped device is inserted. The device contains three ports, the center for the laparoscope, and two lateral ports for operative instruments. Because the operative channels are very close and interfere with each other, the operative instruments for single port access laparoscopy contain a hinge that is flexed inside the peritoneal cavity to allow for manipulation of tissue and operative procedures. There are several case reports in the general surgery literature describing single port access used for laparoscopic appendectomy and cholecystectomy. The gynecology literature includes a few case reports of single port access laparoscopic tubal ligation, adnexal surgery, and laparoscopically assisted vaginal hysterectomy.

Trocars

A disposable shielded trocar has a shield that partially retracts and exposes a sharp tip when it meets the resistance of the abdominal wall; however, once it enters the peritoneal cavity, the shield springs forward to cover the sharp tip. Consequently, the shielded trocars are expected to be safer than traditional trocars. However, their safety record has been shown to be similar to that of traditional trocars.

Greater safety may be achieved with the radially expanding access system that includes a 1.9 mm Veress needle within an expanding polymeric sleeve. The needle and sleeve are inserted through a small skin incision of 3–5 mm, the needle is removed, and the 5–10 mm trocar with the blunt obturator is introduced into the peritoneal cavity through the expanding polymeric sleeve. The initial 1.9 mm incision thus stretches to 5 mm or 10 mm without cutting into tissue. The radial expansion of the defect in the abdominal wall makes the defect approximately 50% smaller and slit-like, separating the tissues rather than cutting them. In a randomized controlled study comparing the radially expanding system with conventional trocars, there was a decreased incidence of trocar site bleeding. However, this system requires a greater force for entry, and it has been shown to have a higher incidence of malfunction when compared with different types of trocars, such as cutting or hybrid types (8, 9).

Some surgeons prefer the visual entry system, which consists of a hollow trocar with a dull, pointed, and transparent tip that is advanced through the abdominal wall under direct visualization from the 5 mm laparoscope placed in the trocar sleeve. As the trocar advances through the abdominal wall and into the peritoneal cavity, the parietal peritoneum is clearly distinguishable and the peritoneal cavity is entered under direct visualization. This system has been found to be particularly useful in obese women, provided they do not have abdominal wall adhesions.

Another trocar is known as an endoscopic threaded imaging port. It consists of a stainless-steel threaded trocar that is advanced by screwing the trocar sleeve through the abdominal wall into the peritoneal cavity under direct visualization with the laparoscope within the trocar sleeve.

An optical trocar with a cutting knife advances 1 mm with each squeeze. This trocar is applied after insufflation and the establishment of an adequate pneumoperitoneum. Although the visual entry achieved by the optical trocar may represent an advantage over traditional trocars, the comparative data are scant.

Insertion of a secondary (accessory) trocar is much less apt to result in injury because prior insertion of the laparoscope allows transillumination of the abdominal wall and direct visualization of these trocars as they are introduced into the peritoneal cavity through the right, left, or middle lower quadrants. The major complications associated with the insertion of accessory trocars include bladder injury, which is less likely with an empty bladder, and injury to the inferior epigastric vessels. The inferior epigastric vessels are located in the abdominal wall of the lower right and lower left quadrants within the triangle formed by the round ligament (laterally) as it inserts into the internal inguinal ring and medially by the obliterated umbilical arteries (ligaments). In thin patients, the inferior epigastric vessels can be visualized by transilluminating the abdominal wall with the laparoscope and inspecting the area lateral to the umbilical artery. In obese patients, the inferior epigastric vessels may not be visible, but they can be avoided by inserting the trocar either lateral to the internal inguinal ring or medial to the umbilical artery because the inferior epigastric vessels always run between these two structures, as shown in Figure 4. The internal inguinal ring may be found by following the round ligament from the uterus to the anterior

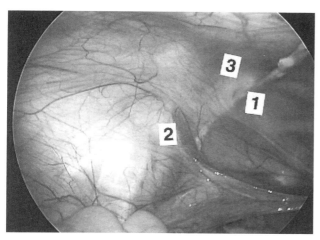

Figure 4. The inferior epigastric vessels **(3)** run between the obliterated umbilical artery medially **(1)** and the internal inguinal ring laterally where the round ligament inserts **(2).**

abdominal wall, where it inserts into the inguinal ring, which is sometimes open. The trocar is placed lateral and superior (cephalad) to the internal inguinal ring and should be directed at a 45-degree angle toward the posterior cul-de-sac. If the trocar is directed vertically, it may go down the pelvic sidewall where it may puncture the deep vessels, such as the external or internal iliac vessels, resulting in profuse hemorrhage or rapidly enlarging retroperitoneal hematoma, both of which require immediate laparotomy and the assistance of a vascular surgeon.

Once all the trocars have been inserted, a thorough diagnostic evaluation is performed that includes evaluating the entire peritoneal cavity, starting with the upper quadrants and examining the liver, gall bladder, diaphragm, stomach, and large and small bowels, including the appendix, before the patients is placed in the Trendelenburg position. Patients with endometriosis or pelvic inflammatory disease may have endometriosis implants or adhesions involving the upper abdominal wall, the liver, and the diaphragm. The patient is then placed in Trendelenburg position allowing the bowel to retract out of the pelvis into the upper abdomen in order to carefully examine the pelvic organs, including the pelvic sidewalls, posterior and anterior cul-de-sacs, all ovarian surfaces, and the course of the ureters. Adhesions should be carefully removed along dissection planes to minimize bleeding and injury to affected organs. When the dissection planes are not obvious and the boundaries of the bladder, rectum, or vagina are unclear, filling the bladder with indigo carmine solution or placing probes in the rectum and the vagina may better delineate the boundaries of these organs in the anterior and posterior cul-de-sacs and better define the planes of dissection in separating these structures from each other. Once all adhesions have been removed and normal anatomy has been restored, the intended surgical procedure should be completed. For deep endometriosis, resection instead of ablation is recommended; for ovarian cysts, especially endometriomas, resection of entire cyst wall instead of just drainage is recommended; and for adhesions, especially of the ovarian cortex, complete removal instead of simply severing them to minimize the risk of disease recurrence is recommended. Hysterectomy also is safer and simpler when performed after adhesiolysis and after restoring the normal anatomy with precise localization of vital structures, including the ureters, the rectum, and the bladder.

After the surgical procedure has been completed, especially in cases where extensive manipulation and dissection of the bladder, rectum, or pelvic sidewalls have occurred, filling the bladder or the rectum with indigo carmine solution will identify any breech of the lumen of these organs. To assess the integrity of the ureters, indigo carmine is administered intravenously and the pelvic sidewalls are inspected for leakage from the ureters; a cystoscopy may be performed to identify the ureteral jets and normal bladder wall.

Complications and Injuries

The complication rates associated with laparoscopic surgery range between 0.3% and 0.6%. Approximately one half of the complications occur during peritoneal access, regardless of the methodology (Box 1).

Vessels

Major vascular injuries are rare, but can be devastating. They occur at rates of 0.01–0.06%, but the associated mortality rates are 12–23% (10, 11). When the injuries involve the aorta, vena cava, or iliac vessels, they should be considered catastrophic events and must be expeditiously managed by laparotomy with an urgent call for the vascular surgical team. Inferior epigastric vessels injuries are more common and more amenable to laparoscopic management, including laparoscopic coagulation with bipolar energy applied from the contralateral lower quadrant port. If this fails, a number 0-absorbable suture on a CT-1 needle can be placed in a figure-of-eight fashion on either side of the trocar; or, a straight needle can be passed transabdomi-

---

Box 1

Complications Associated With Laparoscopy

- Trocar access injuries
- Neurologic injuries
- Pneumoperitoneum complications
- Subcutaneous emphysema
- Trocar site hernia

nally on the distal side of the trocar and passed through the abdominal wall and back into the subcutaneous fascia using laparoscopic forceps, tying the suture within the trocar incision and burying it beneath the skin. In some cases, the trocar incision may need to be extended to identify the bleeding vessel and control it with a ligature.

Bladder

Bladder injury is rare and is most likely to occur in patients with previous surgery, especially cesarean delivery, or patients with extensive endometriosis involving the anterior cul-de-sac where endometriosis may cause dense and cohesive adhesions between the bladder, anterior broad ligament, and anterior abdominal wall. At the time of laparoscopic hysterectomy, if the bladder has not been adequately dissected and pushed down away from the upper vagina, it may be injured during the separation of the cervix from the vagina. When suspected, bladder injury should be confirmed or ruled out by filling the bladder with a solution of indigo carmine and observing for any leakage. Bladder injuries with sharp instruments, such as scissors, usually can be repaired laparoscopically. Thermal injuries with power instruments are more serious and involve resecting the thermally damaged tissue completely and approximating the healthy tissue.

Ureters

Identification of the ureter as it courses along the pelvis is crucial for safe laparoscopic surgery of the reproductive organs. The surgeon should be alert to potential anatomic distortions when nodularity and thickening are present in the area of the uterosacral ligaments, ovarian fossa, and pelvic brim. The ureter can be protected in several ways. When implants of endometriosis are present on the peritoneum overlying the ureter, as is often the case in the ovarian fossa, a small incision is made in the normal peritoneum above the ureter. The ureter is then gently dissected off the peritoneum with the tip of the scissors or with fine forceps placed between the peritoneum and the ureter, displacing it medially to free it from the peritoneum with its endometriosis implant. This procedure is applicable only when the endometriosis does not invade the wall of the ureter. When the ureter is closely involved with the uterosacral or cardinal ligament, the retroperitoneal space is opened to identify and dissect the ureter free of the uterosacral ligaments and uterine arteries. Early recognition of ureteral injury is critical for successful management. Ureteral injuries may be detected by dissecting of the ureter and identifying leakage of blue urine after intravenous administration of indigo carmine solution.

Symptoms of fever, flank pain, and abdominal distention that occur within 48–72 hours of surgery should alert the clinician to possible ureteral injury. Leukocytosis and hematuria also may be present. Establishing the diagnosis may be difficult because the patient may present with symptoms that are indistinguishable from ileus or bowel injury. Imaging is necessary to help establish the correct diagnosis.

Small Bowel

Lacerating intestinal injuries can be produced during sharp dissection with scissors, laser, or electrosurgical instruments. Risk of injury is much greater with dense adhesions and where tissue planes are poorly defined. In addition, traction on the bowel with serrated graspers may result in abrasions and lacerations. Inspection of the bowel after sharp dissection and noting bleeding or hematoma should alert the operator to bowel trauma requiring closer examination. Care should be taken with any manipulation of the bowel, such as retraction and displacement from the pelvis with a blunt metal probe. Blunt dissection of the bowel should be avoided.

Although small injuries to the small bowel, such as those caused by a Veress needle, may not require any special care other than careful follow-up, some experts advocate oversewing the area with a 3-0 delayed absorbable suture to minimize postoperative morbidity. Other injuries will need an extensive repair or possibly even a resection of the damaged segment of the bowel.

Large Bowel

Most injuries to the large bowel occur as a result of sharp or blunt dissection in the presence of severe adhesions and endometriosis in the posterior cul-de-sac. However, colonic injuries from the laparoscopic trocar or burn injuries from lasers or electrosurgical instruments also have been reported. When a difficult pelvic operation is contemplated, the surgeon should assess the likelihood of bowel involvement. If perforation of the rectosigmoid is suspected, a definitive diagnosis should be established before the completion of surgery. A rectal probe may be placed transanally and its advancement into the proximal sigmoid colon monitored under laparoscopic visualization. A more definitive test involves instill 150–200 mL of indigo carmine solution transanally and observation for any intraperitoneal spillage by laparoscopy. Small defects can be treated laparoscopically with two-layer closures. Large defects, especially if they are made with laser or electrosurgical instruments, may require segmental resection and anastomosis.

Shoulder Pain

Often patients report this pain as the most troubling aspect of their laparoscopic surgery. It is believed to be due to the accumulation of carbon dioxide (CO_2) under the diaphragm, when the patient stands up or sits up. The gas combines with the fluid to form carbonic acid, which irritates the diaphragm, and the pain is referred to the shoulder by the phrenic nerve. Complete removal of intraabdominal CO_2 is difficult, but the pain may be improved by maintaining the patient in a Trendelenburg position at the end of the procedure to allow the gas to gravitate toward the lower abdomen. In addition, the anesthetist should be instructed to administer several deep breaths while the surgeon is closing the punctures (12). The severity and frequency of shoulder pain can be further minimized by filling the peritoneal cavity with 500–1,000 mL of lactated Ringer's solution or 4% icodextrin solution, which promotes further removal of entrapped CO_2, dilutes the carbonic acid formed from the entrapped CO_2, and reduces shoulder pain. If, in spite of these measures, shoulder pain still develops, the patient may assume a supine position with a pillow under the buttocks to elevate the lower abdomen allowing gas to gravitate into the pelvis where it is less irritating.

Incisional Hernia

Herniation of either the omentum or small bowel at the umbilical incision site has been reported and is found primarily with trocar incisions of greater than 5 mm.

Patients at increased risk of this complication are obese, have chronic coughs, or have a history of hernias. With trocars of 12 mm or greater, incisional hernias of the small bowel were reported to occur in 1 case per 32 puncture sites after major laparoscopic procedures (13). The clinical signs of small bowel herniation are nausea and vomiting that persist and progressively get worse after 24 hours and beyond, unlike the nausea and vomiting that are common after uneventful laparoscopy and resolve within 6–12 hours postoperatively. Early diagnosis is critical to minimize bowel injury and necrosis. Computed tomography is the preferred test to establish the diagnosis, often revealing fluid-filled distended loops of small bowel and protrusion of part of the small bowel wall (or the entire bowel loop) through the fascia. The classic appearance of Richter hernia is illustrated in Figure 5. To prevent it, the fascia of greater than 5 mm incisions should be closed with deep stitches, approximating the fascia and sometimes the peritoneum.

Robotics

The only robotic system currently approved by the U.S. Food and Drug Administration for use in gynecologic procedures is the da Vinci surgical system. It consists of a robotic cart with three to four arms to control the laparoscopic operative instruments, a three-dimensional

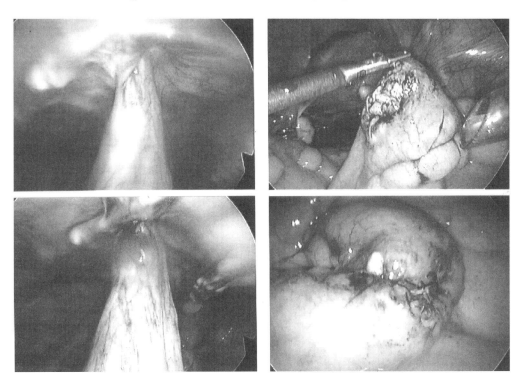

Figure 5. Richter hernia. Small bowel loop stuck in the 12-mm trocar puncture. The fascia was closed at the initial surgery with 2-0 vicryl sutures, but the peritoneum was left open. The bowel had herniated through the peritoneum and into the rectus muscle (left upper and lower panels) from which it was successfully separated without opening the bowel (right upper panel). The serosal abrasions were approximated with 4-0 interrupted vicryl sutures (right lower panel).

camera that projects a highly magnified, high-definition image on a monitor, wristed instruments, and a surgical console remote from the operating table. Sitting at the console, the surgeon can direct three or four robotic arms that control a 12-mm three-dimensional endoscope and the various instruments that allow the surgeon to perform tissue manipulation, dissection, clamping, endosurgery, and suturing. Robotics offer the advantages of three-dimensional visualization, improved dexterity (seven degrees of movement with elimination of tremor and improved tissue manipulation in narrowed spaces), advanced microsurgery in multiplanar views, and decreased surgeon fatigue. These features of robot-assisted laparoscopy have been reported to be especially useful in the more complex gynecologic procedures such as tubal anastomosis, radical hysterectomy with node dissection, myomectomy, delicate ovarian cystectomy, prolapse suspension procedures, and resection of deep rectovaginal endometriosis (14–16). There are disadvantages to robot-assisted laparoscopic surgery, at least with the current system, such as the expense of the robot and the instruments. The equipment is bulky, requires a large operating space, and is difficult to reposition once surgery has begun. The instruments used in the system also are bulkier than those used in traditional laparoscopy and require larger incisions. Also, there is lack of tactile feedback to the surgeon. As with all new technologies, robot-assisted surgery has been compared with non–robot-assisted surgery, mostly in retrospective, poorly conducted studies and with inconclusive results. None of these studies have shown better or worse outcomes with robotics, except for consistently greater expenses associated with robotics versus traditional laparoscopy (17).

References

1. Antibiotic prophylaxis for gynecologic procedures. ACOG Practice Bulletin No. 104. American College of Obstetricians and Gynecologists. Obstet Gynecol 2009;113:1180–9.

2. Barnett JC, Hurd WW, Rogers RM Jr, Williams NL, Shapiro SA. Laparoscopic positioning and nerve injuries. J Minim Invasive Gynecol 2007;14:664–72; quiz 673.

3. Brown CB, Luciano AA, Martin D, Peers E, Scrimgeour A, diZerega GS, et al. Adept (icodextrin 4% solution) reduces adhesions after laparoscopic surgery for adhesiolysis: a double-blind randomized, controlled study. Fertil Steril 2007;88:1413–26.

4. Ahmad G, Duffy JM, Phillips K, Watson A. Laparoscopic entry techniques. Cochrane Database of Systematic Reviews 2008, Issue 2. Art. No.:CD006583. DOI: 10.1002/14651858.CD006583.pub2.

5. Roy GM, Bazzurini L, Solima E, Luciano AA. Safe technique for laparoscopic entry into the abdominal cavity. J Am Assoc Gynecol Laparosc 2001;8:519–28.

6. Nezhat C, Nezhat C, Nezhat F, Ferland R. Laparoscopic access: principles of laparoscopy. In: Nezhat C, Nezhat F, Nezhat C, editors. Nezhat's operative gynecologic laparoscopy and hysteroscopy. 3rd ed. New York (NY): Cambridge University Press; 2008. p. 40–56.

7. Jansen FW, Kolkman W, Bakkum EA, de Kroon CD, Trimbos-Kemper TC, Trimbos JB. Complications of laparoscopy: an inquiry about closed- versus open-entry technique. Am J Obstet Gynecol 2004;190:634–38.

8. Shafer DM, Khajanchee Y, Wong J, Swanstrom LL. Comparison of five different abdominal access trocar systems: analysis of insertion force, removal force and defect size. Surg Innov 2006;13:183–9.

9. Venkatesh R, Sundaram CP, Figenshau RS, Yan Y, Andriole GL, Caylman RV, et al. Prospective randomized comparison of cutting and dilating disposable trocars for access during laparoscopic renal injury. JSLS 2007;11:198–203.

10. Chapron CM, Pierre F, Lacroix PF, Querleu D, lansac J, Dubuisson JB. Major vascular injuries during gynecologic laparoscopy. J Am Coll Surg 1997;185:461–5.

11. Baggish MS. Analysis of 31 cases of major-vessel injury associated with gynecologic laparoscopy operations. J Gynecol Surg 2003;19:63–7.

12. Phelps P, Cakmakkaya OS, Apfel CC, Radke OC. A simple clinical maneuver to reduce laparoscopy-induced shoulder pain: a randomized controlled trial. Obstet Gynecol 2008;111:1155–60.

13. Boike Gm, Miller CE, Spirtos NM, Mercer LI, Fowler JM, Summitt R, et al. Incisional bowel herniations after operative laparoscopy: a series of nineteen cases and review of the literature. Am J Obstet Gynecol 1995;172:1726–31; discussion 1731–3.

14. Falcone T, Goldberg JM, Margossian H, Stevens L. Robotic-assisted laparoscopic microsurgical tubal anastomosis: a human pilot study. Fertil Steril 2000;73:1040–2.

15. Field JB, Benoit MF, Dinh TA, Diaz-Arrastia C. Computer-enhanced robotic surgery in gynecologic oncology. Surg Endosc 2007;21:244–6.

16. Advincula AP, Wang K. Evolving role and current state of robotics in minimally invasive gynecologic surgery. J Minim Invasive Gynecol 2009;16:291–301.

17. Bedient CE, Magrina JF, Noble BN, Kho RM. Comparison of robotic and laparoscopic myomectomy. Am J Obstet Gynecol 2009;201:566.e1–566.e5.

Gynecologic Imaging

Daniel M. Breitkopf

Gynecologic imaging is key in the diagnostic evaluation of many reproductive health conditions in women. The most common symptoms a gynecologist encounters in practice, such as abnormal bleeding and pelvic pain, routinely require pelvic imaging for accurate diagnosis and treatment. Over the past 10 years, imaging technology has improved, resulting in better image quality and wider availability of imaging options. Techniques, such as positron emission tomography (PET) and sonohysterography, will be reviewed in this section. More established modalities, such as ultrasonography, magnetic resonance imaging (MRI) and computed tomography (CT), also are discussed.

Positron Emission Tomography

Technical Considerations

Positron emission tomography involves creating three-dimensional images reconstructed from two-dimensional images of radiation detected in target areas of the patient's body. A positron-emitting radionuclide is administered to the patient and allowed to be absorbed by the target tissue. The photons created by the annihilation of positrons can then be detected by probes placed on the either side of the patient's body. The most common radiopharmaceutical agent used for this type of imaging is fluorine-18 deoxyglucose. This agent is transported into cells in a manner similar to the way glucose is transported into cells; however, when the metabolism is blocked after phosphorylation by hexokinase, fluorine-18 deoxyglucose accumulates intracellularly (1).

In gynecology, PET with fluorine-18 deoxyglucose is used to detect cancer and monitor patients for cancer recurrence. The main advantage of PET over other techniques, such as CT and MRI, is its ability to provide functional imaging of the tissue. The fluorine-18 deoxyglucose uptake by tumor cells is proportional to tumor glucose metabolism. The increased uptake of fluorine-18 deoxyglucose by tumor cells is primarily due to the increased glucose transporter and hexokinase activities in the tumor cells as compared with nontumor cells. Because the nontumor soft tissue has low activity or uptake of fluorine-18 deoxyglucose, the surrounding structures are not well visualized on PET. Thus, anatomical landmarks indicating tumor location are difficult to visualize. This limitation of PET has inspired the development of a hybrid technique, where the functional details from the PET images are combined with the anatomical landmarks from CT scans (1).

Clinical Applications

Positron emission tomography has high sensitivity and specificity in the initial staging of cervical cancer (2). The combination of PET and CT techniques was noted to be more sensitive than MRI in detection of lymph node metastases in cervical cancer in one study (3). Positron emission tomography also is useful in the detection of extrapelvic metastases and the recurrence of cervical cancer (Fig. 6). In ovarian cancer, PET may be helpful in predicting outcome of therapy. In a study of 33 patients with stage IIIC and stage IV ovarian cancer receiving neoadjuvant chemotherapy, quantitative PET imaging results predicted clinical outcome better than those of CA 125 assessment or clinical response criteria (4). Positron emission tomography shows promise in surveillance for the recurrence of endometrial cancer, with sensitivities of 96–100% and specificities of 78–88%. It also appears to have improved perfor-

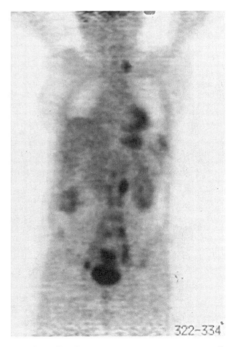

Figure 6. Whole body positron emission tomograhic image of a patient with International Federation of Gynecology and Obstetrics stage IIA cervical carcinoma and evidence of metastasis to pelvic, paraaortic, and left supraclavicular lymph nodes. (Reprinted from Gynecologic Oncology, Vol. 87, Belhocine T, Thille A, Fridman V, Albert A, Seidel L. Nickers P, et al. Contribution of whole-body 18FDG PET imaging in the management of cervical cancer. Pages 90–97, Copyright 2002, with permission from Elsevier.)

mance in the detection of recurrent endometrial cancer when compared with MRI or CT (2).

Computed Tomography

In this technique, images are generated based on the differences in X-ray attenuation. These differences are relatively small between the pelvic organs. However, because pelvic organs are outlined by extraperitoneal fat, administration of intravenous (IV) contrast agents will optimize visualization, making CT useful in imaging the female pelvis.

Computed tomography can be used for imaging of the uterus and adnexa, although ultrasonography and MRI are preferred. Computed tomography of the pelvis and abdomen is useful for visualization of the retroperitoneum to evaluate it for lymphadenopathy. The ureters can be seen throughout their course. The omentum and upper abdominal structures also are well visualized on CT and so is the abdominal wall (for detecting hernias and abdominal wall endometriomas).

Computed tomography plays a role in the evaluation of postoperative complications of gynecologic surgery. It is superior to intravenous urography in detecting ureteral injury and to plain film radiography or barium studies in detecting a small bowel obstruction. Postoperative fluid collection also is best visualized, characterized, and drained with the use of CT (2).

Pelvic Ultrasonography

Transvaginal ultrasound imaging remains the most common modality for evaluation of the female pelvis. Three-dimensional imaging for gynecologic applications has a limited role, mostly for characterization of müllerian anomalies. Sonohysterography has become a useful tool for the evaluation of abnormal uterine bleeding and postmenopausal bleeding.

Transvaginal Ultrasonography

ENDOMETRIAL STRIPE ASSESSMENT

Use of the endometrial stripe thickness for evaluation of postmenopausal bleeding has been extensively studied. In the menopause, the endometrium becomes atrophic and its thickness decreases, remaining relatively constant without hormonal stimulation. Ultrasound evaluation of the endometrial stripe involves the transvaginal technique, measuring the thickest portion of the endometrial echo in the sagittal plane. Women with postmenopausal bleeding may be evaluated initially with transvaginal ultrasonography. Based on most published literature, an endometrial stripe thickness of 5 mm or greater in women with postmenopausal bleeding should be interpreted as abnormal (5). Such cases warrant further evaluation to exclude endome-

trial carcinoma or other endometrial lesions, eg, with sonohysterography, hysteroscopy, or endometrial biopsy. Conversely, if the endometrial stripe thickness is 4 mm or less, endometrial sampling is not required. Transvaginal ultrasound assessment of the endometrial stripe also is useful when insufficient tissue for diagnosis was obtained during endometrial biopsy. The incidence of insufficient tissue for endometrial biopsy ranges from 0% to 54% (5), which favors the use of transvaginal ultrasonography in evaluation of women with postmenopausal bleeding.

ADNEXAL MASSES

Adnexal masses are well characterized by ultrasonography. Transvaginal imaging, in particular, provides high-resolution images of adnexal structures and masses. The criteria for description of adnexal masses on imaging include solid masses versus cystic masses, presence of septations or papillary projections, and the echogenicity of the fluid in the presence of a cystic mass. Cystic masses are characterized as simple or complex: simple masses contain anechoic fluid and are unilocular, smooth walled, and without papillary projections or solid areas, whereas complex cystic masses are those that do not meet the criteria for simple cysts.

For evaluation of adnexal masses, transvaginal ultrasonography is the modality of choice (6). No other imaging technology has superiority over ultrasonography in terms of diagnostic accuracy. Table 1 summarizes the sensitivity and specificity of various imaging modalities for the evaluation of adnexal masses.

Various scoring systems have been developed to discriminate between benign and malignant adnexal masses with ultrasound criteria. However, none of the systems developed to date have been able to consistently exclude the possibility of malignancy. It appears that an accurate method for discriminating between

Table 1. Imaging of Adnexal Masses

Modality	Sensitivity (%)	Specificity (%)
Grayscale transvaginal ultrasonography	0.32–0.91	0.68–0.81
Doppler ultrasonography	0.86	0.91
Computed tomography	0.90	0.75
Magnetic resonance imaging	0.91	0.88
Positron emission tomography	0.67	0.79

Data from Management of adnexal masses. ACOG Practice Bulletin No. 83. American College of Obstetricians and Gynecologists. Obstet Gynecol 2007;110:201–14 and Agency for Healthcare Research and Quality. Management of adnexal mass. Evidence Based Report/Technology Assessment No. 130. AHRQ Publication No. 06-E004. Rockville (MD): AHRQ; 2006.

benign and malignant ovarian masses is by combining the subjective evaluation of both the grayscale and Doppler images (7). In a European multicenter series of 1,066 women with adnexal masses, the accuracy of discriminating between benign and malignant ovarian masses was assessed using ultrasound-based pattern recognition. Pattern recognition was defined as the subjective evaluation of grayscale and Doppler ultrasound findings. Pattern recognition correctly predicted malignancy in 97% of the cases of primary invasive tumors and in 93% of the cases of metastatic tumors.

Benign ovarian masses can be accurately assessed with ultrasonography. Endometriomas and dermoid cysts have characteristic appearances that are easily detected with ultrasonography; thus, these conditions can be diagnosed easily. Endometriomas often are seen as unilocular cystic structures with homogenous internal echoes. In contrast with hemorrhagic cysts, endometriomas do not typically resolve spontaneously and the pattern of internal echoes is more uniform. Dermoid cysts are characterized by a mass with a hyperechoic area that has posterior acoustic shadowing, fluid–fluid levels, and a "mesh" appearance consisting of hyperechoic lines and dots (Fig. 7). The sensitivity of ultrasonography for the diagnosis of endometriomas is 77% and 86% for the diagnosis of benign teratomas and dermoid cysts (7).

POSTMENOPAUSAL OVARIAN CYSTS

The increased resolution of transvaginal ultrasonography allows for accurate characterization of ovarian cysts. Investigators from the University of Kentucky monitored more than 15,000 postmenopausal women with transvaginal ultrasonography as part of an ovarian cancer screening program. More than 3,000 women had an isolated finding of simple ovarian cysts of less than 10 cm and none of them developed ovarian cancer. Most of the cysts (69%) resolved within 3 months.

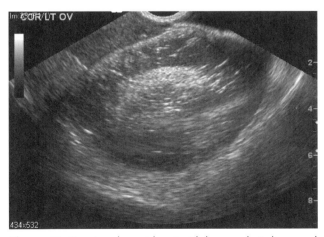

Figure 7. Ovarian dermoid cyst with hyperechoic lines and dots.

Serial transvaginal ultrasonography is a safe alternative to immediate surgical management of simple ovarian cysts less than 10 cm in diameter in menopausal women (6). As long as the cysts do not enlarge or characteristics easily identifiable by ultrasonography do not change, there is essentially no risk of missing an ovarian malignancy.

Three-Dimensional Ultrasonography

Three-dimensional ultrasound imaging offers some potential advantages over conventional two-dimensional technique. The data for three-dimensional imaging are acquired via manual or automatic two-dimensional scanning through the pelvis. The resulting images can be displayed as three-dimensional rendered depictions of the structure of interest or as multiplanar images. For gynecologic applications, the multiplanar views are the most useful. Three-dimensional ultrasonography offers the true coronal view of the uterus, which is not available in two-dimensional imaging. Volume rendered three-dimensional reconstructions of the surface of pelvic organs are less useful because the internal structural details are not well seen. Three-dimensional ultrasonography can be enhanced by adding the dimension of time, allowing for real-time three-dimensional (or four-dimensional) ultrasound images to be acquired. However, this four-dimensional imaging is more useful in obstetric scanning than in gynecologic applications.

In gynecology, three-dimensional sonohysterography is primarily useful for evaluation of müllerian anomalies. The uterine fundal contour is more easily seen by three-dimensional multiplanar imaging than by two-dimensional imaging (8). Delineation of the fundal contour aids in differentiating between a septate uterus and bicornuate uterus. Three-dimensional sonohysterography does not appear to add diagnostic accuracy in the imaging of endometrial cavity lesions, such as polyps and leiomyomas.

Three-dimensional imaging also can be used to improve the efficiency of an imaging practice. The volume data from three-dimensional images can be stored for later retrieval, viewing, and manipulation. Acquisition and storage of a three-dimensional image is rapid, but contains much information that can be manipulated in different planes during subsequent analyses. Thus, several three-dimensional volumes can be obtained by an ultrasound technician in a matter of minutes, and the image acquisition is not as operator dependent as is two-dimensional imaging. The data obtained during three-dimensional imaging also may improve the ability for remote interpretation of gynecologic studies because the interpreting physician can view the entire set of volume images in multiple planes instead of just the static images when two-dimensional techniques are used (9).

Sonohysterography

Sonohysterography involves the transcervical infusion of a sterile fluid (more commonly saline solution) into the endometrial cavity during real-time imaging with transvaginal ultrasonography. The fluid acts as a contrast agent to delineate the endometrium and intracavitary masses (Fig. 8 and Fig. 9). In most cases, less than 10 mL of saline solution is required to adequately visualize the endometrial cavity. A complete list of indications is presented in Box 2. Sonohysterography should not be attempted in patients with pelvic infection, known or suspected pregnancy, or both. In women with regular menstrual cycles, the procedure is best performed soon after menses to avoid interference with artifacts from a thick secretory endometrium. The procedure can be performed in the presence of active vaginal bleeding; however, the interpretation of the findings may be difficult because of retained intracavitary clots (10).

The primary role of sonohysterography is the workup of abnormal uterine bleeding (Fig. 10). Various studies have examined the diagnostic accuracy of sonohys-

terography in identifying endometrial cavity pathology. The sensitivity and specificity for sonohysterography in both premenopausal and postmenopausal women with abnormal uterine bleeding are 95% and 88%, respectively (11). In premenopausal women with abnormal uterine bleeding at low risk of endometrial cancer, sonohysterography may be a more effective first-line test than endometrial biopsy because the former is less painful than endometrial biopsy or diagnostic hysteroscopy performed in an office setting (12).

Sonohysterography may be useful for diagnosing adenomyosis. Fluid tracking into "myometrial cracks" during sonohysterography was associated with adenomyosis in one series (13). The authors postulated that basal endometrial in-growth into the myometrium creates channels through which the instilled fluid tracks during sonohysterography.

Sonohysterography also can be used to guide endometrial biopsy. In one series of 80 cases, sonohysterographic-guided endometrial biopsy was significantly more accurate in the detection of focal endometrial lesions and malignancy than blind endometrial biopsy (14). Another report comparing blind endometrial biopsy with a novel device designed to obtain sonohysterographic-directed samples indicated that the two techniques were equivalent in reliably establishing overall histologic diagnosis (15). However, the sonohysterographic-directed biopsy detected more focal lesions, such as polyps, than did the blind biopsy. Sonohysterographic-directed endometrial biopsy appears to be as effective as hysteroscopic-directed biopsy in diagnosing premalignant and malignant endometrial lesions (16).

A potential for inadvertent spill of malignant cells into the peritoneal cavity during sonohysterography has been studied in the medical literature. Several studies have attempted to address the issue of transtubal spillage of endometrial cancer cells and the effect on stag-

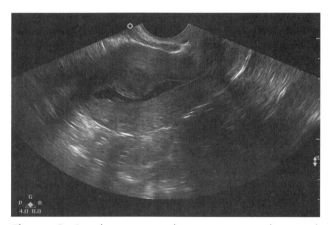

Figure 8. Sonohysterogram demonstrating a submucosal leiomyoma.

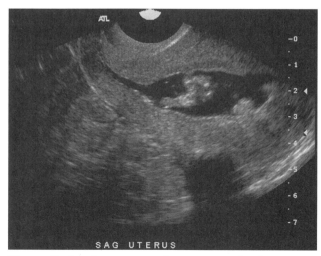

Figure 9. Sonohysterogram showing several polyps.

Box 2

Indications for Sonohysterography

- Abnormal uterine bleeding in premenopausal and postmenopausal women
- Infertility and habitual abortion
- Congenital abnormalities of the uterine cavity
- Suspected uterine myomas, polyps, and synechiae
- Abnormalities detected on transvaginal ultrasonography, including focal or diffuse endometrial or intracavitary abnormalities
- Suboptimally imaged endometrium by transvaginal ultrasonography

Sonohysterography. ACOG Technology Assessment No. 5. American College of Obstetricians and Gynecologists. Obstet Gynecol 2008;112:1467–9.

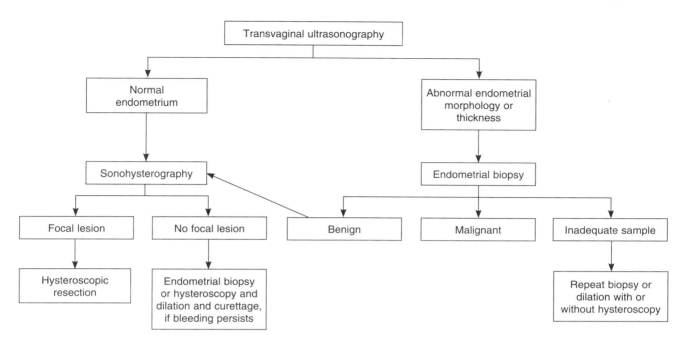

Figure 10. Algorithm for sonographic based triage of premenopausal and postmenopausal bleeding. (Shi AA, Lee SI. Radiological reasoning: algorithmic workup of abnormal vaginal bleeding with endovaginal sonography and sonohysterography [published arratum appears in AJR Am J Roentgenol 2009;192 (suppl):S62]. AJR Am J Roentgenol 2008;191:S68–73. Reprinted with permission from the American Journal of Roentgenology.)

ing of endometrial cancer. One study found transtubal spillage in 31% of patients (n = 16) who underwent sonohysterography for endometrial carcinoma (17). One patient had nonviable carcinoma cells in the fluid that spilled from the tube during sonohysterography. Another study evaluated women with endometrial cancer who underwent dilation and curettage (D&C) alone or a combination of D&C and sonohysterography and compared surgical staging between these groups (18). The D&C and sonohysterography were performed, on average, 27 and 11 days before hysterectomy, respectively. No differences were found in positive peritoneal cytology between the groups or in upstaging of the cancer. In another series, malignant or suspicious cells were present in fluid that spilled from fallopian tubes during sonohysterography in 25% of women with endometrial cancer (19). Based on the data available, the significance of transtubal spillage of endometrial cells during sonohysterography is not clear. Thus, sonohysterography should not be used in patients with known endometrial cancer. However, in women with abnormal uterine bleeding and no known endometrial malignancy, the risk of malignant cell dissemination is outweighed by the diagnostic information gained by accurate ultrasound assessment of the endometrial cavity.

Training, Certification, and Accreditation

Box 3 contains Internet resources for information regarding accreditation and training standards for ultra-

sonography. Obstetrician–gynecologists receive training in ultrasonography during residency. Current Accreditation Council for Graduate Medical Education residency program requirements for obstetrics and gynecology stipulate education in gynecologic ultrasonography. Residents are required to document experience in transvaginal ultrasonography during their training programs.

The American Institute of Ultrasound in Medicine (AIUM) and the American College of Radiology (ACR) have established standards for accreditation of ultra-

---

Box 3

Internet Resources for Training and Accreditation in Ultrasonography

American Institute of Ultrasound in Medicine Standards and Guidelines for the Accreditation of Ultrasound Practices
www.aium.org/publications/viewStatement. aspx?id=26

American College of Radiology
Ultrasound Accreditation Practice Requirements
www.acr.org/accreditation/ultrasound/ultrasound_reqs.aspx

Accreditation Council for Graduate Medical Education Program Requirements for Graduate Medical Education in Obstetrics and Gynecology
www.acgme.org/acWebsite/downloads/RRC_prog Req/220obstetricsandgynecology01012008.pdf

sound practices. Accreditation has become more important because some third-party payers are requiring accreditation in order for health care providers to be reimbursed for imaging services. The American Institute of Ultrasound in Medicine and ACR accreditation processes involve peer review of qualifications for physicians and ultrasound technicians, quality assurance and control, record keeping, and case studies. Specific accreditation can be obtained in obstetric ultrasonography, gynecologic ultrasonography, or both.

Both the ACR and AIUM have requirements for physician training and experience, mostly based on performance of supervised examinations in residency, fellowship, or practice. Other than board certification, there are no existing certification programs for obstetrician–gynecologists specifically targeting ultrasonography. The American Registry for Diagnostic Medical Sonography (ARDMS) offers credentials to individual ultrasound technicians. The American Institute of Ultrasound in Medicine accreditation guidelines indicate that ARDMS certification is required for ultrasound technicians in the practice if a physician is not immediately available at the time of the examination. The American College of Radiology accreditation requires that all ultrasound technicians are ARDMS certified.

Magnetic Resonance Imaging

Technical Considerations

Magnetic resonance imaging plays a major role in gynecologic imaging because of its increased accessibility, greater clinical application, and clinical studies demonstrating its utility. Multiple image planes can be evaluated, including the sagittal and coronal planes, which are not available in CT imaging. Magnetic resonance imaging maintains an advantage over other imaging technologies in its ability to accurately distinguish between fat and blood (20). Imaging techniques include the use of T1 and T2 weighted images in the axial and sagittal planes. T1 weighted images show fat planes and they are useful for visualizing lymph nodes that are usually surrounded by fat. T1 images with fast spin echo imaging and fat saturation are useful in characterizing adnexal masses. T1 images also can show hemorrhage within organs. T2 weighted images are best for demonstrating contrast in the soft tissues and, thus, are useful for visualizing the endometrium, myometrium, and cystic structures in the ovaries. Contrast enhancement with gadolinium is primarily used for characterization of endometrial and ovarian pathology.

Several advances in MRI technology have improved resolution and the speed of acquiring images. The magnet strength of newer equipment has doubled from 1.5 T to 3 T, which improves resolution, particularly of smaller structures. The time of acquisition of images has decreased with the advent of parallel imaging. Older MRI equipment contained only one receiver of the MRI signal. Newer equipment includes multiple receivers that allow for simultaneous acquisition of signals from tissue, increasing the speed of the examination twofold to threefold (20). Faster image acquisition reduces motion artifacts.

Müllerian Anomalies

Magnetic resonance imaging is considered the diagnostic test of choice for imaging of müllerian duct anomalies because its sensitivity and specificity are close to 100% for the diagnosis of these disorders (20). The high accuracy of MRI in the diagnosis of müllerian anomalies is from the clear delineation of the external and internal uterine contours and the contrast between the endometrium and myometrium. Magnetic resonance imaging also can depict vaginal septa clearly and define vaginal anatomy in pediatric patients when clinical examination may be difficult (20).

Adnexal Masses

Magnetic resonance imaging is also useful in the evaluation of adnexal masses because of its ability to identify different tissue types and to delineate soft tissue contrast. Many benign ovarian tumors, such as teratomas, endometriomas, and ovarian fibromas, have characteristic or specific features on MRI. Magnetic resonance imaging is helpful when masses are incompletely characterized by ultrasonography because it provides additional detail on soft tissue composition and can give multiplanar views to aid in the determination of the origin and extent of the pathology (21). Intravenous contrast agents are essential to differentiate between benign and malignant masses with MRI. These agents aid in the characterization of solid components of adnexal masses, peritoneal implants, and omental disease. Papillary projections within adnexal cysts will be enhanced on contrast MRI, whereas clots, debris, and fat will not. The enhancement of papillary projections is an advantage of MRI over ultrasonography in imaging the adnexal mass (21).

Despite some advantages of MRI, pelvic ultrasonography is still recommended as the primary method for evaluation of the adnexal mass (6). The sensitivity and specificity of ultrasonography and MRI for the diagnosis of adnexal masses do not appreciably differ (Table 1). However, ultrasonography costs less. In contrast, the use of MRI is preferred in some cases, eg, for the ultrasound-indeterminate pelvic mass, MRI can provide a noninvasive method to characterize the origin and nature of such lesions.

Uterine Leiomyomas

Although the primary method for evaluation of leiomyomas is ultrasonography, MRI can be helpful in cases where ultrasound imaging results are indeterminate; eg, in distinguishing leiomyomas from other pelvic masses before uterine artery embolization. Magnetic resonance imaging can identify subserosal leiomyomas by visualizing the vascular supply of the mass as arising from the uterus. Magnetic resonance imaging also is accurate in differentiating adenomyosis from leiomyomas, which may be important in selecting therapeutic options. However, MRI cannot distinguish reliably between leiomyomas and their malignant counterparts, leiomyosarcomas (22).

Gynecologic Cancer

Magnetic resonance imaging has some clinical utility in the evaluation of the extent of disease of the uterus and cervix. Determining the extent of regional spread of uterine corpus and cervical cancer is more accurate with MRI than with CT.

The overall accuracy of evaluating uterine cancer by MRI is between 85% and 93%. Use of a dynamic IV contrast agent improves the accuracy in determining the depth of myometrial invasion. The junctional zone between the endometrium and myometrium is disrupted in stage IB tumors as compared with stage IA tumors (Fig. 11). Additionally, disruption of subendometrial enhancement may be seen with stage IB endometrial tumors. The sensitivity of MRI for the detection of myometrial invasion ranges from 69% to 94% and the specificity ranges from 64% to 100%. Large polypoid masses, leiomyomas, and adenomyosis may lead to lower accuracy in determining the depth of invasion. The accuracy of determining cervical invasion in endometrial cancer cases is 92%. Parametrial

involvement indicating stage III disease and invasion into the bladder or rectum indicating stage IV disease also may be imaged with MRI (23).

Leiomyosarcomas remain difficult to diagnose preoperatively. Magnetic resonance imaging cannot reliably distinguish a sarcoma from endometrial carcinoma. Degenerating leiomyomas also may be confused with sarcomas on MRI (23).

Cervical carcinomas are best seen by T2 weighted images. The use of an IV contrast agent does not aid in the staging of cervical cancer. Magnetic resonance imaging is helpful in evaluating parametrial involvement with the tumor, extension into the lower uterine segment, and depth of stromal invasion. Although MRI cannot be used for the clinical staging of cervical cancer, it may have a role in determining the therapeutic approach in cervical cancer. Clinical situations in which MRI may be useful include cervical cancer in pregnancy, endocervical lesions, and clinical stage IB disease where the tumor is 2 cm or greater (Fig. 12). Large stage IB tumors are more likely to involve the parametria and lymph nodes. The rates of accuracy of CT and MRI in staging cervical cancer are similar. Magnetic resonance imaging is better at visualization of the primary lesion and parametrial involvement than CT (24). It also may be useful in the preoperative evaluation of women desiring fertility-sparing treatment for stage I cervical cancer. In these patients, MRI can predict myometrial invasion and determine the relationship of the tumor to the internal os. Magnetic resonance imaging can overestimate the parametrial invasion in large cervical tumors. The stromal edema from inflammation or compression of the surrounding vasculature may mimic parametrial involvement on T2 weighted images (24).

Both MRI and CT have similar rates of detecting metastases involving lymph nodes. The main difficulty in the diagnosis of lymph node metastasis by imaging is the low sensitivity because the criteria are based

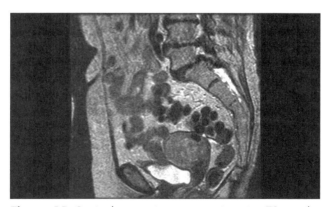

Figure 11. Sagittal magnetic resonance imaging T2 weighted image of a patient with stage IC endometrial carcinoma. The junctional zone is not seen and the tumor extends beyond one half of the myometrial thickness. A small subserosal fibroid is seen as the hypodense area posteriorly.

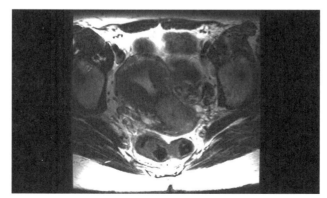

Figure 12. Axial magnetic resonance imaging image of a patient with stage IB cervical carcinoma. Note the bulky mass in the cervix and lower uterine segment inferior to the endometrium.

on the size of the lymph node. Advances in the use of nanoparticle IV MRI contrast agents may allow for improved detection of lymph node metastasis in endometrial and cervical cancer (25).

Dynamic contrast agent enhanced MRI allows for assessment of tumor vascularity and response to radiation therapy and chemotherapy. In a series of 101 patients with advanced cervical cancer, serial dynamic contrast agent enhanced MRI assessment of tumor perfusion status provided early predictive value of primary tumor control and disease-free survival (26). Further study of dynamic contrast agent enhanced MRI is needed to determine its role in the assessment of treatment response in patients with cervical cancer.

High-field strength MRI equipment is becoming more widely available. Increasing field strength improves image quality because of the increased signal-to-noise ratio. Staging of ovarian cancer with a 3 T MRI was comparable in accuracy to surgical staging in one study of 77 patients, using histopathology as the standard diagnostic method (27).

As previously mentioned, PET has an emerging role in the imaging of gynecologic cancer. Although MRI offers great anatomical detail, PET adds detail regarding the function of the tissue. When there is doubt about the clinical significance of a structure imaged on MRI, PET may offer a noninvasive method to assess whether the structure is likely related to the underlying malignancy. Uptake of the labeled deoxyglucose on PET images may indicate that a retroperitoneal lymph node seen on MRI likely represents lymphatic extension of the primary tumor. Magnetic resonance imaging and PET may play an expanding and complementary role in noninvasive evaluation of gynecologic malignancy before and after primary therapy.

References

1. Kim EE. Whole-body positron emission tomography and positron emission tomography/computed tomography in gynecologic oncology. Int J Gynecol Cancer 2004;14:12–22.

2. Gjelsteen AC, Ching BH, Meyermann MW, Prager DA, Murphy TF, Berkey BD, et al. CT, MRI, PET, PET/CT, and ultrasound in the evaluation of obstetric and gynecologic patients. Surg Clin North Am 2008;88:361–90, vii.

3. Choi HJ, Roh JW, Seo SS, Lee S, Kim JY, Kim SK, et al. Comparison of the accuracy of magnetic resonance imaging and positron emission tomography/computed tomography in the presurgical detection of lymph node metastases in patients with uterine cervical carcinoma: a prospective study. Cancer 2006;106:914–22.

4. Avril N, Sassen S, Schmalfeldt B, Naehrig J, Rutke S, Weber WA, et al. Prediction of response to neoadjuvant chemotherapy by sequential F-18-fluorodeoxyglucose positron emission tomography in patients with advanced-stage ovarian cancer [published erratum appears in J Clin Oncol 2005;23:9445]. J Clin Oncol 2005;23:7445–53.

5. The role of transvaginal ultrasonography in the evaluation of postmenopausal bleeding. ACOG Committee Opinion No. 440. American College of Obstetricians and Gynecologists. Obstet Gynecol 2009;114:409–11.

6. Management of adnexal masses. ACOG Practice Bulletin No. 83. American College of Obstetricians and Gynecologists. Obstet Gynecol 2007;110:201–14.

7. Sokalska A, Timmerman D, Testa AC, Van Holsbeke C, Lissoni AA, Leone FP, et al. Diagnostic accuracy of transvaginal ultrasound examination for assigning a specific diagnosis to adnexal masses. Ultrasound Obstet Gynecol 2009;34:462–70.

8. Ghate SV, Crockett MM, Boyd BK, Paulson EK. Sonohysterography: do 3D reconstructed images provide additional value? AJR Am J Roentgenol 2008;190:W227–33.

9. Benacerraf BR, Benson CB, Abuhamad AZ, Copel JA, Abramovicz JS, Devore GR, et al. Three- and 4-dimensional ultrasound in obstetrics and gynecology: proceedings of the American Institute of Ultrasound in Medicine Consensus Conference. J Ultrasound Med 2005;24:1587–97.

10. Sonohysterography. ACOG Technology Assessment No. 5. American College of Obstetricians and Gynecologists. Obstet Gynecol 2008;112:1467–9.

11. de Kroon CD, Jansen FW, Louwe LA, Dieben SW, van Houwelingen HC, Trimbos JB. Technology assessment of saline contrast hysterosonography. Am J Obstet Gynecol 2003;188:945–9.

12. Van den Bosch T, Verguts J, Daemen A, Gevaert O, Domali E, Claerhout F, et al. Pain experienced during transvaginal ultrasound, saline contrast sonohysterography, hysteroscopy and office sampling: a comparative study. Ultrasound Obstet Gynecol 2008;31:346–51.

13. Verma SK, Lev-Toaff AS, Baltarowich OH, Bergin D, Verma M, Mitchell DG. Adenomyosis: sonohysterography with MRI correlation. AJR Am J Roentgenol 2009;192:1112–6.

14. Moschos E, Ashfaq R, McIntire DD, Liriano B, Twickler DM. Saline-infusion sonography endometrial sampling compared with endometrial biopsy in diagnosing endometrial pathology. Obstet Gynecol 2009;113:881–7.

15. Gorlero F, Nicoletti L, Lijoi D, Ferrero S, Pulle A, Ragni N. Endometrial directed biopsy during sonohysterography using the NiGo device: prospective study in women with abnormal uterine bleeding. Fertil Steril 2008;89:984–90.

16. Leone FP, Carsana L, Lanzani C, Vago G, Ferrazzi E. Sonohysterographic endometrial sampling and hysteroscopic endometrial biopsy: a comparative study. Ultrasound Obstet Gynecol 2007;29:443–8.

17. Berry E, Lindheim SR, Connor JP, Hartenbach EM, Schink JC, Harter J, et al. Sonohysterography and endometrial cancer: incidence and functional viability of disseminated malignant cells. Am J Obstet Gynecol 2008;199:240.e1–240.e8.

18. Takac I. Saline infusion sonohysterography and the risk of malignant extrauterine spread in endometrial cancer. Ultrasound Med Biol 2008;34:7–11.

19. Dessole S, Rubattu G, Farina M, Capobianco G, Cherchi PL, Tanda F, et al. Risks and usefulness of sonohysterography in patients with endometrial carcinoma. Am J Obstet Gynecol 2006;194:362–8.

20. Church DG, Vancil JM, Vasanawala SS. Magnetic resonance imaging for uterine and vaginal anomalies. Curr Opin Obstet Gynecol 2009;21:379–89.

21. Rajkotia K, Veeramani M, Macura KJ. Magnetic resonance imaging of adnexal masses. Top Magn Reson Imaging 2006;17:379–97.

22. Sala E. Magnetic resonance imaging of the female pelvis. Semin Roentgenol 2008;43:290–302.

23. Sala E, Wakely S, Senior E, Lomas D. MRI of malignant neoplasms of the uterine corpus and cervix. AJR Am J Roentgenol 2007;188:1577–87.

24. Hricak H, Gatsonis C, Chi DS, Amendola MA, Brandt K, Schwartz LH, et al. Role of imaging in pretreatment evaluation of early invasive cervical cancer: results of the intergroup study American College of Radiology Imaging Network 6651-Gynecologic Oncology Group 183. American College of Radiology Imaging Network 6651; Gynecologic Oncology Group 183. J Clin Oncol 2005;23: 9329–37.

25. Narayanan P, Iyngkaran T, Sohaib SA, Reznek RH, Rockall AG. Magnetic resonance lymphography: a novel technique for lymph node assessment in gynecologic malignancies. Cancer Biomark 2009;5:81–8.

26. Yuh WT, Mayr NA, Jarjoura D, Wu D, Grecula JC, Lo SS, et al. Predicting control of primary tumor and survival by DCE MRI during early therapy in cervical cancer. Invest Radiol 2009;44:343–50.

27. Booth SJ, Turnbull LW, Poole DR, Richmond I. The accurate staging of ovarian cancer using 3T magnetic resonance imaging—a realistic option. BJOG 2008;115:894–901.

Cervical Cytology and Cervical Intraepithelial Neoplasia

Mark Spitzer

The developments in the field of cervical cancer screening and management of cervical cancer precursors along with advances in the technology applied to this field have resulted in changes in the guidelines for managing these conditions. In 2006, the American Society for Colposcopy and Cervical Pathology (ASCCP) revised its consensus guidelines for the management of women with cytologic abnormalities (1) and cervical cancer precursors (2). Significant changes include recommendations for a more conservative approach to the management of adolescents, pregnant women, and women with cervical intraepithelial neoplasia (CIN) grades 1 and 2. The reason for this more conservative approach was the recognition of the risks associated with treatment for CIN, especially the loop electrosurgical excision procedure (LEEP). In 2009, the American College of Obstetricians and Gynecologists (the College) took the first major step in revising its screening guidelines (3). The introduction of the first human papillomavirus (HPV) genotyping assay in 2009 led to a new guideline for the triage of women older than 30 years with normal cervical cytologic results and human papillomavirus (HPV) test results positive for high-risk HPV types (4, 5). Finally, in 2006 and in 2009, two different HPV vaccines were approved for use in women and girls. It is important to note that the approach to cervical cancer screening and the management of cervical cytologic abnormalities should not change in vaccinated women (6).

Screening

Cervical cancer screening modalities currently in use in the United States include conventional cytology, liquid-based cytology, and combination of cytology and HPV testing. In 1999, the Agency for Health Care Policy and Research completed a meta-analysis that reported the sensitivity and specificity of conventional cytology to be 51% and 98%, respectively (7). In 2002, the American Cancer Society (ACS) noted that the available evidence suggests that liquid-based cytology is somewhat more sensitive but less specific than conventional cytology for high-grade lesions and recommended that the screening interval can be increased to every 2 years when liquid-based cytology is used (8). However, more recent evidence questions the conclusion that liquid-based cytology is more sensitive than conventional cytology. A large randomized trial showed that liquid-based cytology did not increase the detection of high-

grade lesions (9). Another large randomized controlled trial showed that the sensitivity and positive predictive value for liquid-based cytology were not better than conventional cytology for the detection of any grade of CIN or cancer (10). One meta-analysis came to the same conclusion (11). Nevertheless, pathologists prefer liquid-based cytology because the slides are easier to read and are more appropriate for use with automatic screening devices. Also, the residual fluid makes cotesting with HPV DNA more convenient (9). Consequently, more than 90% of U.S. obstetrician–gynecologists use liquid-based cytology (3).

When to Begin Screening

Although HPV infections are quite common in adolescents, because of their high rate of sexual activity and reported number of partners (12), cervical cancer is rarely diagnosed in women younger than 20 years (13). Also, one study found that the rate of CIN 3 among study participants referred for cervical cytology reported as atypical squamous cells—undetermined significance (ASC-US) or low-grade squamous intraepithelial lesions (LSIL) was 6.3%, less than one half of that reported in adults (14). Furthermore, young women are less likely to show persistence of HPV infections and those with persistence are less likely to be at risk of invasive cancer (15). With the recognition that there is little to gain from initiating cervical cancer screening in young women, U.S. screening guidelines have been evolving. In 2002–2003 the ACS (8), the College, and the United States Preventive Services Task Force (USPSTF) (16) recommended that rather than screening girls at their sexual debut or age 18 years, the first Pap test should be postponed to approximately 3 years after initiation of sexual intercourse, but no later than age 21 years. The consensus was that cervical cancer screening in adolescents within the first 3 years after initiation of sexual intercourse is not likely to result in the identification of high-grade squamous intraepithelial lesion (HSIL) or cancer but is likely to increase anxiety, morbidity, and expense from increased follow-up procedures. However, by 2006 it became evident that the potential for adverse effects associated with the follow-up of young women with abnormal cytology screening results far exceeded any potential benefits. This prompted the ASCCP consensus meeting to emphasize a much more conservative approach to women younger than 21 years with abnormalities shown on their Pap test (1). This approach was endorsed by the College (17).

In 2009, the College took the logical incremental step in recommending that cytologic screening should begin at age 21 years regardless of the age of onset of sexual intercourse (3). This is based in part on the very low incidence of cancer in young women. It also is based on the potential for adverse effects associated with follow-up of young women with abnormal cytologic screening results. Screening before age 21 years should be avoided because it may lead to unnecessary and harmful evaluation and treatment in women who are at very low risk of cancer. Sexually active adolescents younger than 21 years should be counseled and tested for sexually transmitted infections, and they should be counseled regarding responsible sex and contraception. These measures may be carried out without cervical cytology and, in the asymptomatic patient, without the introduction of a speculum.

When to Discontinue Screening

In the United States, the incidence and prevalence of CIN peak in the mid-reproductive years and begin to decline in approximately the fourth decade of life. Among screened older women, the rates of cytologically detected HSIL are low (16) and cervical cancer is rare especially among women with multiple prior consecutive negative cervical cytologic test results (8). Most new cases of cervical cancer in U.S. women older than 65 years are found in unscreened or infrequently screened women (18). In addition, vaginal atrophy, which is common after menopause, may predispose older women to false-positive cytologic results. Furthermore, it may be difficult to obtain satisfactory samples from older women because of conditions, such as atrophy and cervical stenosis. Older women also are disproportionately more likely to be evaluated for false-positive findings, which results in unnecessary and sometimes harmful interventions (8). Any attempt at setting an upper age for screening must, therefore, take into consideration a woman's past screening history. Although there is general agreement that screening should be discontinued in low-risk older women, the age at which screening may be discontinued is somewhat arbitrary. The ACS set the age at 70 years (8) and the USPSTF set the age at 65 years (16). Although initially the College declined to set an age at which to discontinue screening, by 2009 it noted that because cervical cancer develops slowly and risk factors decrease with age, it is reasonable to discontinue cervical cancer screening at either age 65 years or 70 years in women who have three or more consecutive negative cytologic test results and no abnormal test results in the past 10 years. If screening is discontinued, risk factors should be assessed during the annual examination to determine if reinitiating screening is appropriate (3). Women treated in the past for CIN 2, CIN 3, or cancer remain at risk of persistent or recurrent disease for at least 20 years after treatment and after initial posttreatment surveillance, and they should continue to have annual screenings for at least 20 years (3).

Women whose cervices have been removed (total abdominal hysterectomy or trachelectomy) and have no history of HSIL are at a low risk of developing vaginal cancer. In one study, more than 9,000 Pap tests were performed in women who had had a hysterectomy for benign indications an average of 19 years previously. Only 1.1% had cytologic abnormalities, and none had vaginal intraepithelial neoplasia grade 3 or cancer on biopsy (19). Thus, abnormal test results after hysterectomy are almost always false positive. Continued screening of low-risk women after a total hysterectomy for benign disease is not cost-effective, causes undue anxiety, and leads to overtreatment, so ACS, USPSTF, and the College all recommend that cytologic screening be discontinued in these women (3, 8, 16). Women who have had a total hysterectomy and have a history of CIN 2 or CIN 3 (or in whom a negative history is not documented) should continue to be routinely screened. Extension of the screening interval is acceptable, but there are no data to support discontinuation of screening of this group.

Screening Interval

The recommended interval between cervical cancer screening tests is related to a woman's underlying risk of disease and the sensitivity of the screening test being used. The optimal number of negative cervical cytologic test results needed to reduce the false-negative rate to a minimum has not been determined, but as the number of sequential negative Pap test results increases, the rate of dysplasia decreases. However, in populations with an organized program of cervical cancer screening, annual cytologic examinations offer little advantage over screenings performed at 2- or 3-year intervals (20). Data from the National Breast and Cervical Cancer Early Detection Program, found a prevalence of CIN 2 and CIN 3 to be 0.028% and 0.019%, respectively, with no cases of invasive cancer among those who had three or more consecutive negative Pap test results. Computer modeling in this cohort showed that annual screening would reduce the number of women developing invasive cancer by only 4 women per 100,000 but at great cost for each case of cancer (21). Formal cost-effective analysis of data from this national program showed that the most cost-effective strategy for cervical cancer screening is cytology testing no more often than every 3 years whereas annual Pap testing was never found to be cost-effective (22).

Another consideration is the role that age plays in the sensitivity of screening. Several studies have shown that a negative Pap test result is less reassuring in women younger than 30 years than in older women (20, 21).

In 2002, the ACS noted that the available evidence suggested that liquid-based cytology is somewhat more sensitive but less specific for high-grade lesions than conventional cytology and recommended that in women younger than 30 years, cervical screening should be done annually when conventional cytology is used, but every 2 years when liquid-based cytology is used (8). Although the College initially maintained that screening should be performed annually in this age group regardless of the modality used (23), in 2009 it revised its guidelines and now recommends cervical cytology screening every 2 years for women aged 21–29 years regardless of the modality used (3).

In women aged 30 years and older who have had three consecutive, technically satisfactory normal or negative cytology results, ACS recommends screening every 2–3 years (unless they have a history of in-utero diethylstilbestrol exposure, are HIV positive, or are immunocompromised by organ transplantation, chemotherapy, or chronic corticosteroid treatment) (8). In 2009, the College recommended extending the screening interval in these low-risk women to every 3 years but restricted the recommendation to women who have not had a history of CIN 2 or CIN 3 (3). This places an additional burden on the health care provider to accurately assess a new patient's screening history. Furthermore, it is important to educate patients about the nature of cervical cytology, its limitations, and the rationale for prolonging the screening interval beyond every year. In addition, regardless of the frequency of cervical cytology screening, physicians also should inform their patients that annual gynecologic examinations may still be appropriate even if cervical cytology is not performed at each visit (3).

Screening With Cervical Cytology Plus HPV DNA Testing

Despite the high lifetime risk of acquiring an infection with high-risk HPV, most newly acquired infections clear spontaneously and the prevalence of HPV positivity decreases with age from a peak in adolescents and women in their 20s (24). In women aged 30 years and older, the prevalence of HPV positivity is low enough to make HPV testing cost-effective for routine screening (1). For a combination of high-risk HPV testing and cervical cytology, the sensitivity for CIN 2 and CIN 3 is significantly higher than that for either test alone. The combination has negative predictive values of 99–100% (25, 26). Women who receive negative test results by both cervical cytology and HPV testing have a less than 1 in 1,000 risk of having CIN 2 or greater, and prospective follow-up studies have shown that the risk of developing CIN 3 over a 10-year period is quite low (27). The 2006 ASCCP Consensus Conference recommended that women who receive negative results by both cytology and high-risk HPV testing should not be rescreened before 3 years (1). The College affirmed this recommendation in 2009 (3). Primary screening with cervical cytology plus HPV testing should be limited to women older than 30 years (1, 3). Screening younger women with this method is not useful because the prevalence of HPV is very high in women younger than 30 years. Screening younger women with HPV tests also may result in overtreatment of women who have self-limited disease.

A large study from Kaiser Northern California summarized their 5-year experience with 580,000 women who underwent cotesting using conventional cervical cytology and high-risk HPV DNA testing (28). In cytologically negative women aged 30 years and older from their routine screening population, the prevalence of high-risk HPV positivity was 4%, but ranged from 6.8% in women in their early 30s to less than 4% in women in their 40s and less than 3% in women aged 50 years and older. The risk of having undetected CIN 2 or greater in cytology-negative, HPV-positive women in well-screened populations ranges from 2.4% to 5.1% (29–32). Because of this low risk, the consensus guidelines recommended conservative follow-up with repeat cytology and HPV testing at 12 months for cytology-negative, HPV-positive women. Women should be evaluated with colposcopy if high-risk HPV positivity persists on repeat testing.

In March 2009, the U.S. Food and Drug Administration (FDA) announced approval for clinical use in the United States of two new HPV DNA diagnostic tests. One of these tests is designed to identify 14 types of high-risk HPV (HPV types 16, 18, 31, 33, 35, 39, 45, 51, 52, 56, 58, 59, 66, and 68). The other test is designed to specifically detect HPV 16 and HPV 18. In exploring the significance of positivity for HPV 16 and HPV 18 compared with positivity for the other high-risk HPV types, authors of one study tested 20,810 women who were enrolled in the Kaiser Permanente health plan in Portland, Oregon, for 13 oncogenic HPV strains and monitored them for 10 years (27). At enrollment, 96% of the women had normal cytologic results, and during the follow-up period, 131 (6%) developed CIN 3 or greater. However, when the data were analyzed by HPV type, the cumulative rates for CIN 3 or greater were 17.2% among HPV 16-positive women, 13.6% among HPV 18-positive women, 3% among HPV-positive women with one of 11 other oncogenic HPV types, and 0.8% in HPV-negative women. These data were discussed at the 2006 ASCCP Consensus Conference in anticipation of the FDA's approval of

HPV genotyping. The consensus guidelines recommended that cytologically negative women who test positive for high-risk HPV types may be "reflex" tested for HPV 16 and HPV 18. Those who test positive for HPV 16 or HPV 18 should be referred for immediate colposcopy. Those who test positive for any of the other high-risk HPV types but negative for HPV 16 and HPV 18 could receive repeat cytology and high-risk HPV testing in 12 months.

The 2001 Bethesda System and Management of Abnormalities

The Bethesda System was introduced in 1988 and revised in 1991 and 2001. It was established to standardize the reporting of cervical cytology in the hope that a uniform system of terminology would provide clear guidance for clinical management. By 2001, more than 90% of U.S. laboratories were using some form of the Bethesda System in reporting cytologic results.

Specimen Adequacy

The 2001 Bethesda System uses two terms for specimen adequacy, satisfactory and unsatisfactory. Satisfactory specimens must be properly labeled and arrive with relevant clinical information. They must have an adequate number of interpretable squamous cells and endocervical or squamous metaplastic cells. Unsatisfactory specimens include those that cannot be assessed by the laboratory because the slides are broken and cannot be repaired, they lack proper patient identification, or are processed by the laboratory but determined to be unsatisfactory because of scant cellularity or obscuring background material, such as blood or inflammation.

In 2002, a task force of the ASCCP published a set of guidelines related to Pap test specimen adequacy and patient management. These guidelines were revised in 2007 (33). The recommended management for most women with an unsatisfactory Pap test result is to repeat the Pap test within 2–4 months. If a specific infection is identified as the cause of obscuring inflammation, it should be treated before repeating the Pap test. Women who are symptomatic, who have an abnormal examination results, or whose Pap test is repeatedly unsatisfactory because of obscuring blood, inflammation, or necrosis should undergo additional clinical evaluation as appropriate (eg, colposcopy, biopsy, or both for women with visible lesions, friable cervix, and postcoital or abnormal bleeding). Pap tests that were not indicated according to an established screening protocol do not need to be repeated (eg, a Pap test in a woman after a hysterectomy for benign disease or in an older woman with a low risk [see earlier discussion]). Specimens showing low cellularity may be acceptable in a woman after a hysterectomy

for malignancy, chemotherapy, or radiation therapy because obtaining specimens with higher cellularity may not be possible in these women.

When a routine Pap test analysis reports the lack of an endocervical or transformation zone component or has a notation about another quality indicator (eg, borderline cellularity or partially obscuring blood or inflammation), in women older than 30 years whose HPV status is negative or unknown, the preferred management is to repeat Pap test in 12 months rather than extending the screening interval to 3 years. Women whose HPV test result is positive should have the Pap test repeated at 6 months, and if the repeat Pap test result is negative, they should have the HPV test repeated at 12 months. Other women who may benefit from an early repeat Pap test (at 6 months) are those with a previous squamous abnormality (atypical or worse) without two subsequent negative Pap test results or a negative HPV test results, those with a previous Pap test result showing an unexplained glandular abnormality, those with a positive high-risk HPV test result within 12 months, those in whom the clinician is unable to clearly visualize the cervix or sample the endocervical canal, those with similar obscuring factors in consecutive Pap test results, and those who have insufficient previous screening (33).

Negative Test Result for Intraepithelial Lesions or Malignancy

If the Pap test result shows epithelial cells with no evidence of changes consistent with intraepithelial neoplasia, the specimen is reported as "negative for intraepithelial lesions or malignancy." Benign cellular changes and the presence of organisms, such as *Trichomonas* species, fungus, and actinomycosis or cellular changes associated with herpes simplex virus can be noted, but the specimen is still reported as negative. Changes consistent with estrogen deficiency, radiation therapy, and intrauterine device or tampon use also may be listed separately.

Epithelial Cell Abnormalities

Cellular changes suggestive but not diagnostic of a squamous intraepithelial lesion are included in the category of "atypical squamous cells." If the cellular changes are suggestive of a low-grade lesion, they are characterized as ASC-US. If the cellular changes are suggestive of a high-grade lesion, they are characterized as "atypical squamous cells, cannot exclude high-grade SIL" (ASC-H). Benign cellular changes, reactive, reparative, and inflammatory changes are no longer characterized as atypical, but are reported as negative for intraepithelial lesions or malignancy with a comment describing the changes (see earlier discussion).

Atypical squamous cell—undetermined significance is the most common cervical cytologic abnormality, accounting for 4.4% of all Pap test results. Although the risk of cancer for any individual patient is very low (0.1–0.2%), and the risk of CIN 2 and higher also is low (6.4–11.9%) because there are so many women with this cytologic abnormality, it is the presenting cytologic result for approximately one half of the women with CIN 2 and higher. Although ASC-H is not highly reproducible among pathologies, studies suggest that cytology reported as ASC-H has a positive predictive value for CIN 2 and CIN 3 that is intermediate between ASC-US and HSIL.

Squamous Intraepithelial Lesions

Squamous intraepithelial lesions may be reported as LSIL, which includes cervical HPV infection and mild dysplasia (CIN 1) or HSIL, which includes moderate dysplasia (CIN 2), severe dysplasia (CIN 3) and carcinoma in situ (CIS). Between 1996 and 2003, the rate of LSIL in the United States increased from 1.6% to 2.1% whereas the rates of other cytologic categories did not change (34). This increase was probably due to the widespread use of liquid-based cytology of which the detection rate for LSIL is 2.4% compared with the detection rate of only 1.4% for conventional cytology. Although cytologic LSIL is thought to reflect the cytopathic effects of HPV infection rather than a true premalignant lesion, women with LSIL remain at moderate risk of having CIN 2 and higher. In the ASCUS/LSIL Triage Study for Cervical Cancer (ALTS), 27.6% women with LSIL were found to have CIN 2 and higher either on colposcopically directed biopsies or on close follow-up over the next 2 years (35). This rate is virtually identical with the rate of CIN 2 and higher in women who presented with HPV-positive ASC-US in the same population (26.7%). A study reporting on colposcopically directed biopsies in 46,009 women, found CIN 2 and higher in 15.2% of women with only LSIL cytology (36). As many as 86.1% of women with LSIL test positive for high-risk HPV types (37) with HPV type 16, the most prevalent of the high-risk types found in 24.8%. Young women become infected with HPV very quickly after initiating sexual activity (38). Consequently, there is a high prevalence of high-risk HPV types in women younger than 30 years, and the rate decreases substantially with age.

In the United States, approximately 0.5% of all Pap test results are reported as HSIL (34). The rate of HSIL varies with age decreasing from 0.6% in women aged 20–29 years to 0.1% in women aged 50–59 years (39). Loop electrosurgical excision procedure identifies CIN 2 and higher in 84–97% of women with Pap test results positive for HSIL and in 53–66% of women with HSIL identified on a single colposcopic examination (40).

Approximately 2% of women with HSIL have invasive cancer (41).

Glandular Cell Abnormalities

In the 2001 Bethesda classification system, the description of glandular cellular abnormalities progresses from "atypical glandular cells—not otherwise specified" (AGC-NOS) to "AGC, favor neoplasia" and, finally, to adenocarcinoma in situ (AIS). The risk associated with AGC is dramatically higher than that seen with ASC. Series of articles have reported that 9–38% of women with AGC have significant neoplasia (CIN 2, CIN 3, AIS, or cancer) and 3–17% have invasive cancer (42–44). The rate and type of significant findings in women with AGC varies with age (44). Women younger than 35 years with AGC are more likely to have CIN and less likely to have cancer whereas in older women the risk of glandular lesions, including malignancies, is higher (42). Human papillomavirus testing, cervical cytology, and colposcopy all perform poorly at detecting glandular disease (43).

In premenopausal women, benign-appearing endometrial cells or the presence of endometrial stromal cells or histiocytes are rarely associated with significant pathology (45). However, in postmenopausal women, they may be associated with significant endometrial pathology (46) and may be thought of as microscopic postmenopausal bleeding. Benign-appearing glandular cells derived from small accessory ducts, foci of benign adenosis, or prolapse of the fallopian tube into the vagina are sometimes seen in cytologic specimens after total hysterectomy and have no clinical significance.

Clinical Management

The 2006 ASCCP guidelines for the management of women with cervical cytologic abnormalities (1) and cervical cancer precursors (2) rely primarily on evidence from randomized controlled trials. These management strategies assume that a small level of risk of failing to detect high-grade neoplasia is acceptable. It is unreasonable for patients or clinicians to expect that the risk can be reduced to zero, and attempts to achieve zero risk could result in greater harm than good in the form of overtreatment. When treating an individual patient, guidelines are not a substitute for clinical judgment because it is impossible to develop guidelines that would apply to all situations.

These guidelines were based on some fundamental principles. A triage test that refers more than 75% of women to colposcopy is not helpful and is not an acceptable option. When the guidelines refer to HPV tests, they mean tests for oncogenic HPV types that are analytically and clinically validated with proven acceptable reproducibility, clinical sensitivity, specificity, and positive and negative predictive values for cervical cancer and verified precancer (CIN 2 and CIN 3), as documented by FDA approval, publication in peer-reviewed scientific literature, or both. Using tests that do not meet these criteria could result in outcomes that are not intended by the guidelines (1, 2). There also is increasing recognition that colposcopy is less sensitive than previously thought and that a single colposcopic examination misses approximately one third of women with CIN 2 or CIN 3 (35). Finally, the sensitivity of colposcopy is significantly greater when two or more biopsies are obtained (47). Results from these studies suggest that biopsies of all visible lesions are warranted, regardless of colposcopic impression, and that follow-up should include multiple colposcopies over time for women with abnormal cytologic or histologic results or women who have persistent low-grade abnormalities or persistently test positive for HPV (17).

Management of Adolescents

In 2006, the ASCCP consensus conference recognized the unique challenges of caring for adolescents with cytologic and histologic abnormalities (Fig. 13) (1, 2). Cervical cancer is almost nonexistent in adolescents, yet HPV infection is very common in this population. Consequently, a much more conservative set of guidelines was created for the management of these abnormalities in adolescents intended to minimize the potential negative effect that treatment may have on future pregnancy outcomes, while taking advantage of the natural history of HPV in young women. The guidelines delay colposcopy and use a higher threshold for intervention compared with adults having comparable abnormalities. Furthermore, they advise against HPV testing and recommend against treatment of LSIL or CIN 1. In addition, among adherent adolescents, treatment of CIN 2 also should be deferred. The College affirmed these guidelines (17).

Atypical Squamous Cells—Undetermined Significance

Although the prevalence of CIN 2, CIN 3, and invasive cancer among patients with ASC-US cytology is relatively low, so many women have ASC-US test results that the category will include many women with CIN 2 and CIN 3 (1). The first step in the evaluation of women with ASC-US is to triage those who are at higher risk to more intensive evaluation (colposcopy) while submitting the others to routine follow-up. Premenopausal women older than 20 years with cytologic results positive for ASC-US may undergo immediate colposcopy or may undergo triage testing to determine whether they should be referred for colposcopy. Under the ASCCP consensus guidelines, repeat cytology at 6 months and

Management of Adolescent Women with Either Atypical Squamous Cells of Undetermined Significance (ASC-US) or Low-grade Squamous Intraepithelial Lesion (LSIL)

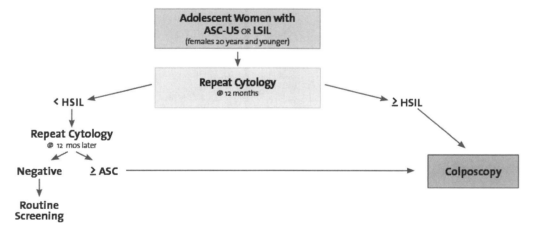

Figure 13. Management of adolescent women with either atypical squamous cells of undetermined significance (ACS-US) or low-grade squamous intraepithelial lesion (LSIL). (Wright TC Jr, Massad S, Dunton CJ, Spitzer M, Wilkinson EJ, Solomon D. 2006 consensus guidelines for the management of women with abnormal cervical screening tests. J Low Gen Tract Dis 2007;11:201– 22. Reprinted from *The Journal of Lower Genital Tract Disease* Vol. 11 Issue 4, with the permission of ASCCP © American Society for Colposcopy and Cervical Pathology 2007. No copies of the algorithm may be made without the prior consent of ASCCP.)

12 months, immediate colposcopy, and HPV testing are all acceptable methods for the triage of women with cytologic results positive for ASC-US. Those with HPV-positive ASC-US results or two consecutive cytologic results positive for ASC-US are referred for colposcopy. Data from ALTS demonstrated that two repeat cytologic examinations at 6 months and 12 months at an ASC-US threshold detected 88% of the CIN 2 or higher grade abnormality while referring 63.6% of the women for colposcopy. Human papillomavirus testing alone detected 92.2% of the CIN 2 and higher while referring 55% of the women to colposcopy. Consequently, in women who had liquid-based cytology or who had an HPV specimen co-collected, reflex testing for high-risk HPV types is preferred (1, 48).

Because recent studies reported a lower prevalence of high-grade disease and HPV DNA positivity than previously thought among immunosuppressed women, the 2006 guidelines recommended that immunosuppressed women be managed similarly to the general population. Also, because HPV DNA positivity rates decrease dramatically as women age, HPV testing actually is more efficient in older women (1). In contrast, using HPV DNA testing to triage adolescents and young women with ASC-US would necessitate referral for colposcopy in large numbers of women who are at low risk of having cervical cancer. Also, many adolescents have multiple sequential HPV infections, so a repetitively positive HPV test in this age group may represent consecutive incident infections rather than a single persistent infection. In adolescents with ASC-US, follow-up with annual cytologic testing is recommended. Testing for HPV and colposcopy are unacceptable for adolescents with ASC-US, and if HPV testing is inadvertently performed, the results should not influence management. In adolescents, the threshold for referral to colposcopy also is different than in adult women (1, 48). At the 12-month follow-up visit, only those with an HSIL or greater result on the repeat cytology should be referred for colposcopy. At the 24-month follow-up, those with an ASC-US or greater result should be referred for colposcopy.

Atypical Squamous Cells—Favor High Grade

Women with ASC-H have a 20–50% risk of having a CIN 2 or CIN 3 lesion and should be evaluated with immediate colposcopy (1, 48). Most women with ASC-H are HPV positive (ranging from 67–84%) (1); therefore, intermediate triage is inappropriate and HPV testing is not recommended. If CIN 2 or CIN 3 is not identified at colposcopy in these women, they should be monitored in a manner similar to HPV-positive women with ASC-US (1, 48).

Low-Grade Squamous Intraepithelial Lesions and HPV-Positive ASC-US

Women with LSIL remain at moderate risk of CIN 2 and higher grade lesions. In ALTS, 27.6% women with LSIL were found to have CIN 2 and higher grade abnormalities either on colposcopically directed biopsies or on close follow-up over the next 2 years (35). This rate is virtually identical to the rate of CIN 2 and higher grade lesions in women who presented with HPV-positive ASC-US in the same population (26.7%). Two thirds of the cases (17.9%) were identified at the initial colposcopy and the remainder in follow-up. Consequently, the consensus guidelines are identical for the management of premenopausal women older than 20 years with HPV-positive ASC-US or two consecutive ASC-US cytologic results or those with LSIL. Colposcopy is recommended in all of these women (1, 48). However, because previously negative postmenopausal women are at low risk of invasive cervical cancer and the prevalence of both HPV positivity and CIN 2 or CIN 3 decrease with age in well-screened women with LSIL, postmenopausal women with LSIL may be screened using HPV testing for triage in the same protocol as is used in reproductive-aged women with ASC-US (1, 48).

When the results of the colposcopically directed biopsy show CIN 2 and higher grade lesions, the patient is treated based on that diagnosis (see later discussion). However, when CIN 2 and higher grade lesions are not identified, additional follow-up is required. In ALTS, the initial colposcopy identified only 58% of the CIN 2 and higher grade lesions. For those women not found to have CIN 2 and higher grade lesions at the initial colposcopy, the rate of CIN 2 and higher grade lesions during follow-up (approximately 10%–13%) was unaffected by the findings at colposcopy (negative findings not worthy of biopsy, negative biopsy, or CIN 1 biopsy). The ASCUS/LSIL Triage Study for Cervical Cancer evaluated different postcolposcopy follow-up strategies and found that HPV testing performed 12 months after the initial colposcopy and two repeat cytologic examinations performed at 6-month intervals were equally effective (49). Because of the additional cost and lack of increased sensitivity, the strategy of combining cytologic and HPV testing was discouraged. In the absence of CIN identified histologically, diagnostic excisional or ablative procedures are unacceptable for the initial treatment of patients with LSIL. Follow-up with either HPV testing at 12 months or cervical cytology at 6 months and 12 months (ASC-US threshold) is acceptable. If the HPV DNA test result is negative or if two consecutive repeat cytologic test results are negative, the return to routine screening is recommended. If either the HPV test result is positive or if the repeat cytologic result is reported as ASC-US or greater, colposcopy is recommended (1, 48).

Atypical Glandular Cells and Adenocarcinoma in Situ

Recommendations for the initial workup of women with glandular cytologic abnormalities are based on the prevalence of squamous intraepithelial neoplasia in many of these women, especially among younger women (42–44). It is further based on the poor sensitivity of cytology and colposcopy for the recognition of glandular disease (43) and the fact that glandular abnormalities also may be associated with noncervical glandular abnormalities that may not be associated with HPV (43). Colposcopy with endocervical sampling is recommended for all of these women with the addition of endometrial sampling in women older than 35 years or those with clinical indications suggesting a risk for neoplastic endometrial lesions (eg, unexplained vaginal bleeding or chronic anovulation or women with atypical endometrial cells) (1, 48). In the latter case, colposcopy can be deferred until the results of the initial biopsies are known. Although triage of these women using cervical cytology or HPV is unacceptable, HPV DNA testing at the time of colposcopy is preferred in women with atypical endocervical cells, endometrial cells, or AGC-NOS. In women with atypical endocervical cells, endometrial cells, or AGC-NOS who do not have CIN 2 or CIN 3 or glandular neoplasia identified histologically, knowledge of the HPV status will allow expedited triage. Women with HPV should have their Pap tests and HPV tests repeated at 6 months and those who do not have HPV should have these tests repeated at 12 months. Those with positive HPV test results or abnormal Pap test results would be referred to colposcopy, whereas those in whom both test results are negative can return to routine cytologic testing. In contrast, if the HPV status is unknown, the Pap test should be repeated every 6 months until there are four consecutive results negative for intraepithelial lesions or malignancy after which the woman can return to routine cytologic testing (1, 48).

In women with atypical endocervical cells, endometrial cells, or AGC-NOS, the evaluation can be concluded and management can be initiated if CIN but no glandular neoplasia is identified histologically. In contrast, women with atypical endocervical or glandular cells "favor neoplasia" or endocervical AIS should undergo a diagnostic excisional procedure unless invasive disease is identified during the initial workup (1, 48).

Endometrial assessment is recommended in postmenopausal women with benign endometrial cells regardless of symptoms. In premenopausal women and in women with a cytologic report of benign glandular cells after a hysterectomy, no further evaluation is required (1, 48).

High-Grade Squamous Intraepithelial Lesions

Cytologic results positive for HSIL carry a high risk of significant cervical disease. A single colposcopic examination identifies CIN 2 or higher in 53–66% of women with HSIL, and CIN 2 or higher grade lesions are diagnosed in 84–97% of women evaluated using LEEP. Because colposcopy can miss a significant number of CIN 2 or CIN 3 lesions and most women with HSIL will eventually undergo a diagnostic excisional procedure, a single-visit strategy ("see and treat") is an acceptable and cost-effective alternative in women in whom future fertility is not desired (1, 48). A diagnostic excisional procedure also is recommended for nonpregnant women with HSIL and an unsatisfactory colposcopy results (1, 48). However, although colposcopic assessment is not required before see-and-treat excision, it may be helpful in tailoring the excision to the size of the lesion and the limits of the transformation zone.

The other alternative to the see-and-treat approach is traditional colposcopy and biopsy. Because some CIN 2 and CIN 3 lesions will regress spontaneously, especially in adolescents and young adults, colposcopic evaluation is more appropriate for the initial evaluation of younger women and those who desire future fertility (1, 48). Colposcopy also affords the opportunity to evaluate the vagina as the source of the high-grade cytologic result. When CIN 2 or higher is not identified on colposcopy, the application of Lugol's solution to the cervix and vagina may identify high-grade lesions not previously detected. However, the sensitivity of colposcopy is limited, and these women may harbor an unsuspected high-grade cervical lesion. A British study found that 44% of women with negative test results after moderate or severe dyskaryosis had CIN found during follow-up (50), whereas a Swedish study found 22% of women with HSIL cytologic results to have CIN during follow-up despite a negative colposcopic result (51). When CIN 2 or higher grade lesions are not identified on a satisfactory colposcopic examination, the alternatives include review of the cytologic, colposcopic, and biopsy results with management after the revised diagnosis, a diagnostic excisional procedure, or observation with cytology and colposcopy. If the next two evaluations (at 6-month intervals) are negative, the woman can return to routine screening. If the results of either test show HSIL, a diagnostic excisional procedure is recommended. Other results are managed according to the guidelines (1, 48).

Finally, cytologic interpretation is subjective, and women with HSIL diagnoses may not have HSIL. In a study of the reproducibility of cervical cytology results,

27% of women with HSIL were found to have LSIL after review of their specimens, whereas 23% had ASC-US, and 3% had negative results (52). Therefore, both the possibility of missed disease and the potential for overtreatment must be considered, and the management must be based on individual patient needs. Ablation is unacceptable when CIN 2 and CIN 3 are not identified histologically or the endocervical assessment identifies CIN of any grade (1, 48).

Histologic Guidelines

It is estimated that each year in the United States, 1 million CIN 1 lesions are diagnosed and CIN 2 or CIN 3 is found in an additional 500,000 women (2). One of the most important factors in the development of the 2006 ASCCP consensus guidelines was the recognition that all treatment for CIN was associated with some increased risk of adverse pregnancy outcome (53, 54). Another important consideration was highlighted by a systematic review that reported that women remained at increased risk of invasive cancer for at least 20 years after treatment (56 per 100,000 women-years compared with 5.6 per 100,000 women-years for the general U.S. population) (55). Therefore, long-term follow-up is essential.

Special populations were identified where treatment would offer little benefit while adding significant risk. Adolescents and young women have a high incidence of CIN lesions but there is a high rate of spontaneous regression of CIN 1 and CIN 2, and the occurrence of invasive cervical cancer is rare. Pregnant women have a low risk of progression of CIN 2 or CIN 3 to invasive cervical cancer during pregnancy, and the incidence spontaneous regression postpartum is relatively high. Furthermore, the complications associated with treatment of CIN during pregnancy are significant and there is a high rate of recurrent or persistent disease after treatment of these women. Therefore, CIN should be managed conservatively in these women.

Cervical Intraepithelial Neoplasia 1

The treatment of women with CIN 1 is dependent on their risk of CIN 2 or CIN 3 and cancer, which, in turn, is related to their presenting cytologic results. Cervical intraepithelial neoplasia 1 is the histologic manifestation of cervical HPV infection. It uncommonly progresses to CIN 2 or CIN 3 or cancer and, therefore, does not need treatment (2, 56). The basis for treating CIN 1 is directly related to the underlying risk of CIN 2 or CIN 3 in these women. Among women enrolled in ALTS who presented with LSIL or HPV-positive ASC-US or two repeat ASC-US Pap test results and were found to have CIN 1 on initial colposcopy, 13% were subsequently found to have CIN 2 or CIN 3 (8.9% CIN 3) and none had cancer during the 24-month follow-up period.

This rate of CIN 2 or CIN 3 on follow-up was similar to that of women whose colposcopic results were completely negative and had no biopsies performed (11.3%) and those whose biopsies were negative for CIN (11.7%). Therefore, a biopsy diagnosis of CIN 1 did not add to the risk of CIN 2 or CIN 3 above the risk inherent to women with the cytologic abnormality alone when referred for colposcopy. The rationale for avoiding treatment in favor of more conservative follow-up is related to the cost, discomfort, and potential morbidity of commonly used treatment modalities. This is especially significant in young women with CIN 1, a group for whom the risk of future pregnancy complications is of concern. Conservative management allows adequate time to identify cases that might have been initially misclassified or to progress to a higher grade lesion while minimizing the risk of developing cancer in the interim.

Adult women with CIN 1 preceded by HPV-positive ASC-US, ASC-H, or LSIL cytologic results should be treated according to the guidelines for those cytologic abnormalities with either HPV testing every 12 months or repeat cervical cytology at 6 months and 12 months (2, 56). The decision to treat is unaffected by whether the colposcopy results are satisfactory or unsatisfactory. Treatment during the first 2 years of follow-up is not recommended (2, 56). Although persistence of CIN 1 beyond 2 years is associated with a higher risk of high-grade dysplasia and the likelihood of regression decreases the longer dysplasia persists, cancer can be effectively prevented with continued follow-up. Thus, it is safe to monitor a patient with semi-annual Pap tests or annual HPV testing with referral to colposcopy for women with positive HPV test results or cytologic results of ASC-US or greater. Some low-grade lesions persist beyond 2 years. Many of these lesions occur in patients who are immunocompromised. Women who smoke also are at increased risk of persistent HPV infection, persistent CIN, and progression to invasive cervical cancer. Counseling efforts to stop smoking are important when caring for patients with CIN. Care should be taken to exclude high-grade CIN. If CIN 1 has not resolved after 2 years, treatment is acceptable with excision or ablation if the colposcopy results remain satisfactory (2, 56). There are no data, however, to preclude continued follow-up beyond 2 years.

The risk of an undetected CIN 2, CIN 3, or AIS lesion is expected to be greater in women with CIN 1 preceded by an HSIL or AGC cytologic result than for women with CIN 1 preceded by ASC or LSIL and is related to the risk associated with the cytologic result for which the patient was referred for colposcopy rather than the CIN 1 histology. Consequently, the management recommendations follow the guidelines for those cytologic abnormalities. The management options are described earlier in the sections on HSIL and AGC (2, 56).

Cervical Intraepithelial Neoplasia 2 and 3

Cervical intraepithelial neoplasia grade 3 is generally considered to be a cancer precursor. The prevalence of CIN 3 peaks between ages 25 years and 30 years, and progression to cancer usually takes at least a decade longer. The risk of progression of CIN 3 is unclear because most experts consider the risk too high to justify observation, and patients are uniformly treated. However, one study found that the cumulative risk of CIN 3 progressing to invasive disease was 13% within 5 years, 20% within 10 years, 26% within 20 years, and 31% within 30 years with the remainder of patients having regressive or stable disease. For those patients whose disease persisted for 6–24 months after the initial diagnosis, the risk of invasion was 20% within 5 years, 31% within 10 years, 42% within 20 years, and 50% within 30 years (57). Smaller lesions with fewer features identifiable on colposcopy are more likely to regress, whereas larger lesions with coarse vascular changes are less likely to regress (58). The malignant potential of CIN 2 is less clear. The risk of progression to CIN 3 and cancer appears greater than for CIN 1. However, many women with CIN 2 will have regression of their lesions without therapy. No accepted tests are available to distinguish between CIN 2 that reflects an exuberant HPV infection from that with true malignant potential. Furthermore, the cutoff between CIN 1 and CIN 2 on the one hand and between CIN 2 and CIN 3 on the other hand is arbitrary. Because of the moderate cancer risk associated with CIN 2, it is often considered the threshold for treatment in the United States. However, in adolescents and young women in whom the risk of progression to invasive cancer is very low and the desire to avoid the pregnancy-related consequences of cervical therapy is high, observation without treatment appears safe and reasonable. Also, because one study found unsuspected cancer in 8% of women with CIN 3 undergoing hysterectomy (59), hysterectomy without prior conization is unacceptable as the primary therapy for CIN 2 and CIN 3.

Adenocarcinoma in Situ

Although the overall incidence of AIS (1.25 per 100,000) is increasing, it remains relatively rare compared with CIN 2 or CIN 3 (41.4 per 100,000). Because cytologic screening and colposcopic detection for AIS are so challenging and the clinical behavior of AIS is so different from CIN 2 or CIN 3, its management principles differ from those in CIN. The colposcopic changes associated with AIS can be minimal or unfamiliar to most colposcopists. Frequently, AIS is multifocal, may have "skip lesions," and frequently extends far into the endocervical canal, making complete excision difficult. Thus, negative margins on a conization specimen do not necessarily mean that the lesion has been completely excised (17).

Although a deep excisional procedure is curative in most of these patients, hysterectomy is the treatment of choice for women with AIS who have completed childbearing (2, 17, 56). Margin status and endocervical sampling at the time of an excisional biopsy (60) are clinically useful predictors of residual disease. Excisional biopsy is required in all women with AIS before making any subsequent management decisions. Conservative management is acceptable if future fertility is desired. If conservative management is planned and the margins of the specimen are involved or endocervical sampling obtained at the time of excision contains CIN or AIS, re-excision is preferred to increase the likelihood of complete excision (2, 56). These women should be reevaluated at 6 months using a combination of cervical cytology, HPV DNA testing, and colposcopy with endocervical sampling. Long-term follow-up after treatment is recommended for all women with AIS.

Positive Margins and Posttreatment Follow-up

Women with CIN 2 or CIN 3 involving the excision margins of a conization specimen and those with CIN 2 or CIN 3 at a postprocedure endocervical sampling are at an increased risk of disease persistence compared with those with clear margins. In a meta-analysis of studies describing more than 35,000 women after an excision, the relative risk of CIN 2 or CIN 3 after incomplete excision was 6.09 compared with that after complete excision (61). Although a positive endocervical margin raises concerns, multiple studies have demonstrated that it alone is not a marker for recurrence (62–64). Independent risks for recurrence or persistence of CIN include old age, large lesions, smoking, immunocompromise, and high-grade disease, with risks as high as 50% for older women with large CIN 3 lesions.

Because most women with positive conization margins do not have residual disease, repeat conization to prevent recurrence usually is not necessary, especially in young women who desire future fertility. However, a repeat diagnostic excisional procedure is acceptable and hysterectomy also is acceptable if a repeat diagnostic procedure is not feasible. The preferred management is observation using the same protocol as for women with negative margins (2, 56).

The risk of recurrent or persistent CIN after treatment is highest during the first year, and most disease is found within the first 1–5 years. However, cancer has been found as long as 20 years after initial therapy (65). The sensitivity of tests to detect recurrent or persistent disease is similar to their sensitivity when used for screening. In one large study of women monitored after treatment for CIN 3, the sensitivity of a single Pap test in identifying recurrent or persistent CIN was only 64%, whereas adding colposcopy improved the sensitivity to 91%, but reduced specificity from 95%

to 88% (66). The sensitivity of cytology improves with repeated testing, and because invasive cancer is rare soon after treatment for CIN 2 or CIN 3, there usually is time for serial cytologic assessment 6 months and 12 months after treatment or a single HPV test at 6 months to 12 months. A combination of HPV testing and cytology is only marginally more sensitive but the least specific and most costly program for identifying persistent or recurrent CIN (67). Colposcopy with endocervical sampling is indicated with cytologic results of ASC-US or greater or a positive HPV test result. After a negative HPV test result or two consecutive negative for intraepithelial lesions or malignancy Pap test results the woman can be returned to routine screening but that screening should continue for at least 20 years (2, 56).

References

1. Wright TC Jr, Massad LS, Dunton CJ, Spitzer M, Wilkinson EJ, Solomon D. 2006 consensus guidelines for the management of women with abnormal cervical cancer screening tests. 2006 American Society for Colposcopy and Cervical Pathology-sponsored Consensus Conference. Am J Obstet Gynecol 2007;197:346–55.

2. Wright TC Jr, Massad LS, Dunton CJ, Spitzer M, Wilkinson EJ, Solomon D. 2006 consensus guidelines for the management of women with cervical intraepithelial neoplasia or adenocarcinoma in situ. 2006 American Society for Colposcopy and Cervical Pathology-sponsored Consensus Conference. Am J Obstet Gynecol 2007;197:340–45.

3. Cervical cytology screening. ACOG Practice Bulletin No. 109. American College of Obstetricians and Gynecologists. Obstet Gynecol 2009;114:1409–20.

4. Food and Drug Administration. FDA approved first DNA test for two types of Human Papillomavirus; Agency also approved second DNA test for wider range of HPV types [press release]. Washington, DC: FDA; 2009. Available at: http://www.fda.gov/NewsEvents/Newsroom/Press Announcements/ucm149544.htm. Retrieved December 7, 2010.

5. American Society for Colposcopy and Cervical Pathology. HPV genotyping clinical update 2009. Hagerstown (MD): ASCCP; 2009. Available at: http://www.asccp.org/pdfs/consensus/clinical_update_20090408.pdf. Retrieved December 7, 2010.

6. Human papillomavirus vaccination. ACOG Committee Opinion No. 344. American College of Obstetricians and Gynecologists. Obstet Gynecol 2006;108:699–705.

7. Agency for Health Care Policy and Research. Evaluation of cervical cytology. Evidence Based Report/Technology Assessment No. 5. AHCPR Publication No. 99–E010. Rockville (MD): AHCPR; 1999.

8. Saslow D, Runowicz CD, Solomon D, Moscicki AB, Smith RA, Eyre HJ, et al. American Cancer Society guideline for the early detection of cervical neoplasia and cancer. CA Cancer J Clin 2002;52:342–62.

9. Ronco G, Cuzick J, Pierotti P, Cariaggi MP, Dalla Palma P, Naldoni C, et al. Accuracy of liquid based versus conventional cytology: overall results of new technologies for cervical cancer screening: randomised controlled trial. BMJ 2007;335:28.

10. Siebers AG, Klinkhamer PJ, Grefte JM, Massuger LF, Vedder JE, Beijers-Broos A, et al. Comparison of liquid-based cytology with conventional cytology for detection of cervical cancer precursors: a randomized controlled trial [published erratum appears in JAMA 2009;302:2322]. JAMA 2009;302:1757–64.

11. Arbyn M, Bergeron C, Klinkhamer P, Martin-Hirsch P, Siebers AG, Bulten J. Liquid compared with conventional cervical cytology: a systematic review and meta-analysis. Obstet Gynecol 2008;111:167–77.

12. Mosher WD, Chandra A, Jones J. Sexual behavior and selected health measures: men and women 15-44 years of age, United States, 2002. Adv Data 2005;362:1–55.

13. Ries LA, Melbert D, Krapcho M, Mariotto A, Miller BA, Feuer EJ, et al, editors. SEER cancer statistics review, 1975-2004. Bethesda (MD): National Cancer Institute; 2007.

14. Moscicki AB, Ma Y, Wibbelsman C, Powers A, Darragh TM, Farhat S, et al. Risks for cervical intraepithelial neoplasia 3 among adolescents and young women with abnormal cytology. Obstet Gynecol 2008 Dec;112:1335–42.

15. Moscicki AB, Schiffman M, Kjaer S, Villa LL. Chapter 5: Updating the natural history of HPV and anogenital cancer. Vaccine 2006;24 Suppl 3:S3/42–51.

16. U.S. Preventive Services Task Force. Screening for cervical cancer: recommendations and rationale. AHRQ Publication No. 03-515A. Rockville (MD): Agency for Healthcare Research and Quality; 2003. Available at: http://www.uspreventiveservicestaskforce.org/3rduspstf/cervcan/cervcanrr.pdf. Retrieved December 7, 2010.

17. Cervical cancer in adolescents: screening, evaluation, and management. Committee Opinion No. 463. American College of Obstetricians and Gynecologists. Obstet Gynecol 2010;116:469–72.

18. Sawaya GF, Kerlikowske K, Lee NC, Gildengorin G, Washington AE. Frequency of cervical smear abnormalities within 3 years of normal cytology. Obstet Gynecol 2000;96:219–23.

19. Pearce KF, Haefner HK, Sarwar SF, Nolan TE. Cytopathological findings on vaginal Papanicolaou smears after hysterectomy for benign gynecologic disease. N Engl J Med 1996;335:1559–62.

20. Sasieni P, Adams J, Cuzick J. Benefit of cervical screening at different ages: evidence from the UK audit of screening histories. Br J Cancer 2003;89:88–93.

21. Sawaya GF, McConnell KJ, Kulasingam SL, Lawson HW, Kerlikowske K, Melnikow J, et al. Risk of cervical cancer associated with extending the interval between cervical-cancer screenings. N Engl J Med 2003;349:1501–9.

22. Kulasingam SL, Myers ER, Lawson HW, McConnell KJ, Kerlikowske K, Melnikow J, et al. Cost-effectiveness of ex-

tending cervical cancer screening intervals among women with prior normal pap tests. Obstet Gynecol 2006;107:321–8.

23. Cervical cytology screening. ACOG Practice Bulletin No. 109. American College of Obstetricians and Gynecologists. Obstet Gynecol 2009;114:1409–20.

24. Dunne EF, Unger ER, Sternberg M, McQuillan G, Swan DC, Patel SS, et al. Prevalence of HPV infection among females in the United States. JAMA 2007;297:813–9.

25. Cuzick J, Clavel C, Petry KU, Meijer CJ,Hoyer H, Ratnam S, et al. Overview of the European and North American studies on HPV testing in primary cervical cancer screening. Int J Cancer 2006;119:1095–101.

26. Human papillomavirus. ACOG Practice Bulletin No. 61. American College of Obstetricians and Gynecologists. Obstet Gynecol 2005;105:905–18.

27. Khan MJ, Castle PE, Lorincz AT, Wacholder S, Sherman M, Scott DR, et al. The elevated 10-year risk of cervical precancer and cancer in women with human papillomavirus (HPV) type 16 or 18 and the possible utility of type-specific HPV testing in clinical practice. J Natl Cancer Inst 2005;97:1072–9.

28. Castle PE, Fetterman B, Poitras N, Lorey T, Shaber R, Kinney W. Five-year experience of human papillomavirus DNA and Papanicolaou test cotesting. Obstet Gynecol 2009; 113:595–600.

29. Ronco G, Segnan N, Giorgi-Rossi P, Zappa M, Casadei GP, Carozzi F, et al. Human papillomavirus testing and liquid-based cytology: results at recruitment from the new technologies for cervical cancer randomized controlled trial. New Technologies for Cervical Cancer Working Group. J Natl Cancer Inst 200;98:765–74.

30. Bigras G, de Marval F. The probability for a Pap test to be abnormal is directly proportional to HPV viral load: results from a Swiss study comparing HPV testing and liquid-based cytology to detect cervical cancer precursors in 13,842 women. Br J Cancer 2005;93:575–81.

31. Cuzick J, Szarewski A, Cubie H, Hulman G, Kitchener H, Luesley D, et al. Management of women who test positive for high-risk types of human papillomavirus: the HART study. Lancet 2003;362:1871–6.

32. Clavel C, Masure M, Bory JP, Putaud I, Mangeonjean C, Lorenzato M, et al. Human papillomavirus testing in primary screening for the detection of high-grade cervical lesions: a study of 7932 women. Br J Cancer 2001; 84:1616–23.

33. Davey DD, Cox JT, Marshall AR, Birdsong G, Colgan TJ, Howell LP, et al. Cervical cytology specimen adequacy: patient management guidelines and optimizing specimen collection. J Low Genit Tract Dis 2008;12:71–81.

34. Davey DD, Neal MH, Wilbur DC, Colgan TJ, Styer PE, Mody DR. Bethesda 2001 implementation and reporting rates: 2003 practices of participants in the College of American Pathologists Interlaboratory Comparison Program In Cervicovaginal Cytology. Arch Pathol Lab Med 2004;128:1224–9.

35. Cox JT, Schiffman M, Solomon D. Prospective follow-up suggests similar risk of subsequent cervical intraepithe-

lial neoplasia grade 2 or 3 among women with cervical intraepithelial neoplasia grade 1 or negative colposcopy and directed biopsy. ASCUS–LSIL Triage Study (ALTS) Group. Am J Obstet Gynecol 2003;188:1406–12.

36. Kinney WK, Manos MM, Hurley LB, Ransley JE. Where's the high-grade cervical neoplasia? The importance of minimally abnormal Papanicolaou diagnoses. Obstet Gynecol 1998;91:973–6.

37. A randomized trial on the management of low-grade squamous intraepithelial lesion cytology interpretations. ASCUS-LSIL Triage Study (ALTS) Group. Am J Obstet Gynecol 2003;188:1393–400.

38. Winer RL, Lee S, Hughes JP, Adam DE, Kiviat NB, Koutsky LA. Genital human papillomavirus infection: incidence and risk factors in a cohort of female university students [published erratum appears in Am J Epidemiol 2003;157:858]. Am J Epidemiol 2003;157:218–26.

39. Insinga RP, Glass AG, Rush BB. Diagnoses and outcomes in cervical cancer screening: a population-based study. Am J Obstet Gynecol 2004;191:105–13.

40. Massad LS, Collins YC, Meyer PM. Biopsy correlates of abnormal cervical cytology classified using the Bethesda system. Gynecol Oncol 2001;82:516–22.

41. Jones BA, Davey DD. Quality management in gynecologic cytology using interlaboratory comparison. Arch Pathol Lab Med 2000;124:672–81.

42. Sharpless KE, Schnatz PF, Mandavilli S, Greene JF, Sorosky JI. Dysplasia associated with atypical glandular cells on cervical cytology [published erratum appears in Obstet Gynecol 2005;105:1945]. Obstet Gynecol 2005;105: 494–500.

43. Derchain SF, Rabelo-Santos SH, Sarian LO, Zeferino LC, de Oliveira Zambeli ER, do Amaral Westin MC, et al. Human papillomavirus DNA detection and histological findings in women referred for atypical glandular cells or adeno-carcinoma in situ in their Pap smears. Gynecol Oncol 2004;95:618–23.

44. DeSimone CP, Day ME, Tovar MM, Dietrich CS 3rd, Eastham ML, Modesitt SC. Rate of pathology from atypical glandular cell pap tests classified by the Bethesda 2001 nomenclature. Obstet Gynecol 2006;107:1285–91.

45. Greenspan DL, Cardillo M, Davey DD, Heller DS, Moriarty AT. Endometrial cells in cervical cytology: review of cytological features and clinical assessment. J Low Genit Tract Dis 2006;10:111–22.

46. Simsir A, Carter W, Elgert P, Cangiarella J. Reporting endometrial cells in women 40 years and older: assessing the clinical usefulness of Bethesda 2001. Am J Clin Pathol 2005;123:571.

47. Gage JC, Hanson VW, Abbey K, Dippery S, Gardner S, Kubota J, et al. Number of cervical biopsies and sensitivity of colposcopy. ASCUS LSIL Triage Study (ALTS) Group. Obstet Gynecol 2006;108:264–72.

48. Wright TC Jr, Massad S, Dunton CJ, Spitzer M, Wilkinson EJ, Solomon D. 2006 consensus guidelines for the management of women with abnormal cervical screening tests. 2006 ASCCP-Sponsored Consensus Conference [published

erratum appears in J Low Genit Tract Dis 2008;12:255]. J Low Genit Tract Dis 2007;11:201–2.

49. Guido R, Schiffman M, Solomon D, Burke L. Postcolposcopy management strategies for women referred with low-grade squamous intraepithelial lesions or human papillomavirus DNA-positive atypical squamous cells of undetermined significance: a two-year prospective study. ASCUS LSIL Triage Study (ALTS) Group. Am J Obstet Gynecol 2003;188:1401–5.

50. Milne DS, Wadehra V, Mennim D, Wagstaff TI. A prospective followup study of women with colposcopically unconfirmed positive cervical smears. Br J Obstet Gynaecol 1999;106:38–41.

51. Trimble CL, Piantadosi S, Gravitt P, Ronnett B, Pizer E, Elko A, et al. Spontaneous regression of high-grade cervical dysplasia: effects of human papillomavirus type and HLA phenotype. Clin Cancer Res 2005;11:4717–23.

52. Stoler MH, Schiffman M. Interobserver reproducibility of cervical cytologic and histologic interpretations: realistic estimates from the ASCUS-LSIL Triage Study. Atypical Squamous Cells of Undetermined Significance-Low-grade Squamous Intraepithelial Lesion Triage Study (ALTS) Group. JAMA 2001;285:1500–5.

53. Jakobsson M, Gissler M, Sainio S, Paavonen J, Tapper AM. Preterm delivery after surgical treatment for cervical intraepithelial neoplasia [published erratum appears in Obstet Gynecol 2008;112:945]. Obstet Gynecol 2007;109: 309–13.

54. Kyrgiou M, Tsoumpou I, Vrekoussis T, Martin-Hirsch P, Arbyn M, Prendiville W, et al. The up-to-date evidence on colposcopy practice and treatment of cervical intraepithelial neoplasia: the Cochrane colposcopy & cervical cytopathology collaborative group (C5 group) approach. Cancer Treat Rev 2006;32:516–23.

55. Wang SS, Sherman ME, Hildesheim A, Lacey JV Jr, Devesa S. Cervical adenocarcinoma and squamous cell carcinoma incidence trends among white women and black women in the United States for 1976-2000. Cancer 2004;100:1035–44.

56. Wright TC Jr, Massad S, Dunton CJ, Spitzer M, Wilkinson EJ, Solomon D. 2006 consensus guidelines for the management of women with cervical intraepithelial neoplasia and adenocarcinoma in situ. 2006 American Society for Colposcopy and Cervical Pathology-sponsored Consensus Conference [published erratum appears in J Low Genit Dis 2008;12:63]. J Low Genit Tract Dis 2007;11: 223–39.

57. McCredie MR, Sharples KJ, Paul C, Baranyai J, Medley G, Jone RW, et al. Natural history of cervical neoplasia and risk of invasive cancer in women with cervical intraepithelial neoplasia 3: a retrospective cohort study. Lancet Oncol 2008;9:425–34.

58. Brewer CA, Wilczynski SP, Kurosaki T, Daood R, Berman ML. Colposcopic regression patterns in high-grade cervical intraepithelial neoplasia. Obstet Gynecol 1997;90:617–21.

59. Kesic V, Dokic M, Atanackovic J, Milenkovic S, Kalezic I, Vukovic S. Hysterectomy for treatment of CIN. J Low Genit Tract Dis 2003;7:32–5.

60. Hwang DM, Lickrish GM, Chapman W, Colgan TJ. Long-term surveillance is required for all women treated for cervical adenocarcinoma in situ. J Low Genit Tract Dis 2004;8:125–31.

61. Ghaem-Maghami S, Sagi S, Majeed G, Soutter WP. Incomplete excision of cervical intraepithelial neoplasia and risk of treatment failure: a meta-analysis. Lancet Oncol 2007;8:985–93.

62. Kalogirou D, Antoniu G, Karakitsos P, Botsis D, Kalogirou O, Giannikos L. Predictive factors used to justify hysterectomy after loop conization: increasing age and severity of disease. Eur J Gynaec Oncol 1997;18:113–6.

63. Lu CH, Liu FS, Kuo CJ, Chang CC, Ho ES. Prediction of persistence or recurrence after conization for cervical intraepithelial neoplasia III. Obstet Gynecol 2006;107: 830–5.

64. Moore BC, Higgins RV, Laurent SL, Marroum MC, Bellitt P. Predictive factors from cold knife conization for residual cervical intraepithelial neoplasia in subsequent hysterectomy. Am J Obstet Gynecol 1995;173:361–6; discussion 366–8.

65. Kalliala I, Anttila A, Pukkala E, Nieminen P. Risk of cervical and other cancers after treatment of cervical intraepithelial neoplasia: retrospective cohort study. BMJ 2005;331:1183–5.

66. Soutter WP, Butler JS, Tipples M. The role of colposcopy in the follow up of women treated for cervical intraepithelial neoplasia. BJOG 2006;113:511–4.

67. Kreimer AR, Guido RS, Solomon D, Schiffman M, Wacholder S, Jeronimo J, et al. Human papillomavirus testing following loop electrosurgical excision procedure identifies women at risk for posttreatment cervical intraepithelial neoplasia grade 2 or 3 disease. Cancer Epidemiol Biomarkers Prev 2006;15:908–14.

Perioperative Care

Thomas E. Snyder

Perioperative care and evaluation begins when the surgeon evaluates a patient and makes a recommendation for a surgical procedure and the patient makes an informed choice to accept that recommendation. It ends when the patient has safely recovered and returned to normal activity. As part of that ongoing care, the surgeon must integrate a plan for identifying, evaluating, and managing not only the surgical procedure and its potential complications but also the comorbidities exhibited by the patient. Today's medical environment demands that this process be performed in a cost-effective fashion. In addition, public awareness of therapeutic options and patient requests for specific forms of therapy (eg, robotic surgery) place increased demands on the gynecologic surgeon regarding technology, informed consent, and patient safety issues.

Medication Management

Management of medications in the perioperative period is challenging, especially when the patient's response to the stress of surgery and other underlying disease states may be affected. A complete list of all medications and remedies taken by the patient is required. Prescription and over-the-counter drugs, such as non-steroidal antiinflammatory drugs (NSAIDs) and complementary and alternative therapies, may have a significant effect on the surgical procedure or the postoperative course. However, most medications are well tolerated through surgery, do not interfere with anesthesia, and may be continued through the morning of the surgery. However, some other medications require dose monitoring and should be checked preoperatively (eg, digoxin or theophylline).

The general considerations for discontinuing and resuming medications in the perioperative period include the following factors (see also Table 2):

- The potential for withdrawal when stopping a medication—medications that have been associated with withdrawal symptoms include selective serotonin reuptake inhibitors (SSRIs), β-blockers, clonidine, statins, and corticosteroids.
- The progression of disease with interruption of drug therapy, especially if the patient is taking a drug with cardiovascular activity
- The potential for interactions with anesthetic agents if the medication is continued—examples include antiplatelet and anticoagulant agents and epidural or spinal anesthesia.

Table 2. Management of Medications in the Perioperative Period

Medication	Risks	Administration
β-blockers	Discontinuation before surgery can cause perioperative infarction in patients with vascular disease	Continue through the day of surgery and throughout hospital stay
		Use parenteral preparations after surgery if necessary
Calcium channel blockers		Continue through day of surgery and postoperatively
ACE inhibitors	Hypotension occurs at anesthesia induction*	Continuation of drug is common†
		Some clinicians recommend discontinuation postoperatively*
Nitrates		Continue up to and including day of surgery
		If therapy cannot be interrupted and patient is not on parenteral feeding, consider transdermal or intravenous administration.
Digoxin		Same as for nitrates
Clonidine		Same as for nitrates
Antiarhythmics		Same as for nitrates
Diuretics		Hold on morning of surgery, especially if the indication is congestive heart failure†§

(continued)

Table 2. Management of Medications in the Perioperative Period (*continued*)

Medication	Risks	Administration
Angiotensin II receptor blockers		Same as for diuretics
NSAIDs	Reversibly inhibit platelet cyclooxygenase and induce renal failure in combination with other medications or hemodynamic stress	Stop short-acting NSAIDs 1 day before surgery Stop long-acting NSAIDs 2–3 days before surgery
	Aspirin increases intraoperative bleeding	Stop aspirin use 1 week before neurosurgery, ophthalmologic, and other surgery with high risk of complications of bleeding Restart postoperatively when risk of bleeding is low
COX-2 inhibitors	Possible increase in cardiac disease	Stop clopidogrel 7 days before surgery
Oral contraceptives	Venous thromboembolism[II]	Stopping 1 month before surgery must be weighed against risk of pregnancy
		For current users, consider heparin prophylaxis
		Discontinuation not necessary before laparoscopic sterilization or other brief procedures
Hormone therapy	Risk of venous thromboembolism increased 6-fold after hip fracture, 18-fold for other lower-extremity fractures, and 5-fold for nonfracture surgery within 90 days of surgery[¶]	Some authors recommend stopping 4 weeks before surgery
Alendronate	Inhibits osteoclast-mediated bone resorption	Patients must be upright for 30 minutes after administration Stop in the perioperative period
Anticholesterol drugs	Myopathy or worsened muscle injury during perioperative period Cholestyramine may cause undesired drug binding	Discontinue 1 day before major surgery Resume when the patient is taking a normal diet

Abbreviations: ACE indicates angiotensin-converting enzyme; COX-2, cyclooxygenase-2; NSAIDs, nonsteroidal antiinflammatory drugs.

*Porterfield WR, Wu CL. Epidural hematoma in an ambulatory surgical patient. J Clin Anesth 1997;9:74–7.

[†]Rao TL, El-Etr AA. Anticoagulation following placement of epidural and subarachnoid catheters: an evaluation of neurologic sequelae. Anesthesiology 1981;55:618–20.

[‡]Coriat P, Richer C, Douraki T, Gomez C, Hendricks K, Giudiulli JF, et al. Influence of chronic angiotensin-converting enzyme inhibition on anesthetic induction. Anesthesiology 1994;81:299–307.

[§]Brabant SM, Bertrand M, Eyraud D, Darmon PL, Coriat P. The hemodynamic effects of anesthetic induction in vascular surgical patients chronically treated with angiotensin II receptor antagonists. Anesth Analg 1999;98:1388–92.

[II] Robinson GE, Burren T, Mackie IJ, Bounds W, Walshe K, Faint R, et al. Changes in haemostasis after stopping the combined contraceptive pill: implications for major surgery. BMJ 1991;302:269–71.

[¶]Grady D, Wenger NK, Herrington D, Khan S, Furberg C, Hunninghake D, et al. Postmenopausal hormone therapy increases risk for venous thromboembolic disease. The Heart and Estrogen/progestin Replacement Study. Ann Intern Med 2000;132:689–96.

Surveys have noted that more than one third of the U.S. population uses some form of alternative medical therapy; however, only 22–32% of patients report their use. Patients are less likely to tell the physician about their use of herbal medicine because they regard them as "natural" and, therefore, safe. Also, they may fear how the physician would respond to self-medication or may feel that the physician is prejudiced against use of these chemicals.

Secondary to this lack of information, complications and morbidity, such as myocardial infarction, stroke, bleeding, inadequate oral anticoagulation, prolonged or inadequate anesthesia, or interference with other medications, may occur (1). Knowledge of the patient's use of herbal medicines in the preoperative setting can avoid these potential problems.

Eight herbs that represent more than 50% of the 1,500–1,800 herbal medications sold in the United

States can cause perioperative complications (Table 3). The literature on anesthesia use suggests that patients discontinue these drugs at least 2–3 weeks before surgery; however, a more targeted approach has been suggested because some are eliminated from the body quickly and others take a significant time to be eliminated (1).

Testing

The clinical utility of preoperative testing on the subsequent management of the patient should be considered for any operation. Reasons for testing include 1) detection of unsuspected abnormalities that might influence the risk of perioperative morbidity or mortality and 2) establishing a baseline for a test that has a high likelihood of being monitored and changed after the surgery is complete. Unnecessary testing is inefficient, expensive, and may lead to surgical delays, cancellations, and a potential increased risk to the patient through additional testing and follow-up.

Hemoglobin

Severe anemia during surgery may cause tissue hypoxia from inadequate oxygen delivery. Many gynecologic surgical procedures are performed for bleeding problems, and a higher incidence of abnormalities might be expected. A baseline hemoglobin level may predict the need for the blood transfusion in procedures associated with significant blood loss. Hemoglobin screening is not indicated in patients undergoing surgery unlikely to result in significant blood loss. Such patients should be screened only if the history and physical examination results suggest severe anemia.

White Blood Cell Count, Platelets, and Coagulation Studies

The prevalence of unanticipated elevations in white blood cell counts not predicted by the history and physical examination is very low; therefore, routine screening is not advised. White blood cell counts should be obtained in patients with histories suggestive of

Table 3. Potential Perioperative Effects of Common Herbal Medicines

Herbal	Effects
Ginseng	Hypoglycemia
	Inhibits platelet aggregation (may be irreversible)
	Inhibits PT–PTT in animals
	Increases anticoagulation effect of warfarin
Ephedra	Myocardial infarction, cerebrovascular accident
	Depletes endogenous catecholamine stores, which can cause intraoperative hemodynamic instability
	Life-threatening interaction with MAO inhibitors
Garlic	Inhibits platelet aggregation (may be irreversible)
	Increases fibrinolysis
	Increases risk of bleeding
	Equivocal blood pressure lowering
Ginkgo biloba	Inhibits platelet-activating factor, leading to increased bleeding risk
Kava	Sedation, anxiolysis
	Increases sedative effect of anesthetics
	Potential for addiction, tolerance, and withdrawal
St John's wort	Many drug–drug interactions from induction of CYP 450 enzymes
Echinacea	Activates cell-mediated immunity
	Allergic reactions
	Immunosuppression
Valerian	Increases sedative effects of anesthesia
	Withdrawal
	May increase anesthesia requirements

Abbreviations: MAO indicates monoamine oxidase; PT–PTT, prothrombin time–partial thromboplastin time.
Data from Ang-Lee MK, Moss J, Yuan C. Herbal medicine and perioperative care. JAMA 2001;286:208–16.

infection, myeloproliferative disease, or leucopenia associated with drug use or disease states. Likewise, the incidence of abnormal platelet counts not anticipated by the history is low. Platelet counts should be obtained for a history suggestive of thrombocytopenia or thrombocytosis, easy bruising, or myeloproliferative disease. Partial thromboplastin time and activated partial thromboplastin time measurements as routine tests also have a low yield when done as routine testing (1% in a review of six studies), and bleeding time is a poor predictor of perioperative bleeding. However, patients who have a history of bleeding disorders or are taking anticoagulants are obviously appropriate candidates for this testing.

Electrolytes

Electrolyte testing also has a relatively low incidence of positive results, and few abnormalities affect management. Even hypokalemia is not a routine risk factor for adverse events. Testing should be obtained in patients with baseline renal insufficiency and congestive heart failure, those taking diuretics, digoxin, angiotensin-converting enzyme inhibitors, or those in whom other conditions or medications may contribute to abnormal results.

Renal and Liver Functions

Preoperative renal insufficiency has been shown to be one of the most important factors predicting complications in both cardiac and noncardiac surgery. The American College of Cardiology (ACC) and the American Heart Association (AHA) classify renal insufficiency as an intermediate clinical risk predictor carrying the same weight as mild angina, previous myocardial infarction, and diabetes. Preoperative testing is recommended in patients older than 50 years with diabetes and hypertension, known cardiac disease, and use of medications that may influence renal function, such as frequently used of NSAIDs, and those undergoing major procedures, including cardiac, vascular, chest, or abdominal surgery. Indications for liver function testing include major surgery in patients with known liver disease or evidence of malnutrition. Liver function tests may include measurements of aspartate transaminase, alanine transaminase, gamma glutamyl transferase, alkaline phosphatase, albumin, and bilirubin levels (2). Serum albumin levels have been shown to predict postoperative morbidity even more than the American Society of Anesthesiologist's patient anesthesia classification, functional status, age, or the fact that the patient had an emergency operation. In one study, a decrease in serum albumin level from concentrations greater than 46 g/L to less than 21 g/L was associated with an increase in morbidity rates from 10% to 65% (3).

Electrocardiography and Chest Radiography

Indications for electrocardiography (ECG) include age older than 50 years and presence of cardiopulmonary disease. It should not be considered a routine test for all patients. It is not necessary for patients undergoing minor procedures under conscious sedation or endoscopic procedures. Electrocardiographic abnormalities, such as the presence of Q waves, are predictive of risk according to the Goldman cardiac risk index. There is little evidence to support chest radiography as a routine preoperative test. A meta-analysis of preoperative chest X-ray results showed 10% to be abnormal, but only in 1.3% were they unexpected, and only 1% resulted in a change in management (4). The medical history should be used to determine functional pulmonary capability, not a test result.

Pregnancy Testing

Pregnancy testing should be obtained in all patients of reproductive age who are at risk of pregnancy before operation. Some hospitals require pregnancy testing of all female patients.

Cardiovascular Evaluation

Guidelines for perioperative cardiovascular evaluation of patients undergoing noncardiac surgery were revised in 2007 (4, 5). However, the guidelines are largely based on studies of male populations, and no gender specific guidelines have been made. The American College of Cardiology and AHA guidelines are organized by steps that determine whether the patient may proceed to surgery or whether further testing is required before the surgery (Fig. 14).

These predictors were developed from the Revised Cardiac Risk Index, which identifies ischemic heart disease, heart failure, cerebrovascular disease, and renal insufficiency as serious comorbidities. If the patient has none of the clinical predictors, she may proceed to surgery; however, if the patient has three or more risk factors, further testing is indicated if it will change management.

A patient with active cardiac disease has a significant risk of major complications and should have surgery only if the condition is emergent. An elective procedure should be postponed until the cardiac condition is stabilized.

Low-risk procedures, such as endoscopy and most ambulatory procedures, carry less than 1% morbidity and mortality, whereas major intraperitoneal surgery is considered an intermediate procedure that carries a cardiac risk of 1–5% (4). The patient should be assessed by her functional status. If the patient is able to perform activity at 4 metabolic equivalent tasks (METs) or greater without chest pain, dyspnea, or fatigue, sur-

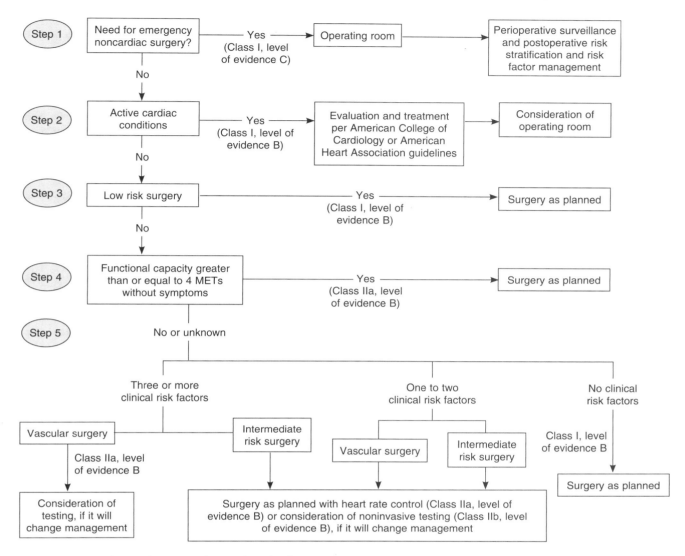

Figure 14. Cardiac evaluation and care algorithm for noncardiac surgery. Guidelines for cardiac evaluation including recommendations for patients with hypertension, heart failure, valvular disease, cardiomyopathies, arrhythmias, conduction abnormalities, pacemakers and implantable cordioverter-defibrillators. (Reprinted from J Am Coll Cardiol, Vol. 50, Fleisher LA, Beckman JA, Brown KA, Calkins H, Chaikof E, Fleischmann KE, et al. ACC/AHA 2007 guidelines on perioperative cardiovascular evaluation and care for noncardiac surgery: a report of the American College of Cardiology/American Heart Association Task Force on Practice Guidelines [Writing Committee to Revise the 2002 Guidelines on Perioperative Cardiovascular Evaluation for Noncardiac Surgery] developed in collaboration with the American Society of Echocardiography, American Society of Nuclear Cardiology, Heart Rhythm Society, Society of Cardiovascular Anesthesiologists, Society for Cardiovascular Angiography and Interventions, Society for Vascular Medicine and Biology, and Society for Vascular Surgery. American College of Cardiology; American Heart Association Task Force on Practice Guidelines [Writing Committee to Revise the 2002 Guidelines on Perioperative Cardiovascular Evaluation for Noncardiac Surgery]; American Society of Echocardiography; American Society of Nuclear Cardiology; Heart Rhythm Society; Society of Cardiovascular Anesthesiologists; Society for Cardiovascular Angiography and Interventions; Society for Vascular Medicine and Biology; Society for Vascular Surgery [published errata appear in J Am Coll Cardiol 2007;50:e242; J Am Coll Cardiol 2008;52:793–4]. Pages e159–241. Copyright 2007, with permission from Elsevier.)

gery may proceed without further testing (one MET is the metabolic equivalent of oxygen uptake while quietly seated; 4 METs are equal to walking on a flat surface, climbing a flight of stairs, or light house work). However, if the patient's functional status is less than 4 METs, further testing is based on clinical risk factors

and the severity of the surgical procedure. Clinical risk factors include the following:

1. History of ischemic heart disease
2. History of compensated or prior heart failure
3. History of cerebrovascular disease (stroke)

4. Diabetes mellitus

5. Chronic kidney disease (creatinine level greater than 2 mg/dL)

For high-risk gynecologic procedures, if the patient has the functional capacity of less than 4 METs and one to three risk factors, further testing is needed. In general, the least invasive and most cost-effective test is the exercise stress echocardiogram (4).

Beginning in the mid-1990s, β-blocker therapy was thought to prevent perioperative cardiac morbidity and mortality for both cardiac and noncardiac operations. The most recent guidelines from ACC and AHA have changed these recommendations (5). If the patient is already receiving β-blocker therapy to treat angina, arrhythmias, hypertension, or other cardiac disease, therapy should be continued (Class I recommendation). The patient with more than one clinical risk factor who is scheduled for intermediate-risk surgery may benefit from β-blocker therapy (Class II recommendation). The POISE (PeriOperative Ischemic Evaluation) trial showed benefit and harm from the use of β-blockers (6). Cardiac death, nonfatal myocardial infarction, and cardiac arrest were reduced with metoprolol compared with placebo; however, overall mortality and stroke increased (6). Noncardiac surgery soon after revascularization is associated with high morbidity and mortality (5.)

Pulmonary Function

The value of perioperative pulmonary function testing has not been established in patients with a history of active pulmonary disease. Testing is used clinically to discover or confirm and then manage obstructive disease.

Endocarditis

The American Heart Association no longer recommends prophylactic antibiotics given only for prevention of bacterial endocarditis for patients undergoing genitourinary procedures. This includes cesarean delivery and hysterectomy.

Deep Vein Thrombosis and Pulmonary Embolism

The prevalence of deep vein thrombosis and pulmonary embolism in patients undergoing gynecologic surgery ranges from 15% to 40% in the absence of prophylaxis (7). Risk factors for venous thromboembolism are listed in Box 4.

Patients are classified by risk categories to determine the appropriate treatment regimen. Recommendations for prevention of venous thromboembolism are listed in Table 4.

Graded compression stockings, intermittent pneumatic compression devices, low-dose unfractionated heparin, and low molecular weight heparin have all been shown to decrease the incidence of thromboembolism. Trials have shown an incidence of 1–6.5% in a gynecologic oncology population treated with one of these modalities (8). Genetic and acquired thrombophilias influence coagulability and contribute to the incidence of thrombosis after an event, such as surgery. Of these, factor V Leiden and prothrombin gene *G20210A* mutation are the most common. Factor V Leiden was described in 1993 and is carried by 5% of Caucasians (9). Heterozygotes have a threefold increased risk of venous thromboembolism, whereas homozygotes have a 50–80-fold increased risk. Prothrombin gene *G20210A* mutation is found almost exclusively in Caucasians and in 6% of patients with a history of thromboembolism. Factor V Leiden and prothrombin mutation may be diagnosed by DNA analysis. Elevated homocystine levels also are correlated with an increase in the risk of venous thromboembolism and can result from both genetic and acquired conditions. Acquired disease is associated with

---

Box 4

Venous Thromboembolism Risk Factors

- Surgery
- Trauma (major or lower extremity)
- Immobility and paresis
- Malignancy
- Cancer therapy (hormonal therapy, chemotherapy, or radiation therapy)
- Previous venous thromboembolism
- Increasing age
- Pregnancy and the postpartum period
- Estrogen-containing oral contraception or hormone therapy
- Selective estrogen receptor modulators
- Acute medical illness
- Heart or respiratory failure
- Inflammatory bowel disease
- Myeloproliferative disorders
- Paroxysmal nocturnal hemoglobinuria
- Nephrotic syndrome
- Obesity
- Smoking
- Varicose veins
- Central venous catheterization
- Inherited or acquired thrombophilia

Geerts WH, Pineo GF, Heit JA, Bergqvist D, Lassen MR, Colwell CW, et al. Prevention of venous thromboembolism: the Seventh ACCP Conference on Antithrombotic and Thrombolytic Therapy. Chest 2004;126(3 Suppl):338S–400S.

Table 4. Risk Classification for Venous Thromboembolism in Patients Undergoing Surgery Without Prophylaxis

Level of Risk	Definition	Successful Prevention Strategies
Low	Surgery lasting less than 30 minutes in patients younger than 40 years with no additional risk factors	No specific prophylaxis; early and "aggressive" mobilization
Moderate	Surgery lasting less than 30 minutes in patients with additional risk factors	Low-dose unfractionated heparin (5,000 units every 12 hours), low molecular weight heparin (2,500 units of dalteparin or 40 mg of enoxaparin daily), graduated compression stockings, or intermittent pneumatic compression device
	Surgery lasting less than 30 minutes in patients aged 40–60 years with no additional risk factors	
	Major surgery in patients younger than 40 years with no additional risk factors	
High	Surgery lasting less than 30 minutes in patients older than 60 years or with additional risk factors	Low-dose unfractionated heparin (5,000 units every 8 hours), low molecular weight heparin (5,000 units of dalteparin or 40 mg of enoxaparin daily), or intermittent pneumatic compression device
	Major surgery in patients older than 40 years or with additional risk factors	
Highest	Major surgery in patients older than 60 years plus prior venous thromboembolism, cancer, or molecular hypercoagulable state	Low-dose unfractionated heparin (5,000 units every 8 hours), low molecular weight heparin (5,000 units of dalteparin or 40 mg of enoxaparin daily), or intermittent pneumatic compression device/graduated compression stockings plus low-dose unfractionated heparin or low molecular weight heparin
		Consider continuing prophylaxis for 2–4 weeks after discharge.

dietary deficiencies in folate, vitamin B_6, and vitamin B_{12} (10). Antiphospholipid syndrome is an acquired thrombophilia associated with both arterial and venous thromboembolism. One half of patients with systemic lupus erythematosus test positive for antibodies. Testing should be considered in patients with venous thromboembolism and other risk factors, such as systemic lupus erythematosus, recurrent pregnancy loss, and early or severe preeclampsia or thrombocytopenia (11).

Prophylactic Options

GRADUATED COMPRESSION STOCKINGS

In addition to early postoperative ambulation and elevating the foot of the bed, graduated compression stockings prevent pooling of blood in the calves. A Cochrane review of randomized trials reported a 50% decrease in DVT formation and greater reduction when the use of stockings was combined with a second prophylactic method (12). Low cost and simplicity are the main advantages of this method. However, the stockings must be fitted properly to avoid a tourniquetlike action at the knee or mid thigh.

PNEUMATIC COMPRESSION

Pneumatic compression devices reduce stasis by compression of the calf with an inflatable pneumatic sleeve. These devices have been shown to be as effective as low-dose unfractionated heparin and low molecular weight heparin in reducing DVT incidence (13); however, most studies are composed of small numbers of patients. The devices should be started at the time of surgery and continued until discharge.

LOW-DOSE UNFRACTIONATED HEPARIN

Numerous trials have shown low-dose unfractionated heparin to be effective in preventing DVT if started 2 hours before surgery and continued every 8–12 hours postoperatively. A two-thirds reduction in the rates of fatal pulmonary embolism with the use of low-dose unfractionated heparin was noted in two large trials compared with the use of placebo or no prophylaxis (14, 15). Patients undergoing gynecologic surgery for benign conditions benefit from low-dose unfractionated heparin given in a preoperative dose and every 12 hours postoperatively; however, this approach was not successful in gynecologic oncology patients (16). Treatment with 5,000 units of heparin 2 hours preoperatively and continued every 8 hours postoperatively did provide good protection in patients with gynecologic cancer (17). Advantages are efficacy and low cost. Blood loss during surgery does not appear to be increased; however, an increase in postoperative hematomas was noted with use of heparin. Use for more than 4 days requires monitoring of platelet counts because of an incidence of thrombocytopenia in 6% of patients.

LOW MOLECULAR WEIGHT HEPARIN

The advantages of low molecular weight heparin use result from longer half-life, more predictable pharmacokinetics, and equivalent efficacy compared with prophylactic use of low-dose unfractionated heparin and include greater bioavailability and once daily dosages. Use of low molecular weight heparin is not associated with thrombocytopenia; however, it is currently more expensive than low-dose unfractionated heparin. Low molecular weight heparin has been shown to be effective for prophylaxis of patients undergoing surgery for gynecologic malignancies. Duration of prophylaxis is important. A 60% reduction in venous thromboembolism was noted for patients treated for 4 weeks versus 1 week with no noted increase in bleeding or thrombocytopenia [18].

DUAL PROPHYLAXIS

A Cochrane review of 19 studies showed that low-dose unfractionated heparin combined with graduated compression stockings was four times more effective than low-dose heparin alone in the prevention of venous thromboembolism [19]. Although no randomized trials exist in the gynecologic literature, if the patient has two of three risk factors (ie, age older than 40 years, cancer, and prior venous thromboembolism), she is in the highest risk category for development of venous thromboembolism. The Seventh American College of Chest Physicians Consensus Conference recommended a combined approach in these patients [7].

Obesity and the Metabolic Syndrome

Obesity and the metabolic syndrome have been shown to have adverse effects on the outcomes of such diverse procedures as coronary artery bypass grafting, percutaneous nephrolithotomy, lumbar and spine surgery, and colorectal surgery. These conditions also increase the risk of postoperative wound infections. Up to 71% of the morbidly obese patients receive the diagnosis of obstructive sleep apnea. Obstructive sleep apnea also has been identified in up to 24% of surgical patients [20]. Detection of obstructive sleep apnea is important because patients with this condition are more sensitive to respiratory depressants, such as benzodiazepines and opiates [21]. Patients who use continuous positive airway pressure for treatment of obstructive sleep apnea should be instructed to bring their positive airway pressure machines for use in the perioperative period.

Obese patients are at a much higher risk of postoperative complications due to the more frequent occurrence of comorbidities, including diabetes mellitus, hypertension, coronary artery disease, sleep apnea, obesity hypoventilation syndrome, and osteoarthritis of the knees and hips. These underlying alterations in physiology result in increased surgical risks and complications, including respiratory failure, cardiac failure, DVT and pulmonary embolism, aspiration, wound infection and dehiscence, postoperative asphyxia, and misdiagnosed intraabdominal complication.

Obesity itself is a risk factor for DVT and pulmonary embolism in apparently healthy patients and hospitalized medical and surgical patients [22]. The perioperative risks of DVT and pulmonary embolism in these patients without specific DVT prophylaxis are estimated at 14% for DVT and 0.5% for pulmonary embolism, respectively. The risk of DVT in these patients may be decreased with the use of pneumatic compression devices and anticoagulants (see earlier discussion).

Venous access poses another problem. Extreme obesity obliterates anatomic landmarks and makes insertion of peripheral lines, as well as central lines, problematic. Adjunctive visualization technology, such as Doppler ultrasound or fluoroscopy, should increase the accuracy and safety of line placement. Arterial line placement facilitates monitoring of pressure and blood gas parameters. Ideally, central venous lines and arterial lines should be placed intraoperatively by the anesthesia team to ensure adequate access in the postoperative period. The intraoperative placement of central lines should be verified for position postoperatively by chest X-ray in the postanesthesia care unit.

The concepts of total body weight as well as ideal body weight require consideration for medication administration. Dosages of certain medications are determined based on ideal body weight (corticosteroids, penicillin, cephalosporins, and β-blockers). Those of others are determined based on total body weight (eg, heparin) and still others on a calculated "dosage weight" (eg, aminoglycosides, fluoroquinolones, and vancomycin). An inpatient pharmacist should be consulted for assistance with proper dosages and to monitor pharmacotherapy.

Anemia

One study showed that anemia with a hemoglobin level of 6 g/dL versus 12 g/dL increases the risk of death 26 times within 30 days after surgery [23]. The risk was even greater if the patient had underlying heart disease and the preoperative hemoglobin level was 10 g/dL or less. None of the patients died if the postoperative hemoglobin level was between 7 g/dL and 8 g/dL; however, there was a significant increase in death among those with a hemoglobin level of less than 5–6 g/dL [23, 24]. A more recent study showed that even mild anemia (hematocrit value of less than 39%) was associated with an increased 30-day morbidity and mortality rate [25].

Treatment

The treatment of anemia may involve pharmacologic and technological options, including iron and erythropoiesis-stimulating agents, autologous blood transfusion, cell salvage, and normovolemic hemodilution (26). Iron deficiency anemia, a common cause of anemia in the gynecologic population, may be treated with iron supplementation. Iron is most easily given in the oral form and is best absorbed in an acidic gastric environment. Reticulocytosis is seen in 7–10 days, and the hemoglobin level should increase by 1 g/dL every 2–3 weeks (24). If the patient does not respond or has conditions, such as inflammatory bowel disease, intestinal malabsorption, or perhaps has undergone cancer chemotherapy, intravenous (IV) iron supplementation may be necessary. An increase in hemoglobin level usually is noted in 1 week with the maximum effect in 2 weeks. Intravenous iron therapy currently is considered safer than blood transfusion (27). Anemia from vitamin B_{12} and folate deficiency also are treated by supplementation. Patients with various chronic diseases, renal insufficiency, forms of human immunodeficiency virus (HIV), or other hematologic diseases may benefit from erythropoietin therapy before surgery (24). Erythropoietin may increase the hemoglobin level enough to avoid transfusion. Only epoetin alfa is approved by the U. S. Food and Drug Administration to be used in patients undergoing major surgery (26). In a randomized trial, the benefit was greatest in patients at the highest risk of transfusion. The target hemoglobin level should be no greater than 12 g/dL to avoid hazard of venous thromboembolism and serious cardiac events associated with erythropoietin. The U.S. Food and Drug Administration has issued a boxed warning to specify an increased risk of DVT in patients not receiving prophylactic anticoagulants.

Transfusion Guidelines

The guidelines of the American Society of Anesthesiology currently recommend transfusion if the hemoglobin level is less than 6 g/dL and that transfusion rarely is necessary, if the hemoglobin level is greater than 10 g/dL (28). If the hemoglobin is between 6 g/dL and 10 g/dL, the clinical decision for transfusion should be made on the basis of organ ischemia, risk of further bleeding, volume status, and susceptibility to complications of inadequate oxygenation (24). Several authorities agree that a transfusion threshold of approximately 7 g/dL can be used if the patient has no underlying heart disease and is asymptomatic. The clinician should evaluate the patient for symptoms and not make the decision for transfusion based solely on the hemoglobin level. Most patients may receive a transfusion at a rate of 1 unit of red blood cells over 1–2 hours. A hemoglobin level increase of 1 g/dL should be expected for every unit of red blood cells transfused (24). A repeat hemoglobin level measurement result should be obtained after each unit transfused.

Perioperative Anticoagulation

Some gynecologic operations are not associated with a significant blood loss (eg, small vulvar biopsies), and do not require interruption of oral anticoagulant therapy (warfarin); however, many will require cessation of therapy secondary to the risk of bleeding, if the patient continues therapy. Whether the patient may benefit from temporary use of a heparin product while warfarin is discontinued perioperatively ("bridging therapy") is determined by the risk of bleeding balanced by the risk of thromboembolism (29). Rapid reversal of anticoagulation is necessary when an emergent procedure is necessary. This usually is accomplished with vitamin K or fresh frozen plasma. There is no dose prediction model available for fresh frozen plasma, and the international normalized ratio (INR) should be monitored after use. If surgery is needed in approximately 24–96 hours, vitamin K is the drug of choice. One study found that 1 mg of IV vitamin K reversed the INR to less than 1.4 in a median time of 27 hours (30). Vitamin K given orally is more convenient, and doses of 1–2.5 mg correct supratherapeutic INRs (of greater than 4.5) to a therapeutic range in 24–48 hours. International normalized ratio values may be decreased to a subtherapeutic value; eg, 1.5, by this method.

Bridging therapy with heparin is used when the patient's risk of thromboembolism necessitates the use of perioperative anticoagulation. The American College of Chest Surgeons has published guidelines for antithrombotic therapy (31). Guidelines for heparin bridging are noted in Box 5. Bridging therapy may be accomplished with either unfractionated heparin or low molecular weight heparin. Low molecular weight heparin has the advantage of improved bioavailability, more predictable response, longer plasma half-life, and less interaction with platelets, endothelial cells, macrophages, and plasma proteins (29). The risk of thrombocytopenia also is lower with low molecular weight heparin. However, unfractionated heparin may have advantages if the patient has compromised renal function, is underweight or overweight, or is pregnant. If using unfractionated heparin for bridging, the patient should be hospitalized for approximately 36 hours after discontinuing warfarin therapy (2–3 days before surgery) and the IV infusion of heparin should be discontinued approximately 4–6 hours before surgery. Figure 15 shows a suggested bridging protocol using low molecular weight heparin. The timing of prophylactic anticoagulation is more complicated if neuraxial anesthesia is used. The American College of Chest Physicians and the American Society of Regional Anesthesiology (ASRA) agree that venous thromboembolism prophylaxis may be used with neuraxial anesthesia as long as precautions are taken to reduce the risk of bleeding (22, 29).

Box 5

Evaluating Perioperative Risk of Thromboembolism:
Who Should Be Bridged?

High risk of thromboembolism—bridging advised

- Known thrombophilia as documented by a thromboembolic event and one of the following: protein C deficiency, protein S deficiency, antithrombin III deficiency, homozygous factor V Leiden mutation, or antiphospholipid antibody syndrome
- Thrombophilia suggested by recurrent (two or more) arterial or idiopathic venous thromboembolic events (not including primary atherosclerotic events, such as stroke or myocardial infarction due to intrinsic cerebrovascular or coronary disease)
- Venous or arterial thromboembolism within the preceding 3 months
- Rheumatic atrial fibrillation
- Acute intracardiac thrombus visualized by echocardiogram
- Atrial fibrillation plus mechanical heart valve in any position
- Older model mechanical valve (single disk or ball-in-cage) in mitral position
- Recently placed mechanical valve (less than 3 months)
- Atrial fibrillation with history of cardioembolism

Intermediate risk of thromboembolism—bridging decision on a case-by-case basis

- Newer model mechanical valve (ie, St Jude) in mitral position
- Older model mechanical valve in aortic position
- Atrial fibrillation without history of cardiac embolism but with multiple risks of cardiac embolism (ie, low ejection fraction [less than 40%], hypertension, older than 75 years, diabetes, history of stroke or transient ischemic attack)
- Venous thromboembolism more than 3–6 months ago*

Low risk of thromboembolism—bridging not advised

- One remote venous thromboembolism (greater than 6 months ago)*
- Intrinsic cerebrovascular disease, such as carotid atherosclerosis, without recurrent strokes or TIAs
- Atrial fibrillation without multiple risks of cardiac embolism
- Newer model mechanical valve in aortic position

Abbreviation: TIA indicates transient ischemic attack.

*For patients with a history of venous thromboembolism undergoing major surgery, consideration can be given to postoperative bridging therapy only (without preoperative bridging)

Reprinted with permission from Jaffer AK, Brotman DJ, Chukumerije N. When patients on warfarin need surgery. Cleve Clin J Med 2003;70:973–84. Copyright © 2003 Cleveland Clinic. All rights reserved.

Renal Dysfunction

The term *acute kidney injury* encompasses the spectrum from small changes in serum creatinine to loss of function requiring dialysis (32). Risks for acute kidney injury include age, history of kidney injury, left ventricular ejection fraction of less than 35%, cardiac index less of than 1.7 (calculated as cardiac output in liters per minute divided by body surface area in square meters [L/min/m²]), hypertension, peripheral vascular disease, diabetes mellitus, emergency surgery, and type of surgery (33).

Acute kidney injury carries a mortality rate of approximately 50% (34). Changes in the serum creatinine level as small as 0.3–0.4 mg/dL were correlated with a 70% increase in risk of death compared with patients with no change in serum creatinine level (35). The goal of therapy to prevent acute kidney injury is to avoid intraoperative hypotension and decreased renal perfusion. Control of blood pressure is important before surgery. Angiotensin-converting enzyme inhibitors and angiotensin II antagonists are commonly used to treat hypertension in patients with chronic kidney disease and also may be associated with intraoperative hypotension with general anesthesia use. These drugs may need to be discontinued approximately 12 hours before administration of general anesthesia to reduce postinduction hypotension (32).

Preoperatively

Ensure patient does not have any contraindications to
LMWH bridging, such as the following therapy factors:
- Allergy to LMWH
- History of HIT
- Severe thrombocytopenia
- Extremes of weight (severely underweight or overweight)
- Creatinine clearance of less than 15 mL/min (weight-based dosage,
  if 15–30 mL/min)
- Poor patient reliability
- Inability to administer injections

Provide the following bridging instructions:
- Stop warfarin therapy 5 days before surgery (if INR 2–3)
- Stop warfarin therapy 6 days before surgery (if INR 3–4.5)
- Start LMWH therapy 36 hours after the last warfarin dose
  (enoxaparin, 1 mg/kg every 12 hours or 1.5 mg/kg every 24 hours,
  or dalteparin, 120 units/kg every 12 hours or 200 units/kg every
  24 hours, or tinzaparin, 175 units/kg every 24 hours)
- Administer the last dose of LMWH 24 hours before procedure
  (full dose if using twice daily LMWH dose; two thirds of a dose
  if using once daily LMWH dose)
- Check INR on morning of surgery to ensure values of less than 1.5
  and, in some cases, less than 1.2

Postoperatively

- Restart LMWH therapy (enoxaparin, 1 mg/kg every 12 hours or
  1.5 mg/kg every 24 hours, or dalteparin, 120 units/kg every 12
  hours or 200 units/kg every 24 hours, or tinzaparin, 175 units/kg
  every 24 hours) approximately 24 hours after the procedure or
  consider thromboprophylactic dose of LMWH on postoperative
  day 1 if patient is at high risk of bleeding (discuss with surgeon)
- Restart warfarin therapy at patient's usual dose on the evening of
  the surgical day
- Check INR daily until patient is discharged and periodically thereafter until INR is therapeutic
- Check complete blood count on postoperative days 3 and 7 to
  monitor platelet count
- Discontinue administration of LMWH when INR is therapeutic for
  2 consecutive days

Figure 15. Perioperative bridging strategy using low molecular weight heparin. Abbreviations: CBC indicates complete blood count; HIT, heparin-induced thrombocytopenia; INR, international normalized ratio; LMWH, low molecular weight heparin. (Grant PJ, Brotman DJ, Jaffer AK. Perioperative anticoagulant managment. Med Clin North Amer 2009;93:1105–21.)

Laparoscopy is also associated with reduction in renal perfusion. Abdominal pressure should be held below 15 mm Hg, and avoidance of hypotension is recommended. Analgesic agents may accumulate in the patient with chronic kidney disease, placing them at risk of respiratory depression. Nonionic contrast agents present a risk to the patient with chronic kidney disease. If these agents must be used, hydration, avoidance of other nephrotoxic agents, and prevention of hypotension are important. Nonsteroidal antiinflammatory drugs are not recommended for patients with chronic kidney disease. The management of patients with renal disease should include communication between the primary care team, nephrologist, surgeon, and anesthesiologist for optimal care.

Endocrine Dysfunction

Diabetes Mellitus

The patient with diabetes mellitus requires a systematic approach to care because the disease affects many organ systems. The goal for this patient is to minimize hypoglycemia, hypovolemia and hypokalemia, and hyperkalemia. The "stress response" to surgery is characterized by hypersecretion of such hormones as glucagon, norepinephrine, cortisol, and growth hormone, which leads to gluconeogenesis, glycogenolysis, and insulin resistance. The end result may be diabetic ketoacidosis in patients with type 1 diabetes mellitus and hyperosmolar hyperglycemic nonketosis in patients with type 2 diabetes mellitus (36). Although there are no guidelines on the perioperative control of diabetes, the American College of Endocrinology recommends maintenance of the blood glucose level at less than 200 mg/dL intraoperatively and less than 150 mg/dL but not less than 80 mg/dL in the postoperative period (37). Box 6 summarizes the recommendations for perioperative management of patients with type 1 diabetes mellitus.

Adrenal Insufficiency

Adrenal insufficiency secondary to suppression of the hypothalamic–pituitary axis by exogenous steroid administration is the most common cause of adrenal suppression in the surgical patient. Any patient who has received the equivalent of 20 mg of prednisone per day for greater than 5 days is at risk. The patient who has been receiving therapy for longer than 1 month may have suppression for up to 6–12 months after stopping the therapy. Likewise, the patient who has received less than 5 mg of prednisone per day for any time period will usually not significantly suppress the hypothalamic–pituitary axis (38). Tests for perioperative adrenal suppression are not very sensitive or specific. Therefore, the decision to administer additional steroids should be based on data in the history and physical examination, and the acuity and severity of the operation. Guidelines for administration of additional steroids are shown in Figure 16. Postoperatively, additional steroids should be administrated for approximately 48 hours. The occurrence of unexplained nausea, hypotension, a change in mental status, hyponatremia, or hyperkalemia should warrant checking thyroxine (T_4), thyroid-stimulating hormone (TSH), and random plasma cortisone levels.

Hyperthyroidism and Hypothyroidism

The cardiovascular system is commonly affected by hypothyroidism, which results in depressed cardiac function and increased systemic vascular resistance. The pulmonary system also may be affected with depressed

response to hypercarbia and hypoxemia. Hypothyroidism is treated with T_4 replacement. Patients should ideally be euthyroid before surgery. Patients who are being treated should monitor their replacement dosages and be aware of increasing hypothyroid symptoms postoperatively. These patients are sensitive to sedation with narcotics and benzodiazepines. Patients with moderate hypothyroidism are not at a significantly increased risk;

Box 6

Perioperative Management of Patients With Type 1 Diabetes*

Night Before Procedure

- Continue usual dose of afternoon glargine or neutral protamine Hagedorn or a mixture (can recommend two thirds of usual dose if tightly controlled) the night before surgery (as long as taking usual oral intake the night before surgery)

- For insulin pump users, continue usual overnight basal rate

Morning of Procedure

- No boluses of short-acting hypoglycemics unless blood glucose level is more than 200 mg/dL and greater than 3 hours preoperatively

- Consider administering insulin drip or usual dose of glargine if routinely taken in the morning

- For insulin pump users, continue usual basal rate and infuse D5–5% throughout operation

- If taking neutral protamine Hagedorn or other insulin mixture:

   —No short-acting insulin within 3–4 hours of the procedure (ie, no mixture preoperatively)

   —Administer one half of the usual intermediate-acting insulin, with D5–5%, at controlled rate throughout procedure

   —If performing operation without continuous D5–5%, administer no insulin preoperatively

Special Situations

- Emergency surgery—Administer no bolus of short-acting hypoglycemics preoperatively. Frequently monitor blood glucose level throughout the operation (every 30–60 minutes). Start insulin infusion if blood glucose level is greater than 200 mg/dL.

- Cardiac surgery—Continue insulin infusion as needed to maintain blood glucose level at 100–150 mg/dL in first 3 postoperative days.

Abbreviation: D5 indicates dextrose containing solution.

*These patients need basal insulin at all times to avoid diabetic ketoacidosis.

Reprinted from Med Clin North Amer, Vol. 93, Kohl BA, Schwartz S. Surgery in the patient with endocrine dysfunction. Pages 1031–47, Copyright 2009, with permission from Elsevier.

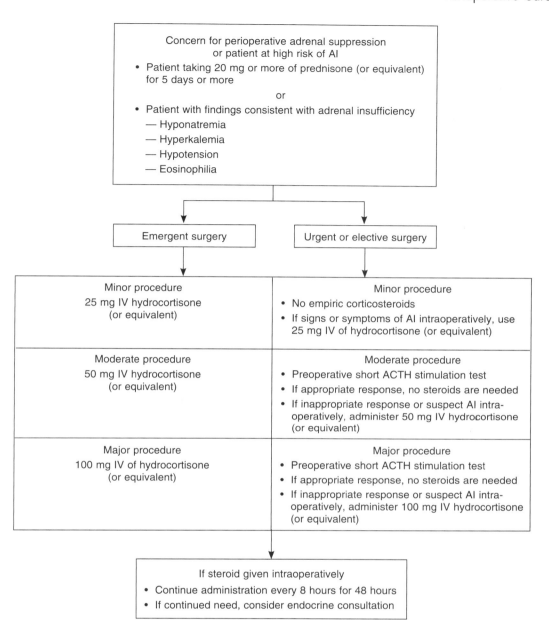

Figure 16. Algorithm for perioperative steroid administration. Minor procedures include those performed under local anesthesia or those less than 1 hour in duration; moderate procedures include most vascular surgeries or orthopedic procedures; major procedures include larger, prolonged operations, such as esophagectomy or those using cardiopulmonary bypass. The short adrenocorticotrophic hormone stimulation involves administration of 250 micrograms intravenous synthetic adrenocorticotrophic hormone followed by a plasma cortisol collection in 30 minutes. A plasma cortisol concentration of more than 18–20 micrograms per deciliter is consistent with normal adrenal function. Abbreviations: ACTH indicates adrenocorticotrophic hormone; AI, adrenal insufficiency; IV; intravenous. (Reprinted from Med Clin North Amer, Vol. 93, Kohl BA, Schwartz S. Surgery in the patient with endocrine dysfunction. Pages 1031–47, Copyright 2009, with permission from Elsevier.)

however, close attention should be devoted to possible airway obstruction. Patients with severe thyroid dysfunction who require surgery may be given intravenous T_4 and triiodothyronine (T_3). These patients also should be considered for steroid replacement (36).

Graves disease, the most common cause of hyperthyroidism, is caused by antibodies directed at TSH receptors causing an increased level of thyroid hormone production. Clinical signs include tachycardia, atrial fibrillation, fever, tremor, goiter, and ophthalmopathy. Some patients are asymptomatic and have normal free thyroid hormone levels and decreased TSH levels. In overt hyperthyroidism, free T_4 and T_3 levels may be mildly elevated and TSH is suppressed. In thyrotoxicosis, free T_4 may be increased. These hormones have inotropic and chronotropic effects on the heart and a direct effect on vascular smooth muscle causing decreased systemic vascular resistance and blood pressure. Patients with hyperthyroidism should take their medication on the morning of surgery. If the patient requires urgent surgery, the anesthesiologist should use medications that block the systemic effects of excess thyroid hormone, including β-blockers and antithyroid medications. The worst complication of hyperthyroidism is thyroid storm that may occur anytime in the perioperative period, but usually in the first 48 hours postoperatively. The mortality rate is 10–75%; thus, the patient must be carefully monitored and observed for symptoms of hyperpyrexia, tachycardia, and delirium. Treatment includes thioamides, β-blockers, and antipyretics. Acetaminophen is preferred over salicylates secondary to their tendency to decrease thyroid-binding protein, thus increasing T_3 and T_4.

Perioperative Bowel Preparation

Until recently, preparation of the bowel before colorectal surgery was major surgical dogma. However, a randomized trial questioned this recommendation, suggesting that mechanical bowel preparation was unnecessary (39). Although there are no randomized clinical trials in open or vaginal surgery, one randomized trial examined the use of bowel preparation in gynecologic laparoscopy (40). In this study, the authors randomized 162 patients scheduled for gynecologic laparoscopy to a bowel preparation with oral sodium phosphate or no bowel preparation. Surgical difficulty, operating time, and postoperative complications were recorded. The authors concluded that mechanical bowel preparation offered no advantages and increased preoperative discomfort (40). A meta-analysis of fourteen trials, including 5,000 patients showed no statistical difference noted for anastomotic leakage, pelvic or abdominal abscess, and wound sepsis (39). When all surgical site infections were considered, the meta-analysis favored no mechanical bowel preparation. In addition, the use of sodium phosphate has been associated with perioperative renal failure in patients with decreased renal function. In view of the available literature, it appears that the routine use of bowel preparation is unnecessary in general gynecologic surgery.

Older Patients

The life expectancy of American women continues to increase. In addition, as the "baby-boomer" generation ages, an increasingly larger population of older women will develop gynecologic problems that will require surgery. In the past, major surgery was avoided in older women. However, surgery can be safely and successfully accomplished despite a patient's age, if the patient is fully evaluated and determined to be a surgi-

cal candidate (41). There is no doubt that older patients have poorer presurgical performance statuses and more intercurrent medical problems than younger patients.

Perioperative management is the key to success when treating older woman. Cardiac and pulmonary complications are the two most common serious problems encountered postoperatively. Careful preoperative assessment of cardiac status should include assessment for underlying coronary artery disease, valvular heart disease, and chronic congestive heart failure. There are several risk assessment algorithms that may be applied to estimate risk of major surgery. Because more than 40% of older women have hypertension, optimal blood pressure control should be achieved preoperatively. Intraoperative hypotension is one of the most common causes of myocardial ischemia and infarction. Pulmonary complications occur in nearly 40% of older women after a major abdominal surgery. Because physiologic changes of aging diminish vital capacity, lung compliance, reduced expiratory flow rates, and increased residual volume, the elderly patient is more likely to have pulmonary complications after general anesthesia. These women may be at an even higher risk if they have chronic obstructive pulmonary disease or asthma. Preoperative assessment may include assessment of pulmonary function by performing spirometry and obtaining an arterial blood gas measurement. Patients with underlying pulmonary disease should have their medical regimen maximized preoperatively, including the use of bronchodilators and steroids. Conduction anesthesia should be strongly considered in consultation with the anesthesiologist in order to avoid the pulmonary complications more frequently encountered with general anesthesia.

Avoiding perioperative hypothermia and hypoxemia are extremely important to avoid additional cardiac oxygen consumption. Invasive monitoring and planned intensive care unit admission should be considered in any circumstance where there is an increased risk of cardiac or pulmonary complications. Care also must be taken when ordering pharmacologic agents because older patients may have altered gastrointestinal absorption and decreased renal or hepatic clearance of specific drugs. Consultation with a clinical pharmacist is advised in order to establish the correct dose of drugs for patients with altered renal or hepatic function.

References

1. Ang-Lee MK, Moss J, Yuan CS. Herbal medicines and perioperative care. JAMA 2001;286:208–16.

2. Smetana GW, Macpherson DS. The case against routine preoperative laboratory testing. Med Clin No Amer 2003;87:7–40.

3. Gibbs J, Cull W, Hederson W, Daley J, Hur K, Khuri SF. Preoperative serum albumin level as a predictor of opera-

tive mortality and morbidity: results from the National VA Surgical Risk Study. Arch Surg 1999;134:36–42.

4. Johnson B, Porter J. Preoperative evaluation of the gynecologic patient. Considerations for improved outcomes. Obstet Gynecol 2008;111:1183–94.

5. Swietzer BJ, Preoperative screening, evaluation, and optimization of the patient's medical status before outpatient surgery. Curr Opin Anaesthesiol 2008;21:711–8.

6. Devereaux PJ, Yang H, Yusuf S, Guyatt G, Leslie K, Villar JC, et al. POISE Study Group. Effect of extended-release metoprolol succinate in patients undergoing non-cardiac surgery (POISE trial): a randomised controlled trial. POISE Study Group. Lancet 2008;371:1839–47.

7. Geerts WH, Pineo GF, Heit JA, Bergqvist D, Lassen MR, Colwell CW, et al. Prevention of venous thromboembolism: the Seventh ACCP Conference on Antithrombotic and Thrombolytic Therapy. Chest 2004;126:338S–400S.

8. Clarke-Pearson DL, Dodge RK, Synan I, McClelland RC, Maxwell GL. Venous thromboembolism prophylaxis: patients at high risk to fail intermittent pneumatic compression. Obstet Gynecol 2003;101:157–63.

9. Dahlback B, Carlsson M, Svensson PJ. Familial thrombophilia due to a previously unrecognized mechanism characterized by poor anticoagulant response to activated protein C: prediction of a cofactor to activated protein C. Proc Natl Acad Sci U S A 1993;90:1004–8.

10. Oger E, Lacut K, Le Gal G, Couturand F, Guenet D, Abalain JH, et al. Hyperhomocysteinemia and low B vitamin levels are independently associated with venous thromboembolism: results form the EDITH study: a hospital-based case-control study. EDITH COLLABORATIVE STUDY GROUP. J Thromb Haemost 2006;4:793–9.

11. Bertolaccini ML, Khamashta MA, Hughes GR. Diagnosis of antiphospholipid syndrome. Nat Clin Pract Rheumatol 2005;1:40–6.

12. Sachdeva A, Dalton M, Amatagiri SV, Lees TA. Elastic compression stockings for prevention of deep vein thrombosis. Cochrane Database of Systematic Reviews 2010, Issue 7. Art. No.: CD001484. DOI:10.1002/14651858. CD0011484.pub2.

13. Maxwell GL. Synan IS, Dodge R, Caroll B, Clarke-Pearson DL. Pneumatic calf compression versus low molecular weight heparin in gynecologic oncology surgery: a randomized trial. Obstet Gynecol 2001;98:989–95.

14. Claget GP, Reisch JS. Prevention of venous thromboembolism in general surgical patients. Results of meta-analysis. Ann Surg 1988;208:227–40.

15. Collins R, Scrimgeour A, Yusuf S, Peto R. Reduction in fatal pulmonary embolism and venous thrombosis by perioperative administration of subcutaneous heparin. Overview of results of randomized trials in general, orthopedic, and urologic surgery. N Engl J Med 1988;318:1162–73.

16. Clarke-Pearson DL, Coleman RE, Synan IS, Hinshaw W, Creasman WT. Venous thromboembolism prophylaxis in gynecologic oncology: a prospective, controlled trial of low-dose heparin. Am J Obstet Gynecol 1983;145:606–13.

17. Clarke-Pearson DL, DeLong E, Synan IS, Soper JT, Creasman WT, Coleman RE. A controlled trial of two low-dose heparin regimens for the prevention of postoperative deep vein thrombosis. Obstet Gynecol 1990;75:684–9.

18. Bergqvist D, Agnelli G, Cohen AT, Eldor A, Nilsson PE, Le Moigne-Amrani A, et al. Duration of prophylaxis against venous thromboembolism with enoxaparin after surgery for cancer. ENOXACAN II Investigators. N Engl J Med 2002; 346:975–80.

19. Wille-Joergensen P, Rasmussen MS, Andersen BR, Borly L. Heparins and mechanical methods for thromboprophylaxis is colorectal surgery. Cochrane Database of Systematic Reviews 2004, Issue 1. Art. No.: CD001217. DOI:10.1002/14651858.CD001217.

20. Chung F, Ward B, Ho H, Yuan H, Kayumov L, Shapiro C. Preoperative identification of sleep apnea risk in elective surgical patients, using the Berlin questionnaire. J Clin Anesth 2007;19:130–4.

21. Mickelson SA. Preoperative and postoperative management of obstructive apnea patients. Otolaryngol Clin North Am 2007;40:877–89.

22. Geerts WH, Bergqvist D, Pineo GF, Samama CM, Lassen MR, et al. Prevention of venous thromboembolism: American College of Chest Physicians Evidence-Based Clinical Practice Guidelines (8th Edition). American College of Chest Physicians. Chest 2008;13:381S–453S.

23. Carson JL, Noveck H, Berlin JA, Gould SA. Mortality and morbidity in patients with very low postoperative Hb levels whodecline blood transfusion. Transfusion 2002;42:812–8.

24. Patel MS, Carson JL. Anemia in the preoperative patient. Med Clin North Amer 2009;1095–104.

25. Wu WC, Schifftner TL, Henderson WG, Eaton CB, Poses RM, Uttley G, et al. Preoperative hematocrit levels and postoperative outcomes in older patients undergoing non-cardiac surgery. JAMA 2007;297:2481–8.

26. Kumar A. Perioperative management of anemia: Limits of blood transfusion and alternatives to it. Cleve Clin J Med 2009;76(Suppl 4):S112–18.

27. Beris P, Munoz M, Garcia-Erce JA, Thomas D, Maniatis A, Van der Linden P. Perioperative anaemia management: concensus statement on the role of intravenous iron. Br J Anaesth 2008;100:599–604.

28. American Society of Anesthesiologists Task Force on Perioperative Blood Transfusion and Adjuvant Therapies. Practice guidelines for perioperative blood transfusion and adjuvant therapies: an updated report by the American Society of Anesthesiologists Task Force of Perioperative Blood Transfusion and Adjuvant Therapies. Anesthesiology 2006;105:198–208.

29. Grant PJ, Brotman DJ, Jaffer AK. Perioperative anticoagulant therapy. Med Clin North Am 2009;93:1105–21.

30. Shields RC, McBane RD, Kuiper JD, Li H, Height JA. Efficacy and safety of intravenous phytonadione (vitamin K1) in patients on long-term oral anticoagulant therapy. Mayo Clin Proc 2001;76:260–6.

31. Bonow RO, Carabello BA, Chatterjee K, Kanu C, de Leon AC, Faxon DP, Freed MD, et al. ACC/AHA 2006 guidelines

for the management of patients with valvular disease: a report of the American College of Cardiology/American Heart Association Task Force on Practice Guidelines (writing committee to revise the 1998 Guidelines for the Management of Patients with Valvular Heart Disease): developed in collaboration with the Society of Cardiovascular Anesthesiologists: endorsed by the Society for Cardiovascular Angiography and Interventions and the Society of Thoracic Surgeons. American College of Cardiology/American Heart Association Task Force on Practice Guidelines. Society of Cardiovascular Anesthesiologists. Society for Cardiovascular Angiography and Interventions. Society of Thoracic Surgeons [published erratum appears in Circulation 2007;115:e409]. Circulation 2006;114:e384–231.

32. Jones DR, Lee HT. Surgery in the patient with renal dysfunction. Med Clin North Amer 2009;93:1083–93.

33. Carmichael P, Carmichael AR. Acute renal failure in the surgical setting. ANZ J Surg 2003;73:144–53.

34. Ympa YP, Sakr Y, Reinhart K, Vincent JL. Has mortality from acute renal failure decreased? A systematic review of the literature. Am J Med 2005;118:827–32.

35. Chertow GM, Burdick E, Honour M, Bonventre JV, Bates DW. Acute kidney injury, mortality, length of stay, and costs in hospitalized patients. J Am Soc Nephrol 2005;16:3365–70.

36. Kohl BA, Schwartz S. Surgery in the patient with endocrine dysfunction. Med Clin North Am 2009;93:1031–47.

37. Garber AJ, Moghissi ES, Bransome ED Jr, Clark NG, Clement S, Cobin RH, et al. American College of Endocrinology position statement on inpatient diabetes and metabolic control. American College of Endocrinology Task Force on Inpatient Diabetes Metabolic Control. Endocr Pract 2004;10 Suppl 2:4–9.

38. Hopkins RL, Leinung MC. Exogenous Cushing's syndrome and glucocorticoid withdrawal. Endocrinol Metab Clin North Am 2005;34:371–84, ix.

39. Slim K, Vicaut E, Launay-Savary MV, Contant C, Chipponi J. Undated systematic review and meta-analysis of randomized clinical trials on the role of mechanical bowel preparation before colorectal surgery. Ann Surg 2009;249:203–9.

40. Muzii L, Bellati F, Zullo MA, Manci N, Angioli R, Panici PB. Mechanical bowel preparation before gynecologic laparoscopy: a randomized, single blind, controlled trial. Fertil Steril 2006;85:689–93.

41. Sung VW, Weiten S, Sokol ER, Rardin CR, Myers DL. Effect of patient age on increasing morbidity and mortality following urogynecological surgery. Am J Obstet Gynecol 2006;194:1411–7.

Benign Disorders of the Vulva

Colleen K. Stockdale and Lori A. Boardman

Vulvar symptoms are common, often chronic, and can interfere significantly with women's sexual function and sense of well-being. Remaining aware of the differences in epithelial and glandular structure, hormonal responsiveness, neural distribution, and immune responses that result from the differences in origin is crucial in assessing vulvar symptoms.

Pruritus and pain are two of the most common symptoms in women presenting to vulvar clinics. Pruritus may occur in the presence of obvious dermatologic disease or in conditions with few visible skin changes. Vulvar pain or discomfort can arise in a number of settings, some with clinically obvious signs and others in the presence of normal physical findings. Commonly identified infections (eg, candidiasis), inflammation (eg, lichen planus), neoplasia (eg, squamous cell carcinoma), or neurologic disorders (eg, herpes neuralgia) can be associated with pain. Discomfort and pain, however, can occur in the absence of visible findings or a specific, clinically identifiable neurologic disorder, and in this instance, the term *vulvodynia* is used to describe the patient's condition.

Vulvar Pruritus

Pruritus is the most common symptom of skin disease and may occur in the presence of obvious dermatologic disease or in conditions with few visible skin changes. In evaluating vulvar pruritus, it is helpful to differentiate women with acute symptoms versus women with chronic symptoms. Acute anogenital pruritus often is infectious, with allergic and irritant contact dermatitis playing a role in some cases. Genital infections, such as tinea, bacterial vaginosis, trichomoniasis, uncomplicated candidiasis, and herpes; as well as dermatitis and recurrent candidiasis; should be considered in the differential diagnosis. Chronic pruritus, in general, has a history of gradual onset, examples of which include lichen simplex chronicus, lichen sclerosus, psoriasis, and various manifestations of HPV-related disease. Each disorder will be considered separately.

Dermatitis

The term dermatitis describes a poorly demarcated, erythematous, and usually itchy rash. Burning sometimes can occur in cases of epithelial involvement. Subtypes are numerous and can be classified as either exogenous (irritant or allergic contact dermatitis) or endogenous (atopic or seborrheic dermatitis). Dermatitis is common

and has been reported to occur in 20–60% of patients seen with chronic vulvar symptoms, with atopic dermatitis being by far the most frequently encountered (1). The clinical appearance of the vulva often does not help confirm the diagnosis, and in many cases, more than one process has led to the symptoms the patient reports. A physician also may encounter a mixed picture where endogenous dermatitis or another epithelial disorder has been worsened by use of ointments or creams to which the patient has had an adverse reaction (1, 2) (Fig. 17).

Contact dermatitis is one of the most frequently encountered and often simultaneously avoidable problems seen in vulvar specialty clinics. Many seemingly innocuous behaviors, such as bathing, the use of sanitary or incontinence pads, or exposure to known irritants or allergens in numerous topical medications (Box 7), have the potential to initiate this eczematous process (2). Attention to vulvar hygiene measures can significantly reduce the occurrence of both contact dermatitis and lichen simplex chronicus (Box 8). Confirmation of the diagnosis also should include assessment to rule out candidiasis. Biopsy results are nonspecific and of little use in the evaluation.

Irritant contact dermatitis has been identified in 5–26% of women with diagnosed vulvar dermatitis; often as a result of exposure to irritants; such as detergents, soaps, perfumes, semen, and propylene glycol,

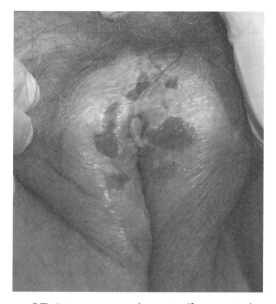

Figure 17. Irritant contact dermatitis (from topical corticosteroids) complicating lichen sclerosus.

an additive found in many topical medications. Allergic contact dermatitis, in contrast, is an immunologically mediated inflammatory reaction (type IV delayed hypersensitivity) to an allergen in a previously sensitized woman. Although distinguishing allergic contact dermatitis from irritant contact dermatitis can be difficult, the intermittent nature of the symptoms and the timing of symptom onset (10–14 days after the exposure but may be less than 24 hours if already sensitized) serve as important keys to establishing the diagnosis of allergic contact dermatitis. A number of topical medications can cause allergic reactions as

well, including a variety of topical medications such as antibiotics (eg, neomycin, bacitracin), antifungals (clotrimazole, miconazole), corticosteroids, and the greatest offenders, topical anesthetics (2).

On examination, clinical signs can range from mild erythema, swelling, and scaling to marked erythema, fissures, erosions, and ulcers (2). For vulvar contact dermatitis, the first line of therapy remains removal of the offending agent or practice, correction of barrier function, elimination of scratching, and reduction of inflammation. Barrier function should be restored through the use of sitz baths, estrogen therapy if indicated, treatment of concomitant infection if present, and application of a thin layer of plain petrolatum. Medications with antihistamine and sedative properties, such as doxepin or hydroxyzine, can be added to control nocturnal itching. A selective serotonin reuptake inhibitor (SSRI) can be used during the day to avoid drowsiness. Antiinflammatory therapy also should begin with a mid- to high-potency corticosteroid for 2–3 weeks. A weaker corticosteroid, such as 1% hydrocortisone, can then be continued as needed. In recalcitrant cases, oral or intramuscular corticosteroids may be necessary (2).

Box 7

Common Vulvar Irritants and Allergens

Irritants
- Topical medications
- Soaps, bubble bath, salts, shampoos, and conditioners
- Laundry detergents, fabric softeners, and dryer sheets
- Sanitary products, including tampons and pads
- Vaginal or vulvar products; especially those containing propylene glycol
- Contraceptive creams, jellies, foams, noxynolol-9, and KY jelly
- Condoms (with lubricant or spermicide)
- Vaginal hygiene products, including perfumes and deodorants
- Adult or baby wipes
- Tea tree oil
- Colored or scented toilet paper

Allergens
- Topical anesthetics (eg, benzocaine, lidocaine, and dibucaine)
- Topical antimycotics (eg, imidazoles and nystatin)
- Topical antibacterials (eg, neomycin, bacitracin, and polymyxin)
- Topical corticosteroids
- Vaginal or vulvar products containing propylene glycol
- Antiseptics (eg, povidone–iodine and hexachlorophene)
- Rubber products (including latex)
- Body fluids (eg, semen)
- Dyes
- Emollients (eg, lanolin, jojoba oil, and glycerin)

Modified from Diagnosis and management of vulvar skin disorders. ACOG Practice Bulletin No. 93. American College of Obstetricians and Gynecologists. Obstet Gynecol 2008; 111:1243–53.

Box 8

Skin Care Guidelines for the Prevention and Control of Vulvar Symptoms

Avoid the Following:
- Vulvar irritants and allergens, many of which are unrecognized as potential causative agents (including detergents and soaps, perfumes, many over-the-counter and prescribed topical medications, such as anesthetics, steroids, antifungals, and antibiotics)
- Douching

Include the Following as Part of Routine Vulvar Care:
- Use of mild soaps for bathing, but avoidance of any soap use on the vulva
- Cleansing of the vulva with water only
- After bathing, gently patting the vulva dry. Application of a preservative-free emollient (such an vegetable oil or plain petrolatum) topically to hold moisture in the skin and improve barrier function
- Use of pericare bottles or rinsing and patting the vulva dry after urination
- Use of 100% cotton menstrual pads
- Use of adequate lubrication for intercourse

Modified from Diagnosis and management of vulvar skin disorders. ACOG Practice Bulletin No. 93. American College of Obstetricians and Gynecologists. Obstet Gynecol 2008; 111:1243–53.

Lichen Simplex Chronicus

Vulvar lichen simplex chronicus is a chronic eczematous disease characterized by intense and unrelenting itching and scratching. In vulvar specialty clinics, lichen simplex chronicus is diagnosed in 10–35% of patients evaluated. Although lichen simplex chronicus occurs primarily in middle to late adult life, it can occur in children. From 65% to 75% of patients will report a history of atopic disease (hay fever, asthma, or childhood eczema), and as such, lichen simplex chronicus can be seen as a localized variant of atopic dermatitis. All patients report pruritus, and most will admit to vigorous scratching or rubbing and often report sleep disturbances as a result of the discomfort.

Clinically, lichen simplex chronicus appears as one or more erythematous, scaling, lichenified plaques. Various degrees of excoriation often are visible. In long-standing disease, the skin appears thickened and leathery, and areas of hyperpigmentation and hypopigmentation may be present. Erosions and ulcers also can develop, most commonly from chronic scratching. Vaginal fungal cultures are helpful in determining the presence of an underlying condition on which lichen simplex chronicus is superimposed. Biopsy (demonstrating marked hyperkeratosis with widening and deepening of the rete ridges) rarely is necessary unless an underlying disease (such as lichen sclerosus or psoriasis) is suspected or the treatment fails.

Lichen simplex chronicus represents an end-stage response to a wide variety of possible initiating processes, including environmental factors (eg, heat, excessive sweating, and irritation from clothing or topically applied products) and dermatologic disease (eg, candidiasis and lichen sclerosus) (3). Treatment consists of identification and removal of the initiating factor, repair of the skin's barrier layer function, reduction of inflammation, and disruption of the itch–scratch cycle. Mid- to high-potency topical corticosteroids (depending on the presence of underlying disease) should be applied nightly until symptoms begin to abate; less frequent use (eg, alternate nights, then twice weekly) should continue until the condition resolves. Medications with antihistamine and sedative properties can be added to control nocturnal itching, an SSRI can be prescribed for daytime use and oral or intralesional steroids can be used for refractory cases (3).

Vulvar Dermatoses

Vulvar dermatoses may manifest themselves in a variety of ways, and may be asymptomatic or disabling. Treatment is not curative and requires long-term maintenance to reduce symptoms and associated anatomic changes. Thus, patient education is imperative and requires ongoing communication.

LICHEN SCLEROSUS

Lichen sclerosus, a chronic disorder of the skin, most commonly is seen on the vulva, with extragenital lesions reported in 5–20% of patients. Although lichen sclerosus may affect any age group, the mean age of onset is 50–60 years. The etiology of lichen sclerosus remains elusive. However, it is most likely a genetic or autoimmune disorder because it is highly associated with other autoimmune disorders, including alopecia, vitiligo, thyrotoxicosis, hypothyroidism, and pernicious anemia (4). The patients with lichen sclerosus are at an increased risk of developing vulvar cancer. Patients presenting with lichen sclerosus most commonly report pruritus, followed by irritation, burning, dyspareunia, and tearing. Because lichen sclerosus may be asymptomatic, its prevalence remains unknown.

On examination, typical lesions of lichen sclerosus are porcelain-white papules and plaques, often with areas of ecchymosis or purpura. The skin often appears thinned, whitened, and crinkling (hence the description "cigarette paper") (Fig. 18). Although the genital mucosa is largely spared with lichen sclerosus, involvement of the mucocutaneous junctions may lead to introital narrowing. Perianal involvement can create the classic "figure of eight" or hourglass shape. Other findings include distortion of the vulvar architecture with fusion of the labia minora, phimosis of the clitoral hood, and fissures (4). Because other vulvar diseases can mimic lichen sclerosus, a biopsy is necessary to confirm the diagnosis. Histology often reveals epidermal atrophy with loss of the rete ridges, hyperkeratosis, and homogenization of dermal collagen with a band-like inflammatory dermal infiltrate. However, histology may be inconclusive even with advanced lichen sclerosus.

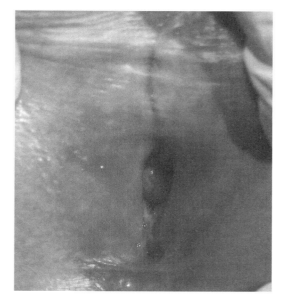

Figure 18. Advanced lichen sclerosus in a postmenopausal woman.

Despite the association between lichen sclerosus and autoimmune-related disorders, there are no recommendations regarding evaluation for coexisting autoimmune-related disorders in women with lichen sclerosus beyond a brief examination for alopecia areata and vitiligo and consideration of thyroid function tests. Additionally, although age and the concomitant presence of squamous hyperplasia did appear to be independently associated with the finding of vulvar carcinoma in women with lichen sclerosus in a case–control study, neither the presence nor duration of symptoms or the loss of vulvar architecture proved to be useful indicators of potential cancer risk (5). Furthermore, despite a greater concern of malignancy with poorly controlled lichen sclerosus, there is no evidence that long-term topical steroid treatment or optimal control of symptoms reduces the risk of malignancy. Persistent or suspicious lesions should be biopsied to exclude intraepithelial neoplasia or invasive squamous cell cancer.

The recommended treatment for lichen sclerosus is a high potency topical steroid ointment, the most studied of which is clobetasol propionate. Although there are no randomized controlled trials to provide evidence regarding the most effective steroid regimen, a reasonable approach is to begin with a once-daily application and taper to alternate days once improvement has been demonstrated. Patients should be monitored closely to confirm improvement and adjust corticosteroid frequency.

Ultrapotent steroid therapy is not without complication (including not only skin changes, but also the possibility of adrenal suppression with overuse of topical therapy), and to this end, topical calcineurin inhibitors have been evaluated and found to be effective in the treatment of lichen sclerosus in several small case studies. Unlike topical steroids, dermal atrophy is avoided with this class of medications. Although promising, subsequent reports of a possible link to skin cancer and lymphoma based on animal studies and case reports in humans limit the use of this medication. Subsequently, the FDA issued a public health advisory in 2005 recommending that health care providers use topical immunosuppressant calcineurin inhibitors, eg, tacrolimus, as second-line agents for short-term and intermittent treatment in patients unresponsive to or intolerant of other treatments. Treatment with other topical therapies, including testosterone and progesterone, has not consistently resulted in improvement in lichen sclerosus and, therefore, is no longer recommended. Surgery, although not curative, is reserved exclusively for the treatment of malignancy and postinflammation sequelae (eg, release of labial adhesions).

Regarding the need for maintenance therapy, the literature is conflicting. Some experts advocate discontinuation of therapy after the initial regimen described earlier with use of therapy for flares or recurrent symptoms, whereas others recommend an ongoing mainte-nance regimen of once-weekly application of either an ultrapotent or moderate strength steroid (4). Initially, monitoring at 3 months and 6 months after the initial therapy is recommended to assess the patient's response to therapy and ensure proper application of the medication. Annual examinations are suggested for patients in whom lichen sclerosus is well-controlled, and more frequent visits for those patients with poorly controlled disease (for whom intralesional steroid injections may also be beneficial), or biopsy may be warranted.

PSORIASIS

Psoriasis is a common skin disorder, occurring in 2–3% of the population, which can frequently affect the genital skin. Vulvar psoriasis, which is usually pruritic, can be seen in girls and women of all ages. The thickened plaques associated with this disorder result from rapid proliferation of the epidermis. What underlies this rapid cellular turnover is unclear, although a genetic predisposition is present and immunologic factors likely play a role.

The typical clinical features of anogenital psoriasis are symmetric "salmon pink" plaques, which can contain silvery scales (Fig. 19). When psoriasis is present on the vulva, the typical silver scaling often is absent. The bright erythema and well-defined outline of the disease, however, tend to remain. The plaques commonly occur on the mons pubis. Although the loss of vulvar architecture is uncommon with psoriasis, it can occur. The differential diagnosis includes tinea cruris, intertrigo, seborrheic dermatitis, and lichen simplex chronicus. Definitive diagnosis is made through biopsy, although in more longstanding cases, biopsy may be nonspecific and interpreted as psoriasiform dermatitis.

When limited to the vulva, local treatment with mid- to high-strength topical corticosteroids is the treatment of choice. If not adequately controlled, calcipotriene may

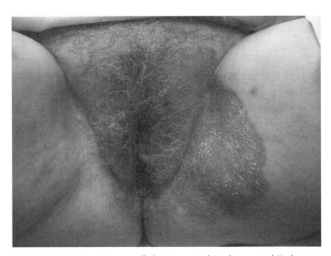

Figure 19. Psoriasis—well demarcated "salmon pink" plaque with silvery scale.

be added, although patients should be cautioned that it may take 1–2 months for improvement to be noted. For disease unresponsive to these measures, systemic therapy with oral methotrexate, retinoids, or cyclosporine should be considered in consultation with a physician experienced with the use of such medications.

LICHEN PLANUS

Lichen planus is an inflammatory, mucocutaneous disorder that exhibits a wide range of morphologies. The most common form and the most difficult to treat is the erosive form that can lead to significant scarring and pain. Most commonly recognized on the skin or oral mucosa, this condition may affect the lower genital tract (vulva and vagina). It is unclear if these variants represent a single underlying etiology or have similar associated conditions. Approximately 1% of the population has oral lichen planus, and of women with oral disease, estimates suggest that 25% have genital vulvovaginal disease (6). Because genital lesions may be asymptomatic and because lesions often go unrecognized during examination, the incidence of genital disease is most likely underestimated (7).

The classic presentation of lichen planus on mucous membranes, including the buccal mucosa, is that of white, reticulate, lacy, or fern-like striae (Wickham striae). On occasion, the skin may appear uniformly white; consequently, lichen planus can be confused with lichen sclerosus. The pruritic, purple, shiny papules typically associated with lichen planus are occasionally found on the genital skin. If present, however, they appear dusky pink in color, without an apparent scale and less well demarcated.

In erosive lichen planus, deep, painful, erythematous erosions appear in the posterior vestibule and often extend to the labia minora, resulting in agglutination and resorption of the labial architecture (Fig. 20). As on the buccal mucosa, Wickham striae may be present. The vaginal epithelium can become erythematous,

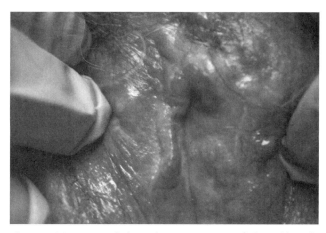

Figure 20. Erosive lichen planus. Scarring of clitoral hood, erosions with Whicham striae present.

eroded, acutely inflamed, and denuded of epithelium. Erosive patches, if present, are extremely friable. Over time, these eroded surfaces may adhere, resulting in synechiae and eventually complete obliteration of the vaginal space (6). Symptoms commonly reported by patients with erosive vulvar lichen planus include dyspareunia, burning, and increased vaginal discharge (8). Examination of the vaginal discharge reveals predominance of inflammatory cells and immature parabasal and basal epithelial cells (these will appear small and round, with relatively large nuclei). The vaginal pH is increased, usually in the range of 5–6. This discharge has often been labeled as desquamative inflammatory vaginitis, but whether desquamative inflammatory vaginitis is a type of erosive lichen planus or a distinct type of vaginitis remains controversial (7).

Among women with erosive vulvovaginal lichen planus, up to 70% have oral disease as well. In one case series of women with vulvovaginal lichen planus, 55% gave a personal history, a family history, or both of an autoimmune disorder, including diabetes mellitus, thyroid disease, and celiac disease (9). In addition, the series also found that the human leukocyte antigen DQB1*0201 allele was present in 80% of women with vulvovaginal lichen planus, suggesting a genetic predisposition to the vulvovaginal form of lichen planus. However, these associations have not been consistently identified in diverse populations. Concern regarding an association with vulvar malignancy and erosive lichen planus has similarly been noted. However, risk of malignancy has been difficult to determine given the rarity of both disorders (8).

The differential diagnosis of lichen planus includes other inflammatory dermatoses. It is commonly confused with lichen sclerosus. However, vaginal involvement is common in erosive lichen planus and is rare in lichen sclerosus.

Biopsy that reveals a band-like infiltrate of lymphocytes and colloid bodies in the basal layers of the epidermis may be relatively nonspecific because of the complete loss of the vaginal epithelium. However, a histologic specimen can help rule out immunobullous diseases, such as cicatricial pemphigoid, bullous pemphigoid, and pemphigus vulgaris that may mimic lichen planus (6). The prognosis for spontaneous remission of vulvovaginal lichen planus is poor.

Treatment, although not curative, can improve patients' symptoms and sense of well-being. Although therapeutic options shown in small trials to be effective include topical and systemic corticosteroids, topical and oral cyclosporine, topical tacrolimus, hydroxychloroquine, oral retinoids, methotrexate, azathioprine and cyclophosphamide, the mainstay of treatment is corticosteroids (6). Ultrapotent topical steroids (ointments will cause less stinging than creams), and at times oral steroids for severe erosions and exudation, may be required. If used intravaginally, care should be taken to monitor the potential side effects of high-dose steroids, including not only atrophy, striae, and steroid dermatitis, but also systemic absorption resulting in adrenal suppression. With frequent use of steroids, infections (eg, yeast and herpes) also should be suspected when symptoms flare (7). To help maintain vaginal patency, the use of vaginal dilators should be encouraged. Surgery in general is not advocated. Despite available therapies for erosive lichen planus, significant control of symptoms and restoration of sexual function remain difficult.

Human Papillomavirus-Related Disease

Genital human papillomavirus (HPV), the most common sexually transmitted viral infection, is associated with a number of vulvar epithelial disorders, including genital warts, vulvar intraepithelial neoplasia, and some vulvar carcinomas. Of the more than 120 HPV subtypes currently identified, more than 40 are specific to the anogenital tract, and of those, approximately 15 are oncogenic. Commercially available probes for HPV DNA typing allow for identification of one half of these anogenital subtypes, including 5 low-risk and 13 or 14 oncogenic subtypes. Although low-risk HPV types 6 and 11 are implicated in the development of genital warts and oncogenic HPV 16 commonly is found in classic (bowenoid) vulvar intraepithelial neoplasia (VIN), routine use of HPV testing for diagnosing vulvar HPV-related disease is not recommended.

Estimates of the prevalence of HPV infection cannot be derived from visible manifestations of disease alone. For example, genital warts have an annual estimated incidence of 2.4 cases per 1,000 individuals, yet the prevalence of the viral types that principally result in warts is significantly greater. The same holds true for HPV-related VIN (10, 11). However, HPV infection is associated with approximately 50% of cases of vulvar cancer (the basaloid and warty types commonly associated with classic VIN).

When clinical manifestations of vulvar HPV infection do occur, they often present as bumps or growths on the vulvovaginal or perianal epithelium. Although commonly asymptomatic, genital warts are as likely to cause itching, burning, pain, or bleeding. On examination, warts can range in morphologic appearance from flat-topped papules to flesh-colored, dome-shaped papules, keratotic warts, or true condylomata acuminata. External genital warts tend to occur on the moist surfaces of the vulva, introitus, and perianal area. Distinguishing warts from vulvar neoplasia based on appearance alone is not always possible. If the diagnosis is uncertain, if lesions appear atypical, do not respond or worsen with treatment, or if the patient is immunocompromised, biopsy should be undertaken

(12). Women with genital warts should undergo routine cervical cancer screening. However, with the use of HPV testing, a change in the frequency of cervical cytologic screening or cervical colposcopy is not indicated in the presence of genital warts. If exophytic cervical warts are detected during examination or if vulvar neoplasia is confirmed by biopsy, referral for colposcopic evaluation is then indicated (12).

Spontaneous regression of genital warts can occur in up to 30% of affected patients. Regression, however, does not necessarily lead to viral clearance because viral genomes can be detected in normal epithelium for months to years after the clearing of visible disease. In immunocompetent women, however, the cell-mediated immunity that resulted in lesion regression most likely controls latent HPV infection. Therefore, disease recurrence is less likely. Women at increased risk of developing HPV-related manifestations include those receiving long-term corticosteroid therapy or chronic immunosuppressive treatment, as well as immunosuppressed women with HIV infection. Antiviral chemotherapies are particularly critical for these populations, if disease recurrences are to be minimized (10).

At present, most currently available treatment options are not targeted antiviral therapies. The goal in general has been physical destruction or removal of visible disease, not eradication of HPV infection, as evidenced by the currently recommended treatment regimens for external genital warts. These include all provider-administered therapies: cryotherapy, podophyllin resin 10–25%, trichloroacetic or bichloracetic acid 80–90%, surgical removal, and laser therapy (12). Although most are equivalent in terms of clearance rates, recurrence rates can be high, particularly for laser therapy, where the rate exceeds 60%. Local irritation (eg, pain, burning, and soreness), erythema, edema, and, at times ulceration, can result from the use of any of the medications. Careless or excessive use can result in extensive burning of the epithelium, with resultant scar formation. Surgical excision or laser vaporization should be reserved for patients with extensive disease.

Newer therapeutic choices include the patient-applied treatments podofilox (keratolytic) and imiquimod (antiviral). Clearance rates for the two treatments are similar and compare favorably with any of the treatments listed previously. The added benefit of imiquimod, as demonstrated in numerous studies, has been its significantly lower recurrence rates (9–19%). The most recent FDA-approved patient applied treatment for external condyloma is sinecatechins, 15% topical ointment. This class of drugs is a mixture of catechins and other green tea components, and has a response rate up to 55% for complete clearance and 78% reduction of external anogenital warts (13). Although the ointment was noted to be well tolerated by patients, long-term follow-up data and recurrence rates are limited (7% recurrence at 12 weeks) (13).

Intralesional interferon, a medication with antiproliferative, antiviral, and immunomodulatory properties, has, unlike imiquimod, demonstrated limited efficacy, and is not recommended for first-line therapy in treating either warts or VIN (10). Its use, however, can be considered an alternative regimen for the treatment of external genital warts (12).

Podofilox and podophyllin, recognized teratogens, as well as imiquimod and sinecatechins, are not recommended for use during pregnancy. Although respiratory papillomatosis is associated with HPV types 6 and 11, the mode of transmission of HPV to fetuses during pregnancy remains uncertain. Thus, routine cesarean delivery is not recommended in women with genital warts (12). However, the Centers for Disease Control and Prevention recommends that pregnant women with genital warts receive counseling regarding the low risk of recurrent respiratory papillomatosis in their infants (12).

Vulvar intraepithelial neoplasia can be unifocal or multifocal. Multifocal VIN most often occurs in young women in their 30s and 40s and is strongly associated with cigarette smoking (11). In older women, VIN is most frequently associated with other epithelial disorders (such as lichen sclerosus) often is HPV negative, and is less common than in young women. Older women account for approximately 2–10% of cases of VIN. Increasing rates of HPV-related VIN and vulvar carcinomas have been reported in women younger than 50 years, with the mean age at diagnosis of VIN 3 decreasing to 33 years. Biopsy of suspicious lesions should be performed to rule out VIN or early invasive carcinoma.

Management of VIN depends on several factors. Observation suffices for VIN 1. Although the risk of invasive malignancy of high-grade VIN is low, high-risk types of VIN (VIN 2 and VIN 3) should be surgically removed or treated and these patients should be appropriately monitored. Observation is initially reasonable for women with high-risk types of VIN who have recently completed a course of corticosteroids, who are temporarily immunocompromised, or who are pregnant. Many of these patients are smokers and should be counseled regarding smoking cessation.

For patients with multifocal or persistent high-risk types of VIN, laser ablation or topical treatment with 5% imiquimod, which acts by activating local immunity, has been used. Imiquimod's efficacy in the treatment of genital warts is well documented, and in a number of recent trials, its use has been associated with encouraging treatment results in the treatment with a greater than 90% response rate (14).

Hidradenitis Suppurativa

Hidradenitis suppurativa, less well known as acne inversa or Verneuil disease, is a common chronic, suppurative, cutaneous process that results from occlusion of follicles and secondary inflammation of apocrine glands. Scarring of the affected sites results from chronic infection and draining abscesses. Unlike acne vulgaris, acne inversa is localized to nonfacial regions, sebum excretion is not increased, and affected areas tend to be rich in apocrine glands that are involved, but not the original source, of the inflammatory process.

The incidence of hidradenitis suppurativa is estimated to be 1 in 300, although hidradenitis suppurativa is most likely underrecognized and underdiagnosed. Women are more likely to be affected then men. Other causal factors in women may include both acquired and genetic characteristics, including onset after puberty and before age 40 years, obesity (with hyperandrogenism), association with other endocrine disorders (eg, diabetes), and an apparent familial predisposition in some patients.

The onset of hidradenitis suppurativa is insidious. Early symptoms consist of pruritus, erythema, burning, and local hyperhidrosis. Occlusion of a hair follicle results in a cyst, similar to the comedones of acne. As the area heals, it becomes scarred and fibrotic. With recurrent cyst formation, induration and inflammation leads to spontaneous rupture and sinus tract formation. Ultimately hyperpigmentation, scaring, pitting, and multiple fistulous sites are noted with associated pain.

Early diagnosis of hidradenitis suppurativa is easily overlooked and often attributed to simple comedones of acne. Although specific diagnostic criteria do not exist, the diagnosis becomes apparent with disease progression; biopsy is neither required nor diagnostic. Clinical criteria suggesting hidradenitis suppurativa include recurrent deep boils in flexural apocrine gland skin sites (typically involving the axilla, inguinal, and anogenital areas), onset after puberty, poor response to

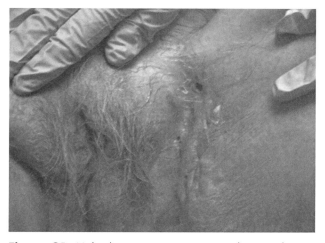

Figure 21. Hidradenitis suppurativa. Late disease characterized by chronic infection, draining abscesses, sinus tracts, and scarring.

conventional antibiotics, and tendency toward relapse and recurrence. Late disease is characterized by chronic infection, draining abscesses, nodules, sinus tracts, scarring, and hyperpigmentation (Fig. 21).

Treatment of hidradenitis suppurativa is challenging and based primarily on anecdotal evidence. Current treatment is directed at prevention of new lesions through medical management and elimination of existing lesions surgically when appropriate. In order to improve the local environment, avoidance of irritants, heat, sweating, and reducing friction (eg, avoidance of tight clothing and limited pad use) is encouraged. Additionally, weight reduction often is helpful. Medical treatment including antibiotics, antiandrogens, corticosteroids, retinoids, and skin care is commonly used with varying success.

The use of long-term antibiotic therapy, however, does not appear to alter the natural history of hidradenitis suppurativa, and recurrence after discontinuation is the rule. Treatment with antiandrogens has produced mixed results in women with hidradenitis suppurativa. For mild hidradenitis suppurativa, both intralesional triamcinolone acetate and low-dose isotretinoin have demonstrated some efficacy.

Surgery is heralded as the primary treatment of severe, extensive hidradenitis suppurativa. However, all treatment options are noted to have a high recurrence rate, including radical surgery.

Bartholin Cysts

The Bartholin cyst is a result of the distal obstruction of the Bartholin gland. The most likely diagnosis in a woman with a unilateral, tender, swollen labial mass is an abscess of the Bartholin gland. Such an abscess should occur in the lower third of the introitus between the vestibule and the labia majora. Diagnosis is based on clinical presentation, with the cyst transected by the labia minor (Fig. 22). Gonococcal infection has been

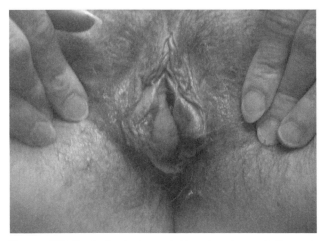

Figure 22. Bartholin duct cyst. Labia minor transects the cyst.

implicated in a number of cases, although the infection is largely polymicrobial. Although abscesses of the Bartholin gland constitute a relatively frequent finding in the ambulatory setting, agreement as to the most efficacious treatment remains unclear. Current treatment modalities include outpatient procedures, such as needle aspiration with antibiotic coverage, incision (on the epithelial surface of the abscess inside the introitus), and drainage with or without placement of a Word catheter, as well as more extensive surgical therapies, such as marsupialization.

Incision and drainage alone or with packing is not generally advocated because the tissue edges tend to reapproximate and lead to recurrence. In contrast, Word catheter placement after incision allows for formation of an epithelialized tract and continued drainage of the gland, thereby reducing recurrences. A small incision is made inside the introitus, the catheter is inserted and inflated, and the catheter end is tucked into the vagina. Removal should not occur until a fistulous tract forms (4–6 weeks) although epithelization may occur as early as 3–4 weeks.

Marsupialization may be used as a first-line therapy or after the failure of the less invasive therapies. Conventional marsupialization consists of incision of the cyst or abscess and suturing of the edges of the cavity to the skin. The procedure has been modified by excising a 2–3-cm oval portion of the vestibular epithelium overlying the cyst or abscess and a smaller oval portion of the cyst wall before suturing of the edges to improve patency of the opening during the healing process and, thus, reduce the likelihood of subsequent recurrence (15).

The management of Bartholin abscesses, the result of polymicrobial infections and occasionally sexually transmitted infections, should also include routine culture for anaerobic and aerobic bacteria as well as testing for *Neisseria gonorrhea* and *Chlamydia trachomatis*. Broad-spectrum antibiotic coverage is warranted when cellulitis is present and it should be tailored to the culture and testing results as they become available. Excision of the entire Bartholin gland and duct, a procedure associated with significant morbidity (excessive bleeding, hematoma formation, and dyspareunia) is the definitive therapy to treat recurrent Bartholin cysts and abscesses.

Bartholin gland carcinoma, although rare, should be considered in the postmenopausal woman presenting with a Bartholin gland enlargement, including cysts (symptomatic or not), or abscesses. Incision or marsupialization with biopsy to rule out an underlying carcinoma will allow for a diagnosis and avoid a possibly unnecessary and potentially morbid procedure. For women older than 40 years with recurrent disease or if a mass persists after the drainage, excision of the gland is recommended.

Vulvodynia

Vulvodynia is an underrecognized and poorly treated multifaceted dysfunction that significantly interferes with intimacy, relationships, and overall quality of life for affected women and their partners. Despite the significant prevalence and negative effect, limited studies have focused on etiology, treatment, and outcome regarding vulvar pain disorders. Management often is based on "trial and error," and is typically frustrating for practitioners, patients, and significant others owing to the complex interrelated medical, psychologic, and psychosexual components.

The International Society for the Study of Vulvovaginal Disease defined vulvodynia as vulvar discomfort, most commonly described as burning pain, occurring in the absence of relevant visible findings (such as infection or inflammation) or a specific, clinically identifiable neurologic disorder (16). Current evidence indicates that the lifetime cumulative incidence of vulvodynia approaches 16%, which suggests that nearly 14 million U.S. women will at some point in their lives experience the symptoms of chronic vulvar burning and pain.

Patients with vulvodynia tend to fall into different groups based on the location of their pain. Generalized vulvodynia is used to describe involvement of the entire vulva by persistent, chronic pain that is burning, stinging, or irritating in nature, whereas localized vulvodynia specifies involvement of only a portion of the vulva, such as the vestibule (termed *vestibulodynia* or *vulvar vestibulitis*). In both generalized and localized vulvodynia, the pain may be provoked (ie, triggered by physical contact of a sexual or nonsexual nature), unprovoked, or both. In the case of provoked pain, common triggers include intromission (resulting in introital dyspareunia), tampon insertion, and the wearing of tight-fitting clothing (16).

Proposed precipitating factors for vulvar pain syndromes are numerous and have included histories of recurrent vaginal infections (most commonly, candidal infections and bacterial vaginosis), use of oral contraceptives (particular early use), and destructive treatments (eg, exposure to irritant agents, such as trichloroacetic acid). Although clinical studies did not initially support the role of past sexual or physical abuse as causative agents, one study demonstrated an increased occurrence of childhood physical and sexual abuse in women with vulvodynia, an association largely confined to those harmed by a primary family member (17). Whether depression, anxiety, and sexual dysfunction are causally related to or are the result of chronic vulvar pain syndromes, remains unclear (16). Both depression and anxiety are, however, common with vulvar pain syndromes. Also, patients with vulvodynia report a higher incidence of irritable bowel syndrome and interstitial cystitis, which may be indicative of aberrant neuronal interactions (ie, irritation of one organ leads to co-sensitization of another).

Although a multifactorial process is most likely involved in the development of vulvar pain, the end result appears to be neuropathically mediated pain manifested predominantly as burning. In general, neuropathic pain is believed to result from damage to and subsequent loss of peripheral afferent elements, a loss that leads ultimately to changes in the central nervous system. For patients with localized pain, the damage has been proposed to result from neurogenic inflammation. This inflammation then leads to sensitization of first the primary afferents (predominantly nociceptors or pain receptors) by inflammatory peptides, prostaglandins, and cytokines and then the spinal cord. Impulses are transmitted along the afferent sympathetics to the central nervous system where a reinforcing signal, returned through efferent fibers, sustains the pain loop. The allodynia (pain to light touch) and hyperalgesia (excessive response to slight pain) seen in women with vestibulodynia can be explained by central nervous system changes (18).

The concomitant role of pelvic floor pathology also should be considered in the assessment of patients with vestibulodynia. The pelvic floor changes seen in women with vestibulodynia appear to be reactive in nature, a conditioned, protective guarding response that results from repeated attempts at vaginal penetration (19). In this study of women with vestibulitis and age-matched controls, significant hypertonicity was observed only at the superficial, and not the deep, muscle layers of the pelvic floor, suggesting that hypertonicity may be the result of and not the cause of vestibulitis. Over time, a protective guarding response to pain is postulated to lead to an increase in the resting tone of the muscle. As a result of the guarding and the increase in resting tone, any pressure applied to the vestibule leads to increased pain, and the cycle becomes self-perpetuating. The pelvic floor hypertonicity seen in women with vestibulitis appears then to both maintain and exacerbate pain.

Management of vulvar pain syndromes is a complex process that begins with identification (diagnosis) and education. Practitioners should have a repertoire of management suggestions for patients with vulvodynia that may be of benefit. Although there are currently no FDA-approved treatments for vulvodynia, treatments have been identified by recognized experts of vulvar pain disorders and include local measures, as well as medical, surgical, and alternative treatments as described earlier. Given the heterogeneous nature of vulvodynia, a multidisciplinary approach based on etiologic factors and the context of the pain should be considered.

The evaluation of patients with vulvovaginal symptoms begins with a thorough history and physical examination. In cases of acute vulvar pruritus, infections and contact dermatitis should be suspected. However, chronic vulvar pruritus should signal a search for underlying dermatoses, such as lichen sclerosus, lichen simplex chronicus, or psoriasis, or neoplasia. Patients presenting with pain should first be evaluated to rule out underlying organic causes, including inflammatory conditions, neoplasias, infections, or neurologic disorders. When organic causes are ruled out, the diagnosis of vulvodynia can be made and attention should then be paid to more fully elucidating the nature of the pain disorder (generalized versus localized and spontaneous versus provoked).

Treatment, if possible, should be evidence-based, although for many vulvar disorders such evidence has not yet been accrued. For a number of disorders, including pain syndromes, health care providers should be aware that often more than one modality will be required, and treatment must be individualized. Patient education in vulvar hygiene measures and avoidance of many common irritants and triggers will help reduce the risk of both development of contact dermatitis and lichen simplex chronicus as well as exacerbation of other underlying vulvar dermatoses.

Consultation with or referral to a specialist in vulvovaginal disorders, if available, can help obstetrician–gynecologists provide comprehensive care and optimal management of their patients' conditions. Also, consultation with health care providers in dermatology, as well as selected use of other specialists, including but not limited to ophthalmologists, dentists, gastroenterologists, and rheumatologists, is often essential to the appropriate diagnosis and management of patients with more complicated disorders.

A proposed diagnostic algorithm (Fig. 23) is particularly useful in approaching the patient presenting with chronic (defined as 3 or more months) vulvar pain (20). First, the pain should be characterized to the best of the patient's ability; use of a targeted pain questionnaire may help facilitate this process and better define the qualities of the pain the patient is experiencing. The health care provider then establishes both the duration and nature (generalized versus localized, unprovoked versus provoked, with versus without spontaneous pain) of the patient's discomfort. During the physical examination, other causes of vulvar discomfort (eg, ulcerations or lesions) are noted and biopsied, cultured, or both as indicated. A vaginal examination is then performed to exclude other common causes of vulvovaginal irritation, including yeast and bacterial vaginosis.

In the absence of abnormal visible findings, the health care provider then performs the cotton swab test, an examination used to specifically localize any painful areas. Using a moistened cotton-tipped swab, the vulva is tested starting at the thighs and moving medially toward the vestibule. The vestibule is systematically palpated using light pressure. The patient is asked to rate the pain. If pain is confirmed, a vaginal fungal culture is obtained in order to definitively rule out a yeast infection because yeast infections caused by atypical *Candida* species often are not obvious on examination. A negative fungal culture, in conjunction with the patient's history and positive findings on the cotton swab test, confirms the diagnosis of vulvodynia (20).

Treatment recommendations, although numerous, rarely have been evidence-based. Although case series demonstrate improvement of symptoms with various treatment modalities, including topical therapies (nitroglycerin, lidocaine, gabapentin cream, and capsaicin), injectable therapies (interferon, steroids, and botulinum toxin type A), systemic therapies, behavioral therapy, and surgery, further evaluation with randomized controlled trials often leads to disappointing results. Several placebo controlled studies have demonstrated a greater response in the placebo group than in the group receiving therapy (21). This clearly demonstrates the need for more rigorous prospective investigations with placebo-control led studies when evaluating potential treatment response. Consequently, the current treatment options for vulvar pain, then, are largely empirical. Tricyclic antidepressants, the most studied of which is amitriptyline, and gabapentin are the most commonly used, largely on the basis of evidence of their efficacy from studies of other pain syndromes, including postherpetic neuralgia and diabetic neuropathy. Data confirming the efficacy of these medications in women with vulvar pain remains sparse. As with other proposed treatments, a recent randomized trial demonstrated amitriptyline with and without a topical steroid was not effective in treating vulvodynia (22). It is important to note that neither tricyclic antidepressants nor anticonvulsants should be abruptly discontinued because significant adverse effects can occur.

The success of treatment interventions using vaginal surface electromyographic biofeedback in this population, coupled with the recent evidence demonstrating increased vaginal hypertonicity and lack of vaginal muscle strength and restriction of the vaginal opening in women with vestibulodynia, suggests that targeting pelvic floor muscle functioning can be successful in relieving the pain these patients experience with intercourse and improving sexual function (19). Physical therapy treatment techniques include, for example, internal (vaginal and rectal) and external soft tissue mobilization and myofascial release, trigger-point pressure application, electrical stimulation, bladder and bowl retraining, and home vaginal dilation (20).

Although physical therapy and biofeedback can clearly be effective in reducing the instability and hypertonicity associated with vestibulitis and improving sexual function, compliance with this treatment option requires repeated visits. For strongly motivated

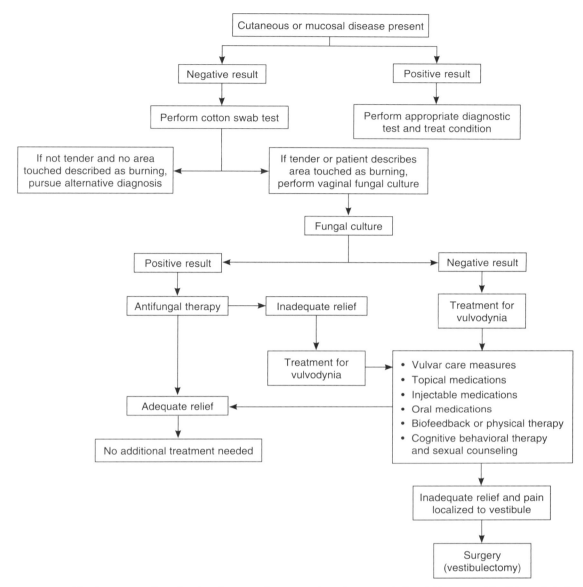

Figure 23. A possible diagnostic algorithm for chronic vulvar pain. (Haefner HK, Collins ME, Davis GD, Edwards L, Foster DC, Hartmann ED, et al. The vulvodynia guideline. J Low Genit Tract Dis 2005;9:40-51.)

patients and patients who wish to avoid the adverse effects of medical or surgical therapy, of which there are many, biofeedback and physical therapy are excellent choices.

Vestibulectomy has the highest reported clinical cure rates in excess of 80% in a number of trials, both controlled and uncontrolled, but is typically reserved for patients with localized pain who have not responded to more conservative therapy. In performing a vestibulectomy and before induction of either spinal or general anesthesia, the health care provider should carefully demarcate and outline the areas of pain. The incision, based on the extent of the patient's pain, may begin anteriorly along the periurethral area (20). As stated previously, surgery is not indicated for women with generalized pain.

Other less well publicized methods of treatment, such as acupuncture and hypnosis, have been used to a lesser extent without any major documentation and may provide comfort for some women. Alternatively, dietary modifications (including a low oxalate diet) have been widely reported with little evidence to support effectiveness.

References

1. Crone AM, Stewart EJ, Wojnarowska A, Powell SM. Aetiological factors in vulvar dermatitis. J Eur Acad Dermatol Venereol 2000;14:181-6.

2. Margesson LJ. Contact dermatitis of the vulva. Dermatol Ther 2004:17:20-7.

3. Lynch PJ. Lichen simplex chronicus (atopic/neurodermatitis) of the anogenital region. Dermatol Ther 2004;17:8-19.

4. Burrows LJ, Shaw HA, Goldstein AT. The vulvar dermatoses. J Sex Med 2008;5:276–83.

5. Jones RW, Sadler L, Grant S, Whineray J, Exeter M, Rowan D. Clinically identifying women with vulvar lichen sclerosus at increased risk of squamous cell carcinoma: a case-control study. J Reprod Med 2004;49:808–11.

6. Diagnosis and management of vulvar skin disorders. ACOG Practice Bulletin No. 93. American College of Obstetricians and Gynecologists. Obstet Gynecol 2008; 111:1243–53.

7. Moyal-Barracco M, Edwards L. Diagnosis and therapy of anogenital lichen planus. Dermatol Ther 2004;17:38–46.

8. Kennedy CM, Galask RP. Erosive vulvar lichen planus: retrospective review of characteristics and outcomes in 113 patients seen in a vulvar specialty clinic. J Reprod Med 2007;52:43–7.

9. Setterfield JF, Neill S, Shirlaw PJ, Theron J, Vaughan R, Escudier M, et al. The vulvovaginal gingival syndrome: a severe subgroup of lichen planus with characteristic clinical features and a novel association with the class II HLA DQB1*0201 allele. J Am Acad Dermatol 2006;55:98–113.

10. Stanley M. Chapter 17: Genital human papillomavirus infections--current and prospective therapies. J Natl Cancer Inst Monogr 2003;31:117–24.

11. Hart WR. Vulvar intraepithelial neoplasia: historical aspects and current status. Int J Gynecol Pathol 2001;20:16–30.

12. Workowski KA, Berman S. Sexually transmitted diseases treatment guidelines, 2010. Centers for Disease Control and Prevention. Division of STD Prevention National Center for HIV/AIDS, Viral Hepatitis, STD, and TB Prevention. MMWR Recomm Rep 2010;59(RR-12):1–110.

13. Kennedy CM, Boardman LA. New approaches to external genital warts and vulvar intraepithelial neoplasia. Clin Obstet Gynecol 2008;51:518–26.

14. Mathiesen O, Buus SK, Cramers M. Topical imiquimod can reverse vulvar intraepithelial neoplasia: a randomised, double-blinded study. Gynecol Onc 2007;107:219–22.

15. Eckert LO, Lentz GM. Infections of the lower genital tract. In: Katz VL, Lentz GM, Lobo RA, Gershenson DM, editors. Comprehensive gynecology. 5th ed. Philadelphia, PA: Mosby Elsevier; 2007. p. 569–606.

16. Moyal-Barracco M, Lynch PJ. 2003 ISSVD terminology and classification of vulvodynia: a historical perspective. J Reprod Med 2004;49:772–7.

17. Harlow BL, Stewart EG. Adult-onset vulvodynia in relatioin to childhood violence victimization. Am J Epidemiol 2005;161:871–80.

18. Gunter J. Vulvodynia: new thoughts on a devastating condition. Obstet Gynecol Surv 2007;62:812–9.

19. Reissing ED, Brown C, Lord MJ, Binik YM, Khalife S. Pelvic floor muscle functioning in women with vulvar vestibulitis syndrome. J Psychosom Obstet Gynaecol 2005; 26:107–13.

20. Haefner HK, Collins ME, Davis GD, Edwards L, Foster DC, Hartmann D et al. The vulvodynia guideline. J Low Genit Tract Dis 2005;9:40–51.

21. Landry T, Bergeron S, Dupuis M, Desrochers G. The treatment of provoked vestibulodynia: a critical review. Clin J Pain 2008;24:155–71.

22. Brown CS, Wan J, Bachmann G, Rosen R. Self-management, amitriptyline, and amitriptyline plus triamcinolone in the management of vulvodynia. J Womens Health (Larchmt) 2009;18:163–9.

Vulvovaginitis

Rudolph P. Galask and Diane Elas

Vulvovaginitis is the most common problem encountered by gynecologists in primary care. It affects all age groups, from young girls to older women, and has many causes (Box 9). The most common causes of vulvovaginitis are bacterial, fungal (candidiasis), parasitic (trichomoniasis), and viral (herpes simples virus [HSV]). Appropriate treatment depends on determining the cause. A significant amount of psychologic stress and sexual dysfunction may occur if a firm diagnosis and treatment plan are not established.

Vaginal Ecosystem

The vaginal flora is a complex group of organisms that display great variability, depending on a multitude of endogenous and exogenous factors. The dominant organisms in the normal flora of women of reproductive age are the lactobacilli. Lactobacilli are facultative gram-positive bacteria that contribute to the maintenance of a low vaginal pH. A pH of 3.5–4.5 is important in suppressing pathogenic organisms. Sixty percent of lactobacilli also produce hydrogen peroxide, which may be a further protective agent against pathogens (1, 2). Other facultative gram-positive bacteria include staphylococci, streptococci, and enterococci. Gram-negative bacteria include *Escherichia coli*, *Proteus* species, and *Klebsiella* species.

Anaerobic bacteria are of particular interest because of their potential role in upper genital tract infections. The normal anaerobic constituents of vaginal flora include *Bacteroides*, *Peptococcus*, *Peptostreptococcus*, *Fusobacterium* species and eubacteria. Some organisms usually thought to be associated with bacterial vaginosis (eg, *Gardnerella vaginalis*) can be normal constituents of the vaginal flora. There may be considerable day-to-day variation in the vaginal flora of an individual woman, which calls into question the significance of organisms usually considered pathogens (3).

Yeast, particularly *Candida albicans*, also can be part of the normal vaginal flora; it has been identified in up to 20% of asymptomatic women. However, a link has been demonstrated between higher percentages of yeast in the vaginal flora and recurrent, symptomatic infection (4).

Endogenous factors play a role in determining the composition of the vaginal flora. The most important endogenous factor is hormonal. Lactobacilli flourish under the influence of estrogen in the reproductive years, and estrogen exerts a lowering effect on pH and

has an inhibitory effect on anaerobic bacteria. Menstruation alters the microbial ecosystem as does genital tract surgery and parturition.

Exogenous factors also are known to contribute to the regulation of the vaginal flora, but the exact roles of some of these factors remain in doubt. It is well recognized that systemic antibiotic therapy alters the delicate equilibrium, as does the presence of semen in the vagina. The presence of a foreign body, such as a retained tampon, may cause infection with pathogenic organisms. Vaginal douching is a practice that is consistently associated with an altered vaginal ecosystem of increased pathogenic organisms and decreased lactobacilli (5).

Evaluation of the Vulva and Vagina

A full history should be obtained regarding the nature and duration of the symptoms, precipitating factors, variation with the menstrual cycle, circadian cycle, and response to any previous treatment. In addition, questions about sexual partners' symptoms and treatment may provide useful information. Specific questions should be asked about potentially irritating or sensitizing substances, such as soap, bath additives, laundry detergent, fabric softeners, douches, moistened wipes, daily pad wear, and sexual aids—particularly in a patient who mentions itching or burning.

Examination of the patient with symptoms of vulvovaginitis includes physical assessment and laboratory testing (Fig. 24). Although general bacterial cultures of the vagina are not useful, specific microbial cultures may be indicated in cases where trichomoniasis or yeast infection is suspected, but the microscopy in not diagnostic. The correct transport medium must be used for the organism in question. A biopsy of the vulvar skin or vulvar–vaginal epithelium may be indicated if an unusual, noninfective cause of vulvovaginitis is suspected (Box 9).

In most cases of infectious vulvovaginitis, clinical presentation and investigative findings are unique for each infection. In cases that do not fit easily into a specific diagnostic pattern, a noninfectious and uncommon cause of vulvovaginitis must be considered (Box 9). Attention to psychologic and psychosexual dysfunction that may accompany vulvovaginitis is important, particularly if the condition is chronic or recurrent. The health care provider should specifically address this issue with the patient because she may be reluctant to volunteer this information.

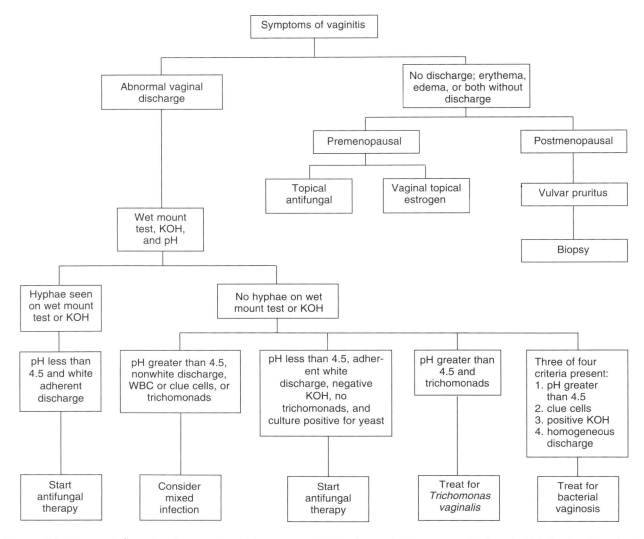

Figure 24. Diagnostic flow chart for vaginitis. Abbreviations: KOH indicates 10% potassium hydroxide; WBC, white blood cells.

Bacterial Vaginosis

Bacterial vaginosis is one of the most common causes of vaginitis in premenopausal women. Its prevalence varies depending on the population studied, as well as from study to study. The condition has been found in 5–15% of women in general gynecologic clinics, in 15–20% of pregnant women, and in 35% of women visiting sexually transmitted disease (STD) clinics (6). As many as 16% of pregnant women have bacterial vaginosis. Its prevalence during pregnancy varies by race or ethnicity and is highest among Hispanics and African Americans (16% and 23%, respectively) and lowest among Asians and whites (6% and 9%, respectively) (7). Up to 50% of women with bacterial vaginosis do not have symptoms. In general, however, the term is reserved for those who are symptomatic.

Once thought of as simply a nuisance, bacterial vaginosis is now believed to be a risk factor for several obstetric and gynecologic complications, includ-ing preterm birth, premature rupture of membranes, chorioamnionitis, postabortion infections, postpartum endometritis, posthysterectomy vaginal cuff cellulitis, and pelvic inflammatory disease. The bacterial vaginosis organisms themselves may be causing salpingitis or they may act as cofactors to facilitate other ascending pathogenic organisms (8, 9). Moreover, bacterial vaginosis may increase the risk of human immunodeficiency virus (HIV) infection and an association with infertility also has been proposed (7, 10).

Pathogenesis

Bacterial vaginosis represents a complex, polymicrobial change in the vaginal ecosystem that results in the absence of *Lactobacillus* species with high concentration of anaerobic bacteria, including *G vaginalis*, *Mobiluncus* species, *Prevotella* species, and *Mycoplasma hominis* (11). The contributory roles of each type of bacteria remain unknown. Symptomatic women typi-

Causes of Vulvovaginitis

Infectious Vulvovaginitis

Common Causes

- Bacterial vaginosis (40–50% of cases)
- Vulvovaginal candidiasis (20–25% of cases)
- Trichomoniasis (15–20% of cases)
- Herpes simplex virus

Uncommon Causes

- Atrophic vaginitis with secondary bacterial infection
- Cytolytic vaginosis
- Foreign body with secondary bacterial infection
- Human immunodeficiency virus-associated idiopathic vaginal ulceration

Noninfectious Vulvovaginitis

- Ulcerative vaginitis associated with staphylococcal toxic shock syndrome
- Atrophic vaginitis
- Irritant contact dermatitis
- Allergic contact dermatitis
- Eczema
- Chronic lichen simplex
- Psoriasis
- Erosive lichen planus
- Traumatic dermatitis
- Reiter disease
- Behçet disease
- Pemphigus vulgaris

cally describe having a malodorous, milky, white to gray vaginal discharge. Frequently, the odor is increased after intercourse. Bacterial vaginosis has been found to be associated with sexual activity, multiple sexual partners, new sexual partner, lack of vaginal lactobacilli, smoking, African American race, and douching (12, 13).

Diagnosis

The most common presenting features of bacterial vaginosis are included in Table 5. Bacterial vaginosis is diagnosed by three or more of Amsel criteria (14), including thin, homogenous vaginal discharge and a vaginal pH greater than 4.5; fishy amine odor upon addition of 10% potassium hydroxide (positive "whiff" test); and on Gram stain, 20% or more of vaginal epithelial cells identified as "clue cells" with the cell borders obliterated with coccobacilli. Another method is the Nugent Gram stain score that evaluates the num-

ber of lactobacilli, *Gardnerella* species, and *Mobiluncus* species per oil immersion field. A score of 0–3 represents normal flora; a score of 4–6, intermediate flora; and a score of 7–10, bacterial vaginosis (15). Culture of vaginal discharge is of no value for diagnosis of bacterial vaginosis. The Pap test also cannot be used to diagnose bacterial vaginosis. Diagnostic aids, such as oligonucleotide probes and kits to detect bacterial metabolic byproducts, are available.

Bacterial vaginosis can be associated with other sexually transmitted genital tract infections. Therefore, a full STD screen should be considered, especially when the patient has recurrent or persistent symptoms.

Treatment

Treatment options for bacterial vaginosis include oral and intravaginal metronidazole and oral and intravaginal clindamycin (Table 6). These treatments have equivalent rates of cure, although recommended dosages and schedules vary. Potential adverse effects of oral clindamycin, especially *Clostridium difficile* enterocolitis, call into question its use as a first-line therapy.

In pregnancy, the use of metronidazole traditionally has been avoided in the first trimester, although meta-analyses do not show evidence of teratogenicity (16). The Centers for Disease Control and Prevention (CDC) recommend that symptomatic pregnant women be treated because bacterial vaginosis has been associated with adverse pregnancy outcomes as described earlier and that those asymptomatic pregnant women who are at high risk of preterm delivery be treated, although the optimal treatment regimen has not yet been established (12). Patients who are HIV positive should receive the same treatment for bacterial vaginosis as other women.

Recurrent disease is common. Approximately 30% of patients will experience relapse within 3 months (17). Women with persistent or multiple recurrences of bacterial vaginosis should be treated in consultation with a specialist.

Candidal Vulvovaginitis

Candidal vulvovaginitis affects up to 75% of women at some time during the premenopausal years. Monitoring trend in the epidemiology of the infection is increasingly more difficult because of widespread self-diagnosis and the availability and use of over-the-counter antifungal medications.

Pathogenesis

Candidal vulvovaginitis generally is sporadic, uncomplicated, and caused by *C albicans* (more than 80% of all cases). *Candida albicans* can be a part of the normal vaginal flora, identified in cultures of some 20% of asymptomatic women. The condition may be more per-

Table 5. Clinical Features of the Three Most Common Causes of Infectious Vulvovaginitis

Clinical Examination Phase	Bacterial Vaginosis	Candidal Vulvovaginitis	Trichomoniasis
History	Malodorous discharge, with odor worse after sexual intercourse May be asymptomatic	Vulvovaginal itching, burning, or both and commonly a thick, white, odorless vaginal discharge resembling cottage cheese	Malodorous, profuse vaginal discharge; itching; burning; dysuria; and dyspareunia May be asymptomatic
Physical examination	Thin, gray-green, homogeneous discharge adherent to vaginal walls and unpleasant, fishy odor	Variable degrees of vulvovaginal edema and erythema with adherent thick white discharge and no abnormal odor May have "satellite" vulvar lesions	Vulvovaginal edema and erythema; copious, malodorous, gray-green, adherent vaginal discharge, which may be frothy; and "strawberry cervix"
Laboratory tests	Elevated pH (greater than 4.5), positive amine "whiff" test result with or without KOH, and the presence of clue cells on microscopy	pH normal and presence of yeast forms on wet-mount microscopy with or without KOH	Elevated pH (greater than 4.5) and presence of motile, flagellated organisms and leukocytes on wet-mount microscopy

Abbreviation: KOH indicates potassium hydroxide.

Table 6. Treatment of Bacterial Vaginosis

Agent	Regimen	
	Nonpregnant Women	*Pregnant Women*
	Recommended	
Metronidazole*	500 mg orally twice daily for 7 days 0.75% gel, 5 g intravaginally once daily for 5 days[†]	500 mg orally twice daily for 7 days 250 mg orally three times daily for 7 days
Clindamycin[‡]	2% cream, 5 g intravaginally at bedtime for 7 days	300 mg orally twice daily for 7 days
	Alternative	
Clindamycin[‡]	300 mg orally twice daily for 7 days	
Clindamycin ovules	100 g intravaginally at bedtime for 3 days	
Tinidazole*	2 g orally once daily for 3 days 1 g orally once daily for 7 days	

*Advise patients to avoid alcohol consumption during treatment and for 24 hours after treatment with metronidazole or tinidazole.

[†]One study has demonstrated that a once-daily dosage with intravaginal metronidazole is as effective as a twice-daily dosage. (Livengood CH 3rd, Soper DE, Sheehan KL, Fenner DE, Martens MG, Nelson AL, et al. Comparison of once-daily and twice-daily dosing of 0.75% metronidazole gel in the treatment of bacterial vaginosis. Sex Transm Dis 1999; 26:137–42.)

[‡]Clindamycin cream is oil-based and might weaken latex condoms and diaphragms.

Note: A new preparation of metronidazole has been approved by the U.S. Food and Drug Administration for treatment of bacterial vaginosis at a dosage of 750 mg once daily for 7 days; however, data comparing its efficacy with conventional treatments are not yet available.

Workowski KA, Berman S. Sexually transmitted diseases treatment guidelines, 2010. Centers for Disease Control and Prevention. Division of STD Prevention National Center for HIV/AIDS, Viral Hepatitis, STD, and TB Prevention. MMWR Recomm Rep 2010;59(RR-12):1–110.

sistent if it occurs in a host with an underlying disease (eg, a woman with poorly controlled diabetes mellitus or immunosuppression).

Complicated vulvovaginitis or a chronic, recurrent infection caused by various *Candida* species occurs in 10–20% of affected women. Recurrent disease, defined as four or more episodes per year, affects less than 5% of healthy women. Underlying disease should be considered, particularly poorly controlled diabetes mellitus or HIV. However, most women with recurrent disease do not have any obvious etiologic factor. The reported incidence of *Candida* species other than *C albicans*, particularly *Candida glabrata*, is increasing. This increase may be the result of increased testing and reporting or it may be a true increase, perhaps caused by the increasingly widespread use of azoles, which may effect the development of the more resistant species. Vaginitis caused by *C glabrata* may occur in older women. Clinical features of this infection may include previous azole exposure (particularly long courses); underlying disease, such as diabetes mellitus; more chronic burning than itching; an often-absent vaginal discharge; and the presence of buds rather than hyphae on microscopy. Furthermore, *C glabrata* infection may coexist with *C albicans* infection.

Diagnosis

Although over-the-counter treatment of potential yeast infections is safe and often effective, misdiagnosis is common. Any woman who either does not respond to such treatment or has a recurrence soon after treatment should be seen by a health care provider for definitive diagnosis. The patient should be advised to discontinue any over-the-counter treatments 3 days before the office visit.

The common clinical features of candidal vulvovaginitis are listed in Table 5. Microscopically, *C albicans* forms spores and hyphae, whereas other *Candida* species may show only budding yeast forms. If microscopy results are positive in a symptomatic patient, a confirmatory culture is not needed before selecting conventional treatment. If microscopy results are negative, but a clinical picture suggests candidal infection, cultures are indicated. A medium specific for yeast, rather than a bacteriology medium, should be used. Positive culture results can be expected after 3–5 days. Culture also may be useful if a patient has recurrent candidal vulvovaginitis after treatment, and it may be used to differentiate between species of *Candida* by sugar assimilation patterns. A diagnosis based on Pap test results needs clinical confirmation because it may represent an asymptomatic carrier rather that a person with vulvovaginitis. In any clinical situation, it is possible that the infection with the *Candida* species is secondary (ie, *Candida* species are present, but the

actual problem causing symptoms is different, such as contact vulvitis).

Treatment

All currently available licensed products are effective in the treatment of uncomplicated, or sporadic, candidal vulvovaginitis, with a cure rate of 80%. Many studies have demonstrated equivalence between different topical and oral azoles (18). When topical agents are chosen, it should be understood that most infections affect both the vulva and vagina, so a combination of vaginal suppositories and cream is appropriate. A meta-analysis of itraconazole and fluconazole has shown azoles to be similarly effective and safe (19). Treatment of women with HIV infection should be the same as that of other women.

In pregnancy, oral azoles are contraindicated. However, if they are inadvertently used as a short-term treatment in early pregnancy, there is no evidence of fetal abnormalities (20). Topical azoles are the treatment of choice (Table 7) (12).

It is important to consider other measures for symptomatic relief. If the skin on the vulva is inflamed, it may be appropriate to use a combined topical steroid and antifungal preparation. Intermittent relief from burning and itching may be achieved using a sitz bath with the addition of bicarbonate of soda. Potential contact irritants, such as soap, perfume, detergents, douches, and pads should be avoided to reduce the chance of simultaneous or subsequent contact dermatitis. Investigation or treatment of male sexual partners is not considered necessary in sporadic candidal vulvovaginitis.

True azole resistance is rare for *C albicans* and usually does not need to be considered. In most recurrent *C albicans* infections, treatment is relatively straightforward. The agent used for short-term, uncomplicated infection can be used for a longer course of therapy for chronic or recurrent candidal infections. This applies to both oral and intravaginal agents. Because hepatotoxicity has been reported, it may be prudent to assess liver function if prolonged therapy (more than 5 days) is considered. Oral regimens of ketoconazole or itraconazole also may be used (21). Clotrimazole is suitable for long-term maintenance intravaginal therapy after initial conventional curative treatment.

In recurrent disease, the usefulness of evaluation and treating sexual partners has been debated; the Centers for Disease Control and Prevention does not recommend treating partners. Evaluation and treatment of partners is an option to be considered. Discontinuation of low-dose combined contraceptive pills also is not necessary. There is no evidence of any benefit from dietary change or from attempts to reduce the gastrointestinal reservoir of *Candida* species.

Table 7. Treatment of Uncomplicated Candidal Vulvovaginitis

Agents	Regimen
Intravaginal Agents	
Butoconazole 2% cream	5 g intravaginally for 3 days*†
	5 g sustained-release single intravaginal application
Clotrimazole 1% cream	5 g intravaginally for 7–14 days*†
Clotrimazole 2% cream	5 g intravaginally for 3 days*†
Miconazole 2% cream	5 g intravaginally for 7 days*†
Miconazole 4% cream	5 g intravaginally for 3 days*† .
Miconazole	100-mg vaginal suppository for 7 days*†
	200-mg vaginal suppository for 3 days*†
	1,200-mg vaginal suppository for 1 day*†
Nystatin	100,000-unit vaginal tablet for 14 days
Tioconazole 6.5% ointment	5 g intravaginally in a single ointment application*†
Terconazole 0.4% cream	5 g intravaginally for 7 days*
Terconazole 0.8% cream	5 g intravaginally for 3 days*
Terconazole	80-mg vaginal suppository for 3 days*
Oral Agent	
Fluconazole	150-mg oral tablet in a single dose

*These creams and suppositories are oil-based and might weaken latex condoms and diaphragms.
†Over-the-counter preparation.
Workowski KA, Berman S. Sexually transmitted diseases treatment guidelines, 2010. Centers for Disease Control and Prevention. Division of STD Prevention National Center for HIV/AIDS, Viral Hepatitis, STD, and TB Prevention. MMWR Recomm Rep 2010;59(RR-12):1–110.

Candida glabrata is resistant to all currently available azoles. Boric acid in the form of intravaginal capsules, 600 mg daily or twice daily for 14 days, achieves a cure in 70% of patients (22). Topical flucytosine as well as gentian violet have been used with success. In recurrent infection, the safety of long-term treatment with boric acid or flucytosine has not been established. After the use of these agents for initial clearance, nystatin intravaginal tablets may be used for maintenance.

Another cause of recurrent yeast infections is a reaction to topical azole therapy. Some women develop symptoms of itching or burning after repeated use of these agents. Repeated use of a topical agent to treat infection will only increase symptoms.

Trichomoniasis

Trichomoniasis is a large problem on a worldwide scale with estimated 174 million cases each year and estimated 7.4 million cases each year in the United States, with a significant portion of these women being asymptomatic (23). Infection with *Trichomonas vaginalis* during pregnancy has been associated with premature rupture of membranes, preterm birth, low birth weight, pelvic inflammatory disease, and endometritis (12, 23). It often coexists with other STDs and with bacterial vaginosis. Of even more concern is the association with HIV because trichomoniasis facilitates HIV transmission (24).

Pathogenesis

Trichomonas vaginalis is a flagellated, motile, anaerobic protozoan organism that colonizes the urethra as well as the vagina. The infection is predominately sexually transmitted; however, the infection may occur by way of fomites, and the organism has been shown to survive in hot tubs and swimming pools.

Diagnosis

Clinical presentation of trichomoniasis ranges from asymptomatic carriage to severe inflammatory disease. The typical presenting features are listed in Table 5. Few cases display a so-called strawberry cervix, caused by punctate intraepithelial hemorrhages.

Motile trichomonads are visualized on microscopy; this method is most effective if the obtained sample is kept warm (body temperature) and microscopy is performed immediately, but has only 60–70% sensitivity. Negative microscopy finding in a symptomatic patient necessitates the use of culture, which has a sensitivity of 95%. The U.S. Food and Drug administration has approved an immunochromatographic capillary flow dipstick technology and a nucleic acid probe test that evaluates for *T vaginalis, G vaginalis,* and *C albicans.* These tests both have a sensitivity of 83% and a specificity of greater than 97% on vaginal secretions (12). The Pap test may detect the infection. It is reasonable to treat on this basis if a patient has symptoms of vaginitis.

Adolescents are at risk of sexually acquired trichomoniasis in conjunction with other sexually transmitted diseases. Point of care rapid antigen tests on vaginal secretions or urine specimens offer the advantage of rapid and sensitive testing for trichomoniasis, chlamydia, and gonorrhea (25, 26). It is important to screen all females for coexistent infections.

Treatment

Metronidazole and tinidazole are the only oral medications available in the United States for treatment of trichomoniasis (Table 8). Recommended regimens produce cure rates of 90–95%. Oral treatment is necessary to eradicate infection from the urethra as well as the

Table 8. Treatment of Trichomoniasis

Agent	Regimen
Recommended Regimen	
Metronidazole	2 g orally in a single dose
Tinidazole	2 g orally in a single dose
Alternative Regimen	
Metronidazole	500 mg twice daily for 7 days
Regimen for Initial Treatment Failure	
Metronidazole	500 mg twice daily for 7days*
Regimen for Repeated Treatment Failure	
Metronidazole	2 g orally once daily for 5 days*
Tinidazole	2 g orally once daily for 5 days*
Recommended Regimen in Pregnancy	
Metronidazole	2 g orally in a single dose

*Ensure that sexual partners have been treated and that intercourse is avoided during treatment.
Workowski KA, Berman S. Sexually transmitted diseases treatment guidelines, 2010. Centers for Disease Control and Prevention. Division of STD Prevention National Center for HIV/AIDS, Viral Hepatitis, STD, and TB Prevention. MMWR Recomm Rep 2010;59(RR-12):1–110.

vagina. It is important to treat sexual partners and to advise against unprotected intercourse during treatment.

Patients who are allergic to metronidazole can be treated by desensitization. Treatment in HIV-positive patients should be the same as in other women.

Vaginal trichomoniasis in pregnancy has been associated with adverse outcomes, such as premature rupture of membranes, low birth weight, and preterm delivery. Treatment of pregnant women with asymptomatic trichomoniasis has not been found to prevent preterm delivery (27). The data are inconclusive that treatment with metronidazole will decrease perinatal morbidity, and the Centers for Disease Control and Prevention recommends counseling individuals regarding risks and benefits of treatment. Previously, there was a concern about the possible teratogenic effect of metronidazole in pregnancy. However, meta-analyses have failed to demonstrate such a link (12). Vaginal clindamycin is a treatment option.

Persistent disease caused by true metronidazole-resistant *T vaginalis* has been reported. Treatments have included a high-dose, prolonged course of oral metronidazole, combinations of oral and intravaginal metronidazole, intravenous metronidazole, oral tinidazole, and intravaginal paromomycin (28–30). Expert advice should be sought in theses cases. Coexistent STDs also must be treated in both the patients and their partners.

Genital Herpes

At least 50 million individuals in the United States live with a genital herpes infection. The two types of HSV are identified as HSV-1 and HSV-2. Symptoms of HSV can range from nonexistent to severe. Once infected, individuals may have a single outbreak or multiple outbreaks of the viral infection throughout their lives. Serologic methods of diagnosis that detect type-specific antibodies are helpful to clarify the true prevalence of the infection. The detection of genital herpes in pregnant women is important because of the risk of transmission to the newborn.

Pathogenesis

Genital herpes infection is caused by HSV-1 or HSV-2. Although most cases of genital infection were known to be caused by HSV-2, genital infection caused by HSV-1 is increasing worldwide. This shift in infection pattern is caused by changes in sexual practice that have led to more unprotected oral–genital contact. Also, the decreasing incidence of oral–labial HSV-1 infection in the developed world has resulted in lower HSV-1 seropositivity and, therefore, some loss of protective immunity. Infection is acquired by skin-to-skin contact or mucous membrane contact during periods of active viral shedding.

After primary infection (which may be entirely asymptomatic), the virus becomes latent in the sacral dorsal root ganglia. From there it can reactivate at any time, producing recurrent infection. Clinical features vary among patients. Herpes simplex virus type 2 reactivates much more frequently than HSV-1, with a 95% recurrence rate for HSV-2 compared with HSV-1 (21). The rate of asymptomatic shedding also is higher for HSV-2. Recurrence is more common in the first few months and years after primary infection.

Neonatal herpes infection can have serious consequences, including death. In pregnancy, it is essential to monitor the women for HSV infection and exposure. Counseling to avoid oral sex with a partner suspected of HSV infection is warranted. Additionally, pregnant women should be advised to use condoms whenever genital contact occurs with a partner with a known or suspected HSV infection. The effectiveness of antiviral therapy and HSV transmission prevention has not been studied in pregnant women (12).

Clinical Features

The clinical presentation of genital herpes covers a wide spectrum of symptoms from entirely asymptomatic infection to painful genital ulceration to rare systemic symptoms and complications. Involvement of only the cervix can occur, resulting in an atypical presentation with profuse vaginal discharge.

Complications may include meningitis and herpetic sacral radiculomyelitis with urinary retention, constipation, and neuralgia. Urinary retention also may occur simply as a result of severe dysuria related to the painful genital ulcerations. In some cases, minor symptoms, such as itching, fissures, or slight discomfort, are the only presenting signs or symptoms of an HSV infection. It is important to teach patients to identify the signs and symptoms of an outbreak in order to start therapy to shorten the duration and decrease the intensity of the viral outbreak. The coexistence of HIV infection or syphilis should be evaluated. Also, immunosuppression results in more severe manifestations of HSV.

Given the variability in clinical presentation, it is no longer possible to state on clinical grounds alone whether a particular episode of genital herpes is primary or recurrent or which virus type is responsible.

Diagnosis

Several methods are available to establish an accurate laboratory diagnosis. Virus isolation by culture is appropriate for genital lesions. Deoxyribonucleic acid polymerase chain reaction is a more sensitive test than a culture and can be used for nonvesicular lesions (eg, late-stage ulcerations or minor lesions). Both methods are type specific for HSV-1 and HSV-2.

Herpes simplex virus type 1 occurs more frequently than HSV-2, although its prevalence is decreasing overall. Worldwide, HSV-1 recurs more frequently than HSV-2; in the United States, HSV-2 recurs more frequently than HSV-1. Accurate diagnosis is more likely in a primary episode than in recurrent episodes, so any patient presenting for the first time with symptoms and signs suspected of an HSV infection should be appropriately tested. Type-specific serologic tests for antibodies to HSV are useful in certain settings, including early pregnancy to ascertain HSV status, in apparently unaffected partners of patients with genital herpes, and as an epidemiologic tool.

Treatment

A number of medications are available for treatment of primary and recurrent disease (Table 9). Topical treatment with acyclovir, although soothing, is not effective. Many studies have compared the efficacy of orally administered acyclovir with valacyclovir and famciclovir; these studies have not demonstrated the superiority of one drug over another (12). The advantage of the newer drugs is a more convenient dosage schedule; the disadvantages are the cost and the lack of long-term safety data.

First Clinical Infection

The patient with a primary infection should be counseled appropriately. A follow-up visit should be arranged to discuss the results of tests and to address the concerns that follow a diagnosis of herpes. Screening for other STDs should be performed at a follow-up visit if the patient was in too much pain at the first visit. The patient's sexual partner(s) should be assessed for HSV as well as other STDs.

Drug treatment of primary infection has been shown to decrease the time to healing and the duration of viral shedding, but not the incidence of recurrence. Symptomatic treatment measures are important. These may include oral analgesia; topical anesthetic agents, such as 2% lidocaine gel; warm saline baths, including urinating in the bath water if dysuria is present; and avoidance of potential contact irritants, such as soap, douches, and perfumes.

Recurrent Infection

There are three approaches to the treatment of a recurrent infection. First, the recurrences may be minor and not particularly troublesome to the patient, in which case symptomatic treatment may be sufficient, along with advice about abstaining from sexual contact while symptomatic.

Second, the recurrences may be infrequent but troubling enough to merit episodic drug therapy. To be effec-

Table 9. Treatment of Genital Herpes

Agent	Regimen
First Clinical Episode	
Acyclovir	400 mg orally three times daily for 7–10 days*
	200 mg orally five times daily for 7–10 days*
Famciclovir	250 mg orally three times daily for 7–10 days*
Valacyclovir	1 g orally twice daily for 7–10 days*
Severe Disease	
Acyclovir	5–10 mg/kg body weight intravenously every 8 hours for 2–7 days or until clinical resolution is attained, followed by oral antiviral therapy to complete at least 10 days of therapy
Episodic Treatment of Recurrent Infection	
Acyclovir	400 mg orally three times daily for 5 days
	800 mg orally twice daily for 5 days
	800 mg orally three times daily for 2 days
Famciclovir	125 mg orally twice daily for 5 days
	1,000 mg orally twice daily for 1 day
	500 mg once, followed by 250 mg twice daily for 2 days
Valacyclovir	500 mg orally twice daily for 3 days
	1 g orally once daily for 5 days
Daily Suppressive Treatment in Recurrent Infection	
Acyclovir	400 mg orally twice daily
Famciclovir	250 mg orally twice daily
Valacyclovir	500 mg orally once daily
	1 g orally once daily

*Treatment may be extended, if healing is incomplete after 10 days of therapy.
Workowski KA, Berman S. Sexually transmitted diseases treatment guidelines, 2010. Centers for Disease Control and Prevention. Division of STD Prevention National Center for HIV/AIDS, Viral Hepatitis, STD, and TB Prevention. MMWR Recomm Rep 2010;59(RR-12):1–110.

tive, episodic drug therapy should be stared at the earliest possible opportunity. Therefore, it should be patient initiated and the patient should have a supply of medication at home.

Third, the recurrences may be frequent or severe enough to require daily long-term suppressive therapy. Although the standard indication for daily long-term therapy is six or more episodes per year, other factors need to be taken into account, such as the severity of the episodes and the psychologic effects on the patient. Generally, it is not advisable to begin suppressive treatment in the first year after primary infection because the rate of recurrence may decrease after the first year without intervention. There is no doubt that suppres-

sive treatment can improve dramatically the patient's quality of life (ie, reduce the frequency of outbreaks by at least 75%) (31). Suppressive therapy reduces the frequency of asymptomatic viral shedding and has not been associated with the development of significant acyclovir resistance. The patient's treatment should be reassessed at regular intervals.

Advice about reducing transmission to sexual partners is vitally important and should include information on the use of condoms and total abstinence during an outbreak. It is not possible to ensure that the patient can avoid transmitting the virus altogether because the wide area of potential genital viral shedding means that a condom cannot provide total coverage. In any case, even with all possible available advice and suppressive therapy for affected patients, transmission cannot be prevented because of the large reservoir of subclinical infection in the population. The greatest hope for reducing transmission of HSV is the development of effective and safe vaccines.

Infection in Pregnancy

Most infection with HSV in pregnancy is asymptomatic, whether primary or recurrent. No antiviral agent has been proved safe in pregnancy, although acyclovir has not shown evidence of teratogenicity. Therefore, acyclovir should be used if treatment is required during pregnancy for symptomatic primary or recurrent episodes (12).

The highest risk of neonatal transmission occurs from primary infections acquired close to the time of delivery, when the mother cannot produce an antibody response in time to protect the fetus. Some clinicians routinely administer acyclovir in suppressive doses during the last few weeks of pregnancy in a woman known to carry HSV; however, this practice has not been proved effective and is not recommended. The American College of Obstetricians and Gynecologists supports the use of cesarean delivery in cases of primary and recurrent lesions (32). Infants of women who acquired primary HSV infection close to term should be considered for immediate treatment with acyclovir, but according to available data, treatment is not recommended routinely for infants exposed to recurrent disease.

Atrophic Vaginitis

As the life expectancy is increasing, so is the proportion of postmenopausal women. In addition, as more information is available about the risks and benefits of hormone therapy, many women are electing not to use it. Therefore, atrophic vaginitis is likely to become more prevalent. It is estimated that 40% of postmenopausal women experience some degree of symptoms of vaginal atrophy, but only 20–25% of these women see a physician for this problem (33). The condition can cause significant reduction in quality of life because of discomfort, sexual dysfunction, and urinary symptoms.

Pathogenesis

Between puberty and menopause, the vaginal epithelium is under the influence of estrogen. Before and throughout menopause, however, the effect of estrogen is diminished. The epithelium becomes thin and dry, and the glycogen content of the cells is reduced, resulting in lower level of lactic acid and an increased pH, which in turn alters the vaginal ecosystem. There is associated loss of elasticity in the connective tissue, resulting in shortening and narrowing of the vagina. The urinary tract also is affected with atrophic changes in the urethra and occasionally the development of a urethral caruncle.

Clinical Features and Diagnosis

Symptoms of atrophic vaginitis vary widely in severity, from minor dryness with intercourse to severe burning, dyspareunia, and urinary incontinence. Typical vaginal symptoms are dryness, itching, burning, a thin, grayish discharge, a serosanguineous discharge, spotting, and dyspareunia. Typical urinary symptoms are urgency, frequency, dysuria, recurrent urinary tract infections, and incontinence.

Examination should start with the vulva. There may be evidence of atrophy. It also is important to keep in mind that other conditions may cause symptoms similar to trophic vaginitis in this age group, such as erosive lichen planus, secondary yeast infection, and vulvar intraepithelial neoplasia. Therefore, if there is any doubt about the signs and symptoms, a biopsy should be obtained and microscopic studies, cultures, or both should be performed. The introitus should be inspected for clinical signs or atrophy, such as a paling of the mucus or the presence of a urethral caruncle. The vagina should be evaluated with the smallest speculum possible to avoid trauma to the delicate tissue. The epithelium may appear pale, shiny, and dry or it may be erythematous with petechiae, erosions, and contact bleeding. Microscopy may demonstrate loss of superficial epithelial cells and an increase in parabasal cells along with an increase in polymorphonuclear leukocytes.

Treatment

Atrophic vaginitis is treated with estrogen administered topically or systemically. The goal of treatment is to alleviate the symptoms of vaginal atrophy with the lowest effective dose of estrogen. Topical vaginal treatment regimens commonly prescribed include commercially available vaginal estrogen creams, such as conjugated estrogen or estradiol cream, vaginal estradiol tablet, or an estradiol-containing vaginal ring. Systemic estrogen replacement includes oral or topical preparations, such as a patch or gel. The choice of the estrogen regimen should be tailored to the individual patient's needs. Systemic replacement is best used in women who are experiencing additional symptoms related to estrogen depletion, such as vasomotor symptoms. In women with a history of breast cancer it is helpful to work with the patient's oncologist in order to balance the risks and benefits of exogenous estrogen exposure with quality of life issues. Some women with mild vaginal dryness may find relief from the use of a lubricant alone. In this situation, the use of vegetable oil can be encouraged because it avoids the risk of contact dermatitis from some commercially available products or further drying from water-based lubricants.

References

1. Hillier SL. The vaginal microbial ecosystem and resistance of HIV. AIDS Res Hum Retroviruses 1998;14 Suppl 1: S17–21.

2. Eckert LO. Clinical Practice. Acute vulvovaginitis [published erratum appears in N Engl J Med 2006;355:2797]. N Engl J Med 2006;355:1244–52.

3. Priestley CJ, Jones BM, Dhar J, Goodwin L. What is normal vaginal flora? Genitourin Med 1997;73:23–8.

4. Giraldo P, von Nowaskonski A, Gomes FA, Linhares I, Neves NA, Witkin SS. Vaginal colonization by Candida in asymptomatic women with and without a history of recurrent vulvovaginal candidiasis. Obstet Gynecol 2000; 95:413–6.

5. Klebanoff MA, Nansel TR, Brotman RM, Zhang J, Yu KF, Schwebke JR, et al. Personal hygienic behaviors and bacterial vaginosis. Sex Transm Dis 2010;37:94–9.

6. Eschenbach DA. History and review of bacterial vaginosis. Am J Obstet Gynecol 1993;169:441–5.

7. Centers for Disease Control and Prevention. Tracking the hidden epidemic: trends in STDs in the United States. Atlanta (GA): CDC; 2010. Available at: http://www.cdc.gov/std/trends2000.pdf. Retrieved December 7, 2010.

8. Soper DE. Gynecologic sequelae of bacterial vaginosis. Int J Gynaecol Obstet 1999;67 Suppl 1:S25–8.

9. Faro S, Martens M, Maccato M, Hammill H, Pearlman M. Vaginal flora and pelvic inflammatory disease. Am J Obstet Gynecol 1993;169:470–4.

10. Wilson JD, Ralph SG, Jackson F, Rutherford AJ. Infertility, preterm birth, and bacterial vaginosis [Letter]. Lancet 1999;354:511.

11. Farage MA, Miller KW, Ledger WJ. Determining the cause of vulvovaginal symptoms. Obstet Gynecol Surv 2008;63: 445–64.

12. Workowski KA, Berman S. Sexually transmitted diseases treatment guidelines, 2010. Centers for Disease Control and Prevention. Division of STD Prevention National Center for HIV/AIDS, Viral Hepatitis, STD, and TB Prevention. MMWR Recomm Rep 2010;59(RR-12):1–110.

13. Cherpes TL, Hillier SL, Meyn LA, Busch JL, Krohn MA. A delicate balance: risk factors for acquisition of bacterial vaginosis include sexual activity, absence of hydrogen peroxide-producing lactobacilli, black race, and positive herpes simplex virus type 2 serology. Sex Transm Dis 2008; 35:78–83.

14. Amsel R, Totten PA, Spiegel CA, Chen KC, Eschenbach D, Holmes KK. Nonspecific vaginitis. Diagnostic criteria and microbial and epidemiologic associations. Am J Med 1983; 74:14–22.

15. Nugent RP, Krohn MA, Hillier SL. Reliability of diagnosing bacterial vaginosis is improved by a standardized method of gram stain interpretation. J Clin Microbiol 1991;29:297–301.

16. Caro-Paton T, Carvajal A, Martin de Diego I, Martin-Arias LH, Alvarez Requejo A, Rodriguez Pinilla E. Is metronidazole teratogenic? A meta-analysis. Br J Clin Pharmacol 1997;44:179–82.

17. Hillier S, Marazzo J, Holmes KK. Bacterial vaginosis. In: Holmes KK, Wasserheit JN, Correy L, Sparling PF, Stamm WE, Piot P, et al, editors. Sexually transmitted diseases. 4th ed. New York (NY): McGraw-Hill; 2008. p. 737–68.

18. Edelman DA, Grant S. One-day therapy for vaginal candidiasis. A review. J Reprod Med 1999;44:543–7.

19. Pitsouni E, Iavazzo C, Falagas ME. Itraconazole vs fluconazole for the treatment of uncomplicated acute vaginal and vulvovaginal candidiasis in nonpregnant women: a metaanyalysis of randomized controlled trials. Am J Obstet Gynecol 2008;198:153–60.

20. Mastroiacovo P, Mazzone T, Botto LD, Serafini MA, Finardi A, Caramelli L, et al. Prospective assessment of pregnancy outcomes after first-trimester exposure to fluconazole. Am J Obstet Gynecol 1996;175:1645–50.

21. Sobel JD. Vaginitis. N Engl J Med 1997;337:1896–903.

22. Sobel JD, Chaim W. Treatment of Torulopsis glabrata vaginitis: retrospective review of boric acid therapy. Clin Infect Dis 1997;24:649–52.

23. Owusu-Edusei K, Tejani MN, Gift TL, Kent CK, Tao G. Estimates of the direct cost per case and overall burden of trichomoniasis for the employer-sponsored privately insured women population in the United State, 2001 to 2005. Sex Transm Dis 2009;36:395–9.

24. Laga M, Manoka A, Kivuvu M, Malele B, Tuliza M, Nzila N, et al. Non-ulcerative sexually transmitted diseases as risk factors for HIV-1 transmission in women: results from a cohort study. AIDS 1993;7:95–102.

25. Simpson P, Higgins G, Qiao M, Waddell R, Kok T. Real-time PCRs for detection of Trichomonas vaginalis beta-tubulin and 18S rRNA genes in female genital specimens. J Med Microbiol 2007;56:772–7.

26. Huppert JS. Trichomoniasis in teens: an update. Curr Opin Obstet Gynecol 2009;21:371–8.

27. Klebanoff MA, Carey JC, Hauth JC, Hillier SL, Nugent RP, Thom EA, et al. Failure of metronidazole to prevent preterm delivery among pregnant women with asymptomatic Trichomonas vaginalis infection. National Institutes of Child Health and Human Development Network of Maternal–Fetal Medicine Units. N Engl J Med 2001;345:487–93.

28. Grossman JH 3rd, Galask RP. Persistent vaginitis caused by metronidazole-resistant trichomonas. Obstet Gynecol 1990; 76:521–2.

29. Coelho DD. Metronidazole resistant trichomoniasis successfully treated with paromomycin. Genitourin Med 1997; 73:397–8.

30. Nyirjesy P, Weitz MV, Gelone SP, Fekete T. Paromomycin for nitroimidazole-resistant trichomonosis [Letter]. Lancet 1995;346:1110.

31. Mindel A, Faherty A, Carney O, Patou G, Freris M, Williams P. Dosage and safety of long-term suppressive acyclovir therapy for recurrent genital herpes. Lancet 1988; 1:926–8.

32. Management of herpes in pregnancy. ACOG Practice Bulletin No. 82. American College of Obstetricians and Gynecologists. Obstet Gynecol 2007;109:1489–98.

33. Bachmann G, Bouchard C, Hoppe D, Ranganath R, Altomare C, Vieweg A, et al. Efficacy and safety of low-dose regimens of conjugated estrogen cream administered vaginally. Menopause 2009;16:719–27.

Pelvic Support Defects

Amy J. Park and Peter L. Rosenblatt

Almost one quarter of U.S. women have a pelvic floor disorder, the prevalence of which increases with age (1). The aging of the U.S. population increases the likelihood that obstetrician–gynecologists will encounter pelvic organ prolapse in their patients. According to one estimate, the number of U.S. women with at least one pelvic floor disorder will increase from 28 million in 2010 to 44 million in 2050, and specifically the number of women with pelvic organ prolapse will increase 46% from 3.3 million to 5 million (2).

Anatomy of the Pelvic Floor

A thorough understanding of the pelvic anatomy is necessary in order to be able to diagnose and treat pelvic floor defects. The pelvic floor consists of the bony pelvis (pubis, ischium, and ilium) in which the viscera, muscles, connective tissue, nerves and vessels reside. In fact, pelvises with a wide transverse inlet and a shorter obstetric conjugate appear to be more predisposed to developing pelvic organ prolapse, possibly due to the neuromuscular and connective tissue injuries incurred during childbirth (3).

Levator Ani Muscle

The levator ani provides an important support mechanism to the vagina. The aponeurosis of the levator ani muscles, or the arcus tendineus fascia pelvis, laterally attaches to the pelvic bones and is located adjacent to the obturator muscles. Anteriorly, it is attached to the pubis, and posteriorly, to the ischial spines. It has three components: 1) the pubococcygeus, 2) iliococcygeus, and 3) puborectalis muscles, which form a U-shape. The urethra, vagina, and rectum exit through openings in the center of the U-shape, called the urogenital diaphragm.

Posteriorly, the puborectalis acts as a sling that closes the potential space of the vagina, as well as the levator hiatus. In a woman with an intact pelvic floor, the puborectalis is in a chronic state of contraction. This contraction closes the vaginal canal and the anterior and posterior vaginal walls are in direct apposition. If there is muscular or neurologic damage to the puborectalis, the levator hiatus widens and the vaginal canal opens.

Perineal Body or Membrane

The perineal membrane is a dense fibromuscular layer that anchors the urethra, distal vagina, and perineal body to the ischiopubic rami. It is approximately 3 cm in length. It includes interlacing muscle fibers of the bulbospongiosus, transverse perineal muscles, and external anal sphincter. The perineal membrane is attached anteriorly to the vaginal epithelium and muscularis. The perineal body refers to the area between the vagina and the anus, and is the central tendinous attachment of the urogenital diaphragm muscles.

Endopelvic Fascia

The pelvic viscera are covered by endopelvic fascia, a connective tissue layer that provides support to the pelvic organs, yet allows for their mobility to permit storage of urine and stool, coitus, parturition, and defecation. Histologically, it is composed of collagen, elastin, adipose tissue, nerves, vessels, lymph channels, and smooth muscle. The endopelvic fascia connects laterally to the aponeurosis of the levator ani muscles at the arcus tendineus fascia pelvis, otherwise known as the White line, located in the space of Retzius, adjacent to the obturator internus muscle.

Vaginal Support

The vagina is a fibromuscular tube that averages 8–10 cm in length. In a standing woman, the axis of the vagina is horizontal. The support of the uterus and vagina can be separated into three levels (4). These levels of support aid in the understanding of normal anatomy and in preoperative planning of the appropriate procedure to address the specific support defect (Fig. 25 and Box 10).

Risk Factors for Developing Pelvic Support Defects

The most consistent risk factors identified for prolapse development have been vaginal childbirth, advancing age, and increasing body mass index. Vaginal childbirth is the factor that has been most consistently associated with prolapse, particularly in the occiput posterior position, or with operative delivery—especially with forceps. The mechanism of pelvic floor injury may be from injury to the levator ani or to the nerves, in particular the pudendal nerve (5). Other factors associated with prolapse are genetic disposition, congenital connective tissue disorders (eg, Marfan syndrome), parity, menopause, prior pelvic surgery, and factors associated

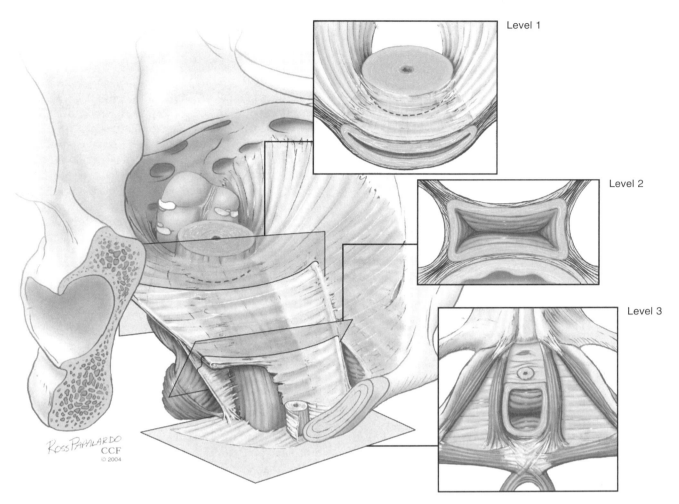

Figure 25. Levels of support. Level I support consists of the cardinal and uterosacral ligaments, which provide apical support to the cervix, uterus, and apex of the vagina. Level II support consists of the pubocervical and rectovaginal fascia, which laterally attach the mid-portion of the vagina to the arcus tendineus fascia pelvis and to the arcus tendineus rectovaginalis. Level III support is the most distal component, consisting of the fusion of the vagina anteriorly to the urethra, posteriorly to the perineal membrane, perineal body, and laterally to the levator ani muscles. (Walters MD, Karam MM. Urogynecology and reconstructive pelvic surgery. Reprinted with permission, Cleveland Clinic Center for Medical Art & Photography © 2004–2010. All Rights Reserved.)

with elevated intraabdominal pressure (eg, obesity and chronic constipation with excessive straining) (6).

Hysterectomy as a risk factor for prolapse remains controversial. Alterations of the connective tissue and injury to the innervation and vascularization to the pelvic floor muscles occur with pelvic surgery. Advocates for supracervical hysterectomy have claimed that preservation of the cervix and the cardinal–uterosacral complex (level I support) would prevent the development of subsequent prolapse. Evidence from randomized clinical trials comparing supracervical with total hysterectomy has not demonstrated a difference in the incidence of prolapse, at least in short term (7). Nevertheless, pelvic organ prolapse can occur many years after hysterectomy. Population-based studies looking at prolapse surgery after hysterectomy have identified risk factors, such as the presence of preoperative pelvic floor disor-

ders, especially grade 2 or greater pelvic organ prolapse, or history of incontinence procedures, chronic pulmonary disease, and increasing parity (8–10).

Diagnosis

In many women, prolapse remains mild and asymptomatic, with the hymen as a cut-off point where prolapse becomes bothersome to many women (11). However, individual variation exists; some women with pelvic support defects are symptomatic, whereas others who may have a similar presentation remain asymptomatic. Increasing severity of prolapse does not necessarily correlate with increased symptomatology (12). If asymptomatic or mildly symptomatic, the woman may be counseled that treatment is appropriate only when her symptoms warrant it.

Box 10

Levels of Vaginal Support

- Level I support consists of the cardinal and utero-sacral ligaments, which provide apical support to the cervix, uterus, and apex of the vagina. The fibers of the uterosacral ligaments extend vertically and posteriorly towards the sacrum, whereas the cardinal ligaments extend laterally. Defects in Level I support result in prolapse of the vaginal apex.

- Level II support consists of the pubocervical and rectovaginal fascia, which laterally attach the mid-portion of the vagina to the arcus tendineus fascia pelvis and to the arcus tendineus rectovaginalis. Defects at this level result in anterior or posterior compartment defects; eg, cystoceles and recto-celes.

- Level III support is the most distal component, consisting of the fusion of the vagina anteriorly to the urethra, posteriorly to the perineal membrane and perineal body, and laterally to the levator ani muscles. A defect in this level posteriorly results in perineal body descent and can contribute to defecatory dysfunction, or anteriorly can cause urethral hypermobility and stress incontinence. Levels I, II, and III are all connected through the endopelvic fascia.

Symptoms

Symptoms associated with pelvic organ prolapse include vaginal bulge, pelvic pressure, splinting (or manually pushing back) the vagina in order to urinate or defecate, sexual dysfunction, and voiding or defecatory dysfunction. The symptoms associated with prolapse, such as bulging of the vagina and pressure, are dynamic and subject to the forces of gravity and, therefore, may worsen by the end of the day or due to long periods of physical exertion, such as lifting and standing, and improve when the patient is lying down. The most specific complaints related to prolapse are the feeling of a vaginal bulge and splinting in order to urinate or defecate (13).

Women with advanced prolapse may report difficulty urinating and incomplete bladder emptying, which may lead to recurrent urinary tract infections due to urinary stasis. Urinary frequency also can occur because incomplete bladder emptying can cause the woman to have the sensation of a full bladder soon after urinating. Some may have a history of stress urinary incontinence in the past that improved or resolved with the worsening of prolapse, and find that they can empty their bladder once their prolapse is reduced. They also may have obstructed defecation. Therefore, it is important that the clinician assess urinary and def-

ecatory function by asking specific questions because many women will not volunteer this information.

Examination

Physical examination should initially take place in the dorsal lithotomy position, performing a Valsalva maneuver. If the patient states that her prolapse is not as evident when lying down as it is when standing, an examination should be performed while straining in the standing position. Valsalva and cough stress testing can be performed in order to elicit stress incontinence. These tests also can be performed with the prolapse reduced in order to elicit occult (or potential) stress incontinence. Urinary function also should be assessed by measuring the patient's voided volume and an evaluation of postvoid residual volume by either catheterization or ultrasonography. Urethral hypermobility testing also can be performed to determine the extent of urethral movement from the resting position compared to Valsalva maneuver, with cotton swab inserted into the urethra with the tip at the bladder neck and measured against a protractor to determine the degree of change. If stress incontinence is present, urethral hypermobility can influence the type of antiincontinence procedure selected. The patient's sensory and neurologic function should be checked by stroking along the labia majora with a cotton swab or a plastic applicator with cotton tuft in order to elicit the bulbocavernosus and anal wink reflexes and to assess for any altered perineal sensation; eg, paresthesias or numbness that may have resulted from a pudendal neuropathy or sacral nerve root injury.

Several systems are currently in use to describe and classify pelvic organ prolapse. The Baden–Walker system is in widespread clinical use, and uses the hymen as a reference point (Box 11). The Pelvic Organ Prolapse Quantification system was developed in order to describe the prolapse more precisely in all compartments and assess change over time (Box 12 and Fig. 26). Familiarity with both classification systems is advised because both are in use in the current literature. The Baden–Walker system probably is adequate for clinical practice as long as all pelvic compartments (anterior, apical, and posterior) are assessed. It can be difficult to distinguish between anterior, apical, or posterior defects if each compartment is not considered on its own (Fig. 27).

Therefore, after the speculum examination to visualize the cervix or vaginal apex and measure the total vaginal length, the patient should bear down in a Valsalva maneuver in order to assess the descent of the vaginal vault. An apical support defect can be diagnosed by using the posterior blade of the speculum or plastic applicators with cotton tuft, to elevate the vaginal apex or cervix and to evaluate if an apical

Box 12

Stages of Pelvic Organ Prolapse

Stages are based on the maximal extent of prolapse relative to the hymen, in one or more compartments.

Stage 0   No prolapse; anterior and posterior points are all –3 cm, and C (cervix) or D (posterior fornix) is between –TVL (total vaginal length) and –(TVL – 2) cm.

Stage I   The criteria for stage 0 are not met, and the most distal prolapse is more than 1 cm above the level of the hymen (less than – 1 cm).

Stage II   The most distal prolapse is between 1 cm above and 1 cm below the hymen (at least one point is –1, 0, or +1).

Stage III   The most distal prolapse is more than 1 cm below the hymen but no further than 2 cm less than TVL.

Stage IV   Represents complete procidentia or vault eversion; the most distal prolapse protrudes to at least (TVL – 2) cm.

Pelvic Organ Prolapse Quantification System

• Six vaginal sites are used in staging prolapse
  —Points Aa and Ba anteriorly
  —Points Ap and Bp posteriorly
  —Point C for the cervix or vaginal apex
  —Point D for the posterior fornix (not measured after hysterectomy)
• Three additional measurements are used
  —genital hiatus (GH)
  —perineal body (PB)
  —total vaginal length (TVL)

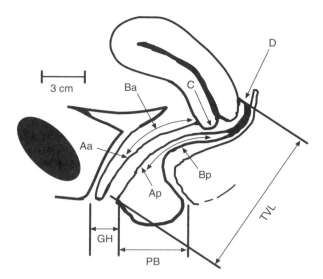

Figure 26. Six sites (points Aa, Ba, C, D, Bp, and Ap), genital hiatus (GH), perineal body (PB), and total vaginal length (TVL) used for pelvic organ support quantitation. (Reprinted from Am J Obstet Gynecol, Vol 175, Bump RC, Mattiasson A, Bo K, Brubaker LP, DeLancey JO, Klarskov P, et al. The standardization of terminology of female pelvic organ prolapse and pelvic floor dysfunction. p. 10-7, Copyright 1996, with permission from Elsevier.)

suspension procedure is necessary. In order to isolate compartment defects, one can use the posterior blade of the speculum to push down the posterior wall in order to fully evaluate the anterior compartment during the Valsalva maneuver. The posterior speculum blade then should support the anterior vagina and the posterior wall should be evaluated for descent of the posterior wall. The measurement of the genital hiatus and perineal body can be performed either before or after this speculum examination. The patient should then contract her levator muscles in order to assess levator muscle strength and then a bimanual examination can be performed.

Assessment of the anal sphincter also is important because many women have fecal incontinence, which can result from an overt or occult anal sphincter laceration from childbirth or from prior anal surgery; eg, hemorrhoidectomy. A rectovaginal examination should assess for rectal tone and rectal squeeze and the presence of a rectocele. Detachment of the rectovaginal septum to the perineal body also can be assessed during the rectovaginal examination.

Imaging

Imaging studies for prolapse do not accurately predict the location of pelvic viscera and in general, are not necessary for the routine management of pelvic organ prolapse (14). Certain ancillary studies, such as dynamic magnetic resonance imaging or defecating

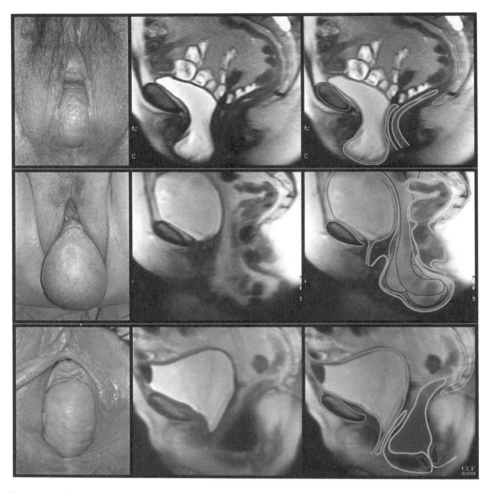

Figure 27. This illustration shows an anterior compartment defect in the top row, with a large cystocele, and a sagittal magnetic resonance imaging scan of the pelvis. The middle row illustrates a large apical defect, or enterocele, where the bowel is filling this vaginal herniation. The last row depicts a posterior compartment defect, or rectocele. Because of the difficulty in distinguishing whether the defect is an anterior or posterior defect, it is imperative to perform a careful speculum examination and document the prolapse on each compartment. (Reprinted from the Lancet, Vol. 369, Jelovsek JE, Maher C, Barber MD. Pelvic organ prolapse. Pages 1027–38, Copyright 2007, with permission from Elsevier.)

proctogram, may be useful in assessing for an intussusception or sigmoidocele if these entities are clinically suspect. Endoanal ultrasonography can elucidate if an anal sphincter defect is present in the patient with fecal incontinence and renal ultrasonography may be ordered if an obstructive uropathy is suspected to assess for hydronephrosis or hydroureter.

Nonsurgical Management

Nonsurgical management should be discussed as an option for all women with prolapse. Pelvic floor physical therapy, lifestyle changes and symptom-directed therapy, and pessary placement are all options for women who cannot or do not wish to have surgery. Appropriate candidates for nonsurgical management are those women who are able to cooperate and understand instructions in order to achieve any degree of success.

Symptom-Directed Therapy and Lifestyle Changes

Treatment options include maintaining a normal weight because overweight is associated with progression of pelvic floor disorders (15). Voiding and defecatory dysfunction also should be addressed. For example, women who have urinary incontinence can be treated with behavioral modification (timed voiding), restricting excessive fluid or caffeine intake, and pelvic muscle physical therapy. Those who have defecatory dysfunction can increase their dietary fiber intake; use stool softeners, laxatives, or enemas; and splint in order to completely empty and avoid straining. Vaginal estrogen can be used in order to treat vaginal dryness, especially in the case of keratinized epithelium that results from the exposed prolapsed vagina. Other lifestyle modifications that may decrease the progression of prolapse include smoking cessation, good nutrition, and avoiding increased abdominal pressure (eg, straining in order to urinate or defecate, heavy lifting, or activity).

Pessaries

Pessaries have traditionally been used in patients who have medical contraindications to undergo surgery, ie, pregnancy or serious medical comorbidities. However, pessaries can be used in any woman who prefers a nonsurgical treatment for prolapse. They also may be used diagnostically to see if a patient's nonspecific symptoms, such as pelvic pressure, resolve with prolapse reduction. The appropriate candidate should be able to present for follow up on a regular basis because neglected pessaries can lead to vaginal ulcerations, erosions, or fistulas into the bladder or rectum. Pessaries can be fitted in most women with prolapse, regardless of site of predominant prolapse or stage, although pessaries tend not to alleviate symptoms related to posterior compartment defects as well.

Pessaries are made of inert, soft silicone, and are available in a variety of shapes and sizes (Fig. 28). They can be categorized as supportive (eg, ring pessary) or space occupying (eg, donut pessary). The most commonly used pessaries are ring (with and without support and incontinence rings), Gellhorn, donut, and cube pessaries. Ideally, the woman should be able to insert and remove the pessary on her own and be able

to use vaginal estrogen, although inability to do so is not a contraindication to pessary use (Fig. 29).

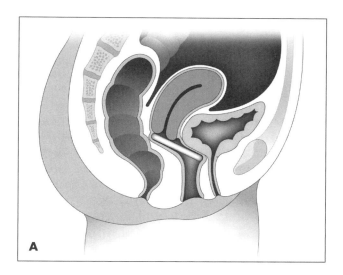

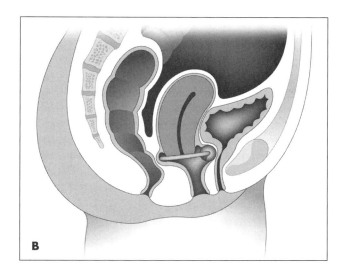

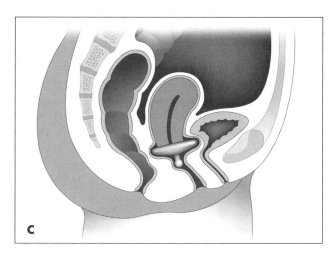

Figure 29. Pessaries in place: **A.** ring, **B.** ring with support, and **C.** Gellhorn.

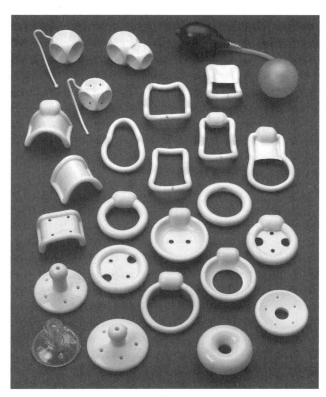

Figure 28. Various types of pessaries. (Photo courtesy of CooperSurgical, Inc., Trumbull, CT.)

Approximately 75% of women can be successfully fitted with a pessary in one to two office visits, but only one half of women maintain pessary use after 6 months (16). Prolapse stage has not been found to be a factor in successful pessary fitting. However, the type of pessary that can be fitted is probably related to the severity of prolapse. In one study protocol, ring pessaries were inserted first and followed by Gellhorn pessaries if the ring did not stay in place. Ring pessaries were more successful in stage II prolapse (100%) whereas stage III prolapse (71%)and stage IV prolapse (64%) more frequently required Gellhorn pessaries. In those patients with successful pessary fitting, more than 90% were satisfied with their pessaries, nearly all prolapse symptoms were alleviated, and one half of urinary symptoms had resolved (17). Sexual activity is not a contraindication to pessary use (18). Factors affecting pessary fitting for pelvic organ prolapse are outlined in Table 10 and those affecting continued pessary use, in Table 11.

The pessary used should be the largest one that is comfortable and will stay in place, yet will still allow the breadth of one finger between the pessary and pelvic sidewall. Evaluation of the levator hiatus using the examiner's fingers to measure the diameter between the lateral fornices of the vagina can aid in choosing the pessary size by comparing this measurement to the diameter of the pessary. If the patient can feel the pessary, then a smaller size should be tried.

Once fitted, the patient should bear down in order to make sure she does not expel the pessary and, before leaving the office, demonstrate that she is able to urinate. The patient also should be taught how to remove and reinsert the pessary, if possible, and to alert the physician if vaginal bleeding occurs. Follow-up visits should then be performed at 2 weeks and then every 3 months to ensure there is not a vaginal erosion or ulceration. In postmenopausal women, the use of vaginal estrogen is encouraged to prevent vaginal erosions through thickening the vaginal epithelium. If need be, a home health care worker or family member can be trained to provide the needed help to either remove and clean the pessary or to ensure that the patient returns for routine checkups.

Surgical Management

Pelvic organ prolapse is a common indication for gynecologic surgery, with more than 186,000 procedures performed in 2006 in the United States. (19). It has been estimated that a woman has an 11% estimated lifetime risk of having at least one surgical procedure for pelvic organ prolapse (20). Up to 40% of these patients will undergo reoperation for procedure failure within 3 years (21). Of these recurrences, 60% occur at the site of the original defect, whereas 32% occur at different sites (22).

Candidates for Surgery

Surgery for pelvic support defects may be indicated for those symptomatic women who prefer to avoid using a vaginal pessary. Patients with pelvic support defects should be evaluated on an individual basis to determine the most appropriate approach to surgery. Factors that may influence the surgeon's choice of sur-

Table 10. Factors Affecting Pessary Fitting for Pelvic Organ Prolapse

Percentage of Study Population With Successful Pessary Fit	Factors Associated With Successful Pessary Fitting	Factors Not Associated With Successful Pessary Fitting
Clemons et al, 2004*: 73 of 100 women (73%)	Longer vaginal length (more than 7 cm) Narrower vaginal introitus (less than the breadth of four fingers)	Age Parity Estrogen use Sexually active Previous hysterectomy Previous prolapse surgery Pelvic organ prolapse stage Predominant prolapse compartment Genital hiatus size
Mutone et al, 2005†: 288 of 407 women (71%)	(not stated)	(not stated)

*Clemons JL, Aguilar VC, Tillinghast TA, Jackson ND, Myers DL. Risk factors associated with an unsuccessful pessary fitting trial in women with pelvic organ prolapse. Am J Obstet Gynecol 2004;190:345–50.
†Mutone MF, Terry C, Hale DS, Benson JT. Factors which influence the short-term success of pessary management of pelvic organ prolapse. Am J Obstet Gynecol 2005:193:89–94.

Table 11. Factors Affecting Continued Pessary Use for Pelvic Organ Prolapse

Percentage of Study Population With Continued Pessary Use	Factors Associated With Continued Pessary Use	Factors Not Associated With Continued Pessary Use
Brincat et al, 2004*: 82 of 136 women (60%)	Sexually active vs not sexually active Pessary use for prolapse vs for stress incontinence	Age Parity Menopausal status Surgical history
Mutone et al, 2005†: 168 of 407 women (41%)	No previous hysterectomy No previous surgery for prolapse Normal weight vs obesity	Age Levator ani strength Pelvic organ prolapse stage Predominant prolapse compartment Genital hiatus size Perineal body length Total vaginal length

*Brincat C, Kenton K, Fitzgerald M, Brubaker L. Sexual activity predicts continued pessary use. Am J Obstet Gynecol 2004;191:198–200.

†Mutone MF, Terry C, Hale DS, Benson JT. Factors which influence the short-term success of pessary management of pelvic organ prolapse. Am J Obstet Gynecol 2005:193:89–94.

gery include the patient's age, body habitus, medical comorbidities, her desire to preserve sexual function, and the surgeon's own experience with various operative techniques (Box 13). A common dilemma faced by the gynecologic surgeon is whether to operate on an asymptomatic or minimally symptomatic patient with significant prolapse. Although it is impossible to make an asymptomatic patient feel better, the surgeon and patient should discuss the potential risks and benefits of expectant management versus surgical correction. If the patient does not have evidence of urinary retention, defecatory dysfunction, vaginal erosions from exteriorization of the prolapse, or other complications resulting from the prolapse, then expectant management with serial examinations is appropriate.

Box 13

Considerations in Choosing the Surgical Approach to Pelvic Reconstructive Surgery

- Age
- Body habitus
- Patient's medical condition and comorbidities
- Associated pelvic relaxation
- Intraabdominal pathology
- Desire to preserve sexual function
- Previous surgery and pelvic adhesions
- Surgeon experience
- Success rates of different procedures

Prolapse that extends to or beyond the hymen may mask signs and symptoms of urinary incontinence. Women with this degree of prolapse should be tested preoperatively to determine whether they have stress incontinence. A simple cough stress test with careful prolapse reduction to avoid any urethral compression may be performed to rule out this condition. If stress incontinence is observed with prolapse reduction, consideration should be given to performing more extensive urodynamic testing (to rule out conditions, such as intrinsic sphincter deficiency and detrusor overactivity) and a continence procedure at the time of surgery, if indicated. The Colpopexy and Urinary Reduction Efforts trial demonstrated that in women with prolapse undergoing abdominal sacrocolpopexy who did not have symptoms of stress urinary incontinence, concomitant Burch colposuspension significantly reduced the postoperative development of stress incontinence without increasing the risks of other urinary tract symptoms (23).

Choice of Approach

Surgical management of pelvic support defects may be performed by a variety of techniques and approaches. The common goal of reconstructive pelvic surgery is to restore the normal depth, axis, and function of the vaginal canal. Previous abdominal surgery or history of pelvic infection (eg, ruptured appendicitis or pelvic inflammatory disease) may suggest the presence of adhesions, which might make an abdominal or laparoscopic approach more difficult. Patients with morbid obesity may not tolerate general anesthesia with steep Trendelenburg position needed for abdominal or laparoscopic reconstructive surgery. The vaginal approach to prolapse surgery has been advocated by many gynecologic surgeons because of advantages, such as reduced hospital stay and postoperative pain and a faster return to normal activities. Long-term outcome studies in recent years, however, have suggested that vaginal approaches to prolapse may result in higher recurrence rates than with abdominal surgery and the subsequent need for reoperation (24). This is especially true of anterior colporrhaphy, using the patient's own native endopelvic fascial tissue to plicate together on the anterior vaginal wall. Depending on the specific technique used, failure rates of up to 50% have been reported in randomized trials at 5-year follow-up (25). However, abdominal approaches to pelvic organ prolapse have the disadvantage of requiring a laparotomy incision, with potential associated morbidity, including wound infections, extended hospital stay, slower return to normal activities, and cosmetic drawbacks. To mitigate these disadvantages, laparoscopic approaches to pelvic reconstructive surgery have been developed (26). Impediments to widespread adoption of these techniques include the technical difficulty with laparoscopic suturing and knot tying and the long learning curves associated with these complex procedures. Laparoscopy is associated with a number of advantages, including shorter hospital stays, decreased postoperative pain, and reduced time to resume normal activities. Another advantage of the laparoscopic approach is improved surgical visualization, which may increase the accuracy of suture placement and possibly improve long-term outcomes. One of the primary goals of the laparoscopic approach is to duplicate proven abdominal techniques, without compromising safety or efficacy, in an effort to perform these procedures in a minimally invasive fashion. More recently, robotic surgery has been applied to pelvic floor reconstructive surgery, with a number of series of robotic sacrocolpopexy reported in the literature (27, 28). Advantages of robotic assistance include three-dimensional vision, articulation of instruments, and a quicker learning curve compared with traditional "straight stick" laparoscopic surgery. Disadvantages of robotic surgery for pelvic floor reconstruction include increased costs (including capital equipment and disposable instruments), increased operating time, and limited availability of robotic units in many communities.

The Use of Grafts

Graft materials have been used to augment various reconstructive procedures in an effort to lower the recurrence rates associated with poor innate fascia. The use of graft materials may be of benefit in some clinical situations, such as recurrent prolapse and extreme prolapse, and in cases where the surgeon cannot find strong endopelvic fascia intraoperatively. Currently, it is difficult to compare the results of studies because surgical techniques and graft materials vary. The use of autologous fascia, allografts, xenografts, and synthetic mesh has been reported for pelvic reconstructive surgery (Box 14). Offsetting the advantages of global reinforcement of potentially weak host fascia are the disadvantages of added cost of the graft, increased surgical complexity and operative times, and potentially increased complications, including mesh exposure, infection, and dyspareunia. The American College of Obstetricians and Gynecologists published a review of the current treatment options (29). Although the current literature does not provide definitive conclusions as to the risk-to-benefit ratio of these techniques, this publication encouraged surgeons to closely monitor emerging literature and to remain knowledgeable as to which procedures should be avoided and which may prove beneficial to patients.

Most experts agree that the physical characteristics of synthetic mesh are important to encourage tissue ingrowth and reduce the risk of complications, such as exposure, erosion, and infection. Although the ideal mesh has yet to be developed, the most commonly used materials are lightweight, macroporous, and monofilament polypropylene (30) because they have better macrophage penetration and less bacterial adherence thereby leading to lower infection and rejection rates.

In November 2007, the Society of Gynecologic Surgeons Systematic Review Group published a review of the literature for transvaginal graft use in pelvic recon-

---

Box 14

Graft Materials for Prolapse Surgery

Organic
- Allografts
  - Fascia lata
  - Dermis
- Xenografts
  - Porcine dermis
  - Porcine small intestinal submucosa
  - Bovine dermis

Synthetic
- Absorbable
  - Polyglactin mesh
  - Polyglycolic mesh
- Nonabsorbable
  - Polypropylene
  - Polyester
  - Polytetrafluoroethylene

structive surgery (31). Although there was an abundance of case series reviewed by this group, the authors noted a paucity of randomized, controlled trials addressing traditional versus mesh-augmented prolapse repairs. Only one out of six randomized controlled trials provided support for increased efficacy of nonabsorbable mesh, and only in the anterior compartment.

Although there has been a growing trend towards mesh augmentation for some cases of vaginal reconstructive surgery, there has also been increasing concern with potential overuse of mesh and possible complications that may occur. In October, 2008, the U.S. Food and Drug Administration issued a Public Health Notification regarding the use of mesh for pelvic floor reconstruction, including prolapse and stress incontinence. More than 1,000 reports had been received by the FDA from medical device manufacturers of complications resulting from mesh use, including erosion through the vaginal epithelium (ie, exposure), chronic pain, dyspareunia, voiding difficulties, infection, hemorrhage, and perforation of organs (eg, bladder and bowel) from the insertion tool used to place the mesh. The U.S. Food and Drug Administration made several recommendations to surgeons who use mesh for pelvic floor reconstruction regarding proper counseling of patients and postoperative vigilance and management of potential complications (Box 15). It should be noted that the FDA Public Health Notification did not discourage the use of synthetic mesh in the pelvis by surgeons, but rather was intended to stress the need for proper counseling of patients and monitoring for problems postoperatively. In addition, the Public Health Notification did not attempt to estimate the rates of these complications.

Box 15

U.S. Food and Drug Administration's Public Health Notification: Recommendations for Physicians

- Obtain specialized training for each mesh technique
- Be vigilant for potential adverse events
- Watch for complications associated with tools
- Inform patients that surgical mesh is permanent
- Counsel patients that complications may require additional surgery
- Inform patients about potential for serious complications
- Provide patients with a written copy of the patient labeling

Food and Drug Administration. FDA Public Health Notification: serious complications associated with transvaginal placement of Surgical Mesh in repair of pelvic organ prolapse and stress urinary incontinence. Washington (DC): FDA; 2008. Available at: http://www.fda.gov/MedicalDevices/Safety/AlertsandNotices/PublicHealthNotifications/ucm061976.htm. Retrieved December 7, 2010.

Surgical Repair

Surgery for pelvic organ prolapse can be divided into the anterior, posterior, and apical vaginal compartments. It is common for several procedures to be required for any individual case because multiple defects in the pelvic floor often occur, resulting in symptomatic and clinically evident prolapse.

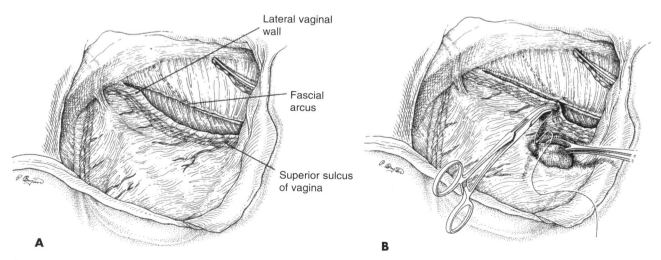

A   **B**

Figure 30. A. Paravaginal defect. Detachment of the pubocervical fascia from the arcus tendineous fascia pelvis results in a paravaginal defect. **B.** Paravaginal repair. (Richardson AC. Paravaginal repair. Oper Tech Gynecol Surg 1996;1:66–75. Copyright A.C. Richardson. Courtesy of A.C. Richardson and P. Bryan, illustrator.)

The goal of site-specific reconstructive surgery is to identify and repair specific defects in the endopelvic fascia that lead to pelvic support disorders. One of the most common defects resulting in cystocele, or anterior vaginal wall prolapse, is paravaginal detachment of the pubocervical fascia from the pelvic sidewall (Fig. 30) at the level of the arcus tendinous fascia pelvis, a condensation of fascia overlying the obturator internus muscle (32). Carefully resupporting the lateral margins of the anterior vaginal wall in the office with an instrument, such as ring forceps, will reduce the cystocele when the etiology is a paravaginal defect. A transverse defect between the pubocervical fascia and the apical vaginal support (pericervical fascial ring, uterosacral ligaments, or both) also may be present and should be investigated preoperatively so that both defects can be corrected at the time of surgery. Women with transverse defects often have a large proximal (or "high") cystocele with a well supported urethra and bladder neck. Paravaginal defect repair of cystocele may be performed abdominally or laparoscopically after gaining access to the space of Retzius, or retropubic space. Paravaginal repair involves placing a series of interrupted permanent sutures between the arcus tendinous fascia pelvis and the detached pubocervical fascia (Fig. 31), starting near the ischial spine and working distally toward the pubic bone (32). In the laparoscopic procedure, the retropubic space usually is entered through a transperitoneal approach using sharp dissection with electrocautery or other energy source. In a series of laparoscopic pelvic floor reconstructions in 73 women, 32 women underwent a standard laparoscopic paravaginal repair (33). Another five women had a modified paravaginal repair,

in which a third bite was placed in the iliopectineal (Cooper) ligament, although nonanatomic elevation was avoided in these patients. In addition, another 17 patients underwent transvaginal anterior colporrhaphy for midline defects. They reported an objective success rate of 87.5%, with a mean follow-up of 8 months (range, 0–26). Vaginal paravaginal repair also may be performed through a midline incision with access gained to the space of Retzius bilaterally. Permanent sutures are placed around the arcus tendinous fascia pelvis and are then attached to corresponding positions on the bladder fascia and anterior vaginal wall (Fig. 32). Although excellent success rates have been reported, this approach may be associated with significant blood loss and other morbidity, including recurrent midline cystocele and development of enterocele (34). In an effort to improve surgical success rates for anterior compartment defects, natural and synthetic grafts have been used to augment the patients' own fascial support, although their use remains controversial. A recent review of prolapse surgery found that the rate of recurrent cystocele could be reduced by augmenting an anterior repair with polyglactin absorbable mesh (24). As mentioned earlier, evidence also exists that nonabsorbable mesh may have a role in reducing recurrent anterior wall prolapse. In a prospective study, authors randomized 202 women to receive anterior colporrhaphy with or without augmentation using a low weight polypropylene mesh. They demonstrated a lower recurrence rate for prolapse (defined as stage 2 or greater) at 1 year with the mesh augmentation (35). Various points of graft attachments have been described in the literature. Apically, grafts have been attached to the

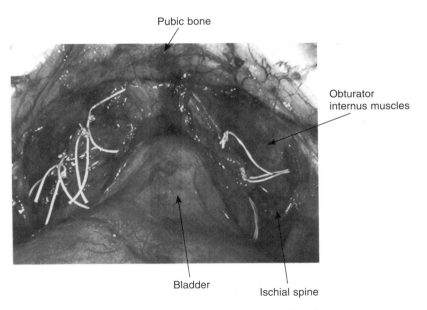

Pubic bone

Obturator internus muscles

Bladder

Ischial spine

Figure 31. Laparoscopic paravaginal repair, completed. (Photo courtesy of Peter L. Rosenblatt.)

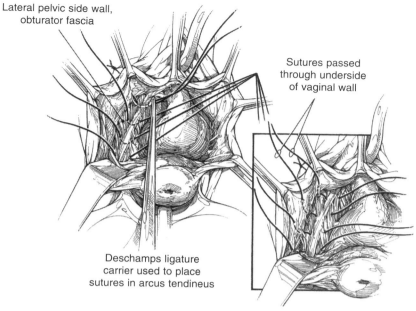

Lateral pelvic side wall, obturator fascia

Sutures passed through underside of vaginal wall

Deschamps ligature carrier used to place sutures in arcus tendineus

Figure 32. Vaginal paravaginal repair. Placement of permanent sutures between the lateral pubocervical fascia and the arcus tendinous fascia pelvis repairs the paravaginal defect. (Nichols DH, Randall CL. Anterior colporrhaphy. Vaginal surgery. 4th ed. Baltimore (MD): Williams & Wilkins; 1996. p. 218–56.)

sacrospinous ligament and the iliococcygeus muscle and fascia. Laterally, the arcus tendinous fascia pelvis has been used for graft fixation. Distally, grafts have been attached to the pubourethral ligaments, the distal arcus tendinous fascia pelvis, and the obturator membrane using a transobturator approach. The concept of transobturator passage of mesh strips to secure synthetic grafts in position has resulted in the introduction of a plethora of techniques and mesh kits that are used to treat anterior defects. Several case series have been published in the literature that report on the efficacy and safety of these novel procedures (36, 37). Despite these reports, however, potential complications from the synthetic mesh, as well as from the tools used to place the mesh, have raised concern among many surgeons, and the proper use of these techniques remains controversial.

Vaginal Vault Prolapse

Although support for the vaginal apex may be accomplished at the time of vaginal hysterectomy (McCall culdoplasty or high uterosacral ligament plication), these procedures may be performed for vaginal vault prolapse remote from the time of hysterectomy as well. Although the classic McCall culdoplasty procedure involves plication of the uterosacral ligaments and incorporates the posterior peritoneum and vaginal wall as well, a high uterosacral ligament suspension involves reuniting the anterior (pubocervical) fascia, the posterior (rectovaginal) fascia, and the proximal uterosacral

ligaments. Transvaginal sacrospinous ligament suspension or sacrospinous colpopexy most often is performed through a posterior vaginal incision, although the procedure also has been described using an anterior or apical approach. Permanent or delayed absorbable sutures are placed in the sacrospinous ligament, which lies within the coccygeus muscle, and these sutures are then secured to the underside of the vaginal apex. The procedure may be performed bilaterally if the width of the proximal vaginal vault allows, although it is most commonly performed unilaterally. In one randomized study, vaginal sacrospinous colpopexy was found to be as successful as abdominal sacrocolpopexy for the treatment of vaginal vault prolapse (38). If preoperative assessment reveals that the vaginal vault is foreshortened and does not reach the sacrospinous ligament, the surgeon has the option of using a graft material to bridge the distance because most experts recommend not leaving suture bridges between these two structures. In addition, some experts have advocated using an iliococcygeus suspension for the foreshortened vagina, although the fascia overlying this muscle group lacks the strength of the sacrospinous ligament. An alternative to sacrospinous colpopexy for vaginal vault suspension is the McCall culdoplasty, which involves suspension of the vaginal apex to the proximal uterosacral ligaments (Fig. 33). This procedure is most often performed at the time of hysterectomy, although it can be performed at any time, as long as the uterosacral ligaments can be identified and are found to be intact proximally.

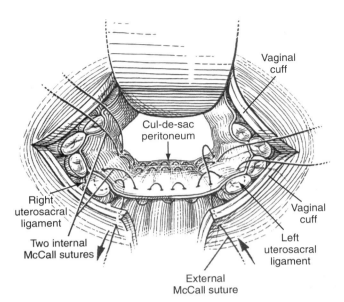

Figure 33. McCall culdoplasty. Sutures are placed through the posterior vaginal cuff and uterosacral ligaments for transvaginal vault suspension and obliteration of the cul-de-sac. (Lee RA. Uterus: vaginal hysterectomy for uterine procidentia with associated cystocele, enterocele, and rectocele. In: Atlas of gynecologic surgery. Philadelphia (PA): Saunders; 1992. p. 131–50. Used with permission of Mayo Foundation for Medical Education and Research.)

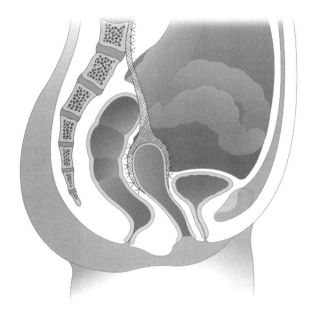

Figure 34. Sacrocolpopexy. Cross-section of the pelvis demonstrating the Y-shaped mesh sutured to the pubocervical fascia anteriorly and to the posterior endopelvic fascia. The mesh then is attached to the anterior longitudinal ligament of the sacral promontory.

Abdominal sacrocolpopexy (Fig. 34) is considered by many gynecologic surgeons to be the standard procedure for the surgical management of vaginal vault pro-

lapse. A review of published studies on sacrocolpopexy reported a success rate of 78–100%, when considering postoperative apical support (39). In one commonly used technique, a Y-shaped mesh is sutured to the anterior and posterior endopelvic fascia with multiple attachment points and then to the anterior longitudinal ligament of the sacrum (Fig. 35A). The mesh usually is buried under the peritoneum to reduce the chance of internal intestinal hernia (Fig. 35B). Synthetic mesh erosions are uncommon, occurring in 0.5–5% of cases, and usually require reoperation to remove the areas of eroded mesh. In an effort to reduce the pain and morbidity associated with laparotomy, laparoscopic sacrocolpopexy has been reported in a number of small series (40, 41) as a reasonable approach, as long as the basic steps of the procedure can be performed in a manner that does not compromise patient outcome.

Developments in the field of synthetic grafts have led to the introduction of new techniques and products for the management of vault prolapse. Posterior intravaginal slingplasty, or infracoccygeal sacropexy, is a minimally invasive technique that involves the use of a narrow strip of polypropylene tape between the perineum and the vaginal vault (Fig. 36). An introducer needle is inserted inferior and lateral to the anus into the ischiorectal fossa and pierces the levator ani muscle near the ischial spine. The needle is then guided by the surgeon's finger through the previously dissected pararectal space and the tape is pulled through this tunnel. The procedure is performed bilaterally and the tape is sutured to the posterior vaginal apex. Vaginal vault suspension is accomplished by a tension-free fixation of the tape to the levator ani fascia and underlying muscles. Although initial results of this procedure seemed promising (42), more recent studies have demonstrated a propensity for mesh erosion and infection (43, 44), which is felt to be due to the unique characteristics of this product because it is a tightly-woven, multifilament polypropylene mesh.

Uterine Prolapse

In the past, hysterectomy was almost universally recommended when contemplating surgery for uterine prolapse. Improvements in the treatment of dysfunctional uterine bleeding, leiomyomas, and other benign uterine conditions have led to a paradigm shift in the management of uterine prolapse. There has been renewed interest in uterine preservation at the time of prolapse surgery (45). Uterine suspension can be performed abdominally or laparoscopically by attaching the cervix to the proximal uterosacral ligaments, or by plicating the uterosacral ligaments in the midline using permanent sutures. In one recent study of laparoscopic suture hysteropexy, 16% of women required further surgery for recurrent uterine prolapse. Transvaginal sacrospinous

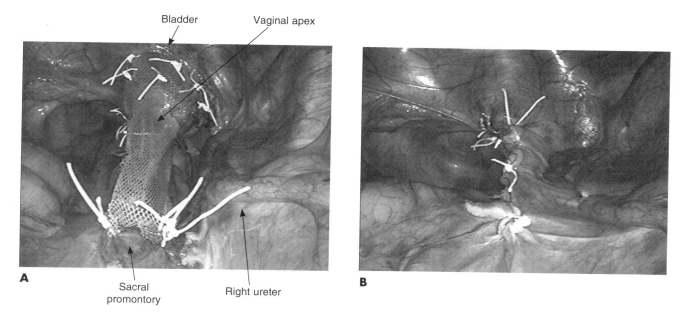

Figure 35. Laparoscopic sacrocolpopexy. **A.** The synthetic mesh has been sutured to the anterior and posterior endopelvic fascia and attached to the anterior longitudinal ligament of the sacrum. **B.** The mesh has been buried under the peritoneum to prevent internal intestinal hernia. (Photos courtesy of Peter L. Rosenblatt.)

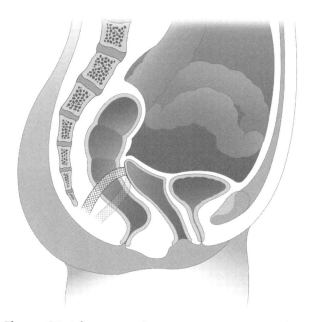

Figure 36. Infracoccygeal sacropexy. Cross-section of the pelvis demonstrating the position of the tape placed through the ischiorectal fossa and supporting the vaginal apex laterally to the levator ani muscle and fascia.

hysteropexy involves suturing the uterosacral ligaments, near their insertion to the cervix, to the sacrospinous ligament through a posterior vaginal incision. In one recent study, 70 eligible women with stage 3 or stage 4 uterovaginal prolapse were offered either sacrospinous hysteropexy or vaginal hysterectomy with sacrospinous vault suspension (46). Objective (74% versus 72%,

respectively) and subjective (78% versus 86%, respectively) success rates were similar for the two groups.

Sacrocervicopexy is performed in a manner similar to sacrocolpopexy, whereby a natural or synthetic graft material is sutured to the cervix and the posterior vaginal endopelvic fascia and is then attached to the anterior longitudinal ligament of the sacrum (Fig. 37). This procedure differs from traditional sacrocolpopexy in that the graft is not attached to the anterior pubocervical fascia. Sacrocervicopexy may be performed abdominally or laparoscopically, usually when the surgeon feels that the uterosacral ligaments are of insufficient strength to perform an uterosacral ligament uterine suspension (Fig. 38). In a retrospective case series, 40 women with advanced prolapse underwent laparoscopic sacrocervicopexy with synthetic mesh. There were no apical failures noted at 12 months. Complications included a rectal injury in one patient and a minor mesh exposure in another patient that was managed conservatively (47). For those women with significant anterior vaginal wall prolapse as well as uterine prolapse, another alternative is combining a supracervical hysterectomy with sacrocolpopexy. By removing the uterine fundus, the surgeon may use a "Y-shaped" mesh, in order to support the anterior and posterior vaginal endopelvic fascia. This procedure may be performed open or laparoscopically, depending on patient characteristics and surgeon preference and experience. Although the idea remains controversial, it has been suggested that compared with total hysterectomy, maintaining the cervix may reduce the incidence of mesh exposure at the time of sacrocolpopexy (39).

Although uterine suspension by round ligament plication has been advocated by some experts, theoretical disadvantages of this technique include the inherent weakness of the round ligaments and the resulting anterior displacement of the vagina, which may expose the posterior cul-de-sac to increased abdominal forces, leading to posterior wall defects. Laparoscopic uterine suspension by a combination of uterosacral ligament shortening and round ligament plication has been reported for women with symptomatic uterine retroversion and mild uterine descensus (48). After a mean follow-up of 3 years, all patients had an anteverted uterus, less chronic pelvic pain and dyspareunia, and greater vaginal length. Theoretically, there may be fewer ureteral and infectious complications, as well as reduced blood loss, associated with uterine-sparing procedures. At this time, however, there is a lack of well-designed studies comparing the success rates of prolapse surgery involving hysterectomy to surgery that provides uterine preservation.

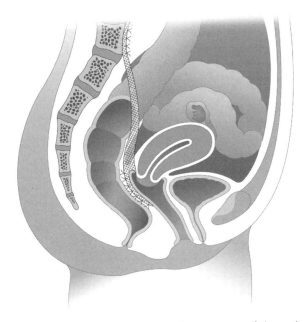

Figure 37. Sacrocervicopexy. Cross-section of the pelvis demonstrating the mesh supporting the posterior endopelvic fascia and cervix to the sacral promontory.

ENTEROCELE

An enterocele is defined as a defect in the endopelvic fascia, where the peritoneum is in direct contact with the vaginal epithelium. Therefore, the traditional approach to enterocele repair, which involves placement of a purse-string suture in the peritoneum around the defect, would be ineffective in reestablishing continuity of the endopelvic fascia. A more appropriate repair of true enteroceles is the reapproximation of the anterior and posterior endopelvic fascia. The vaginal approach to enterocele repair should involve dissection and identification of substantial anterior and posterior endopelvic fascia with excision of redundant, and usually attenuated, vaginal epithelium. Because enteroceles often are discovered in association with a vaginal vault pro-

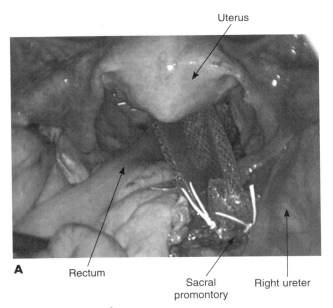
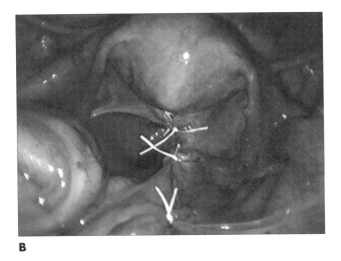

Figure 38. Laparoscopic sacrocervicopexy. **A.** The synthetic mesh has been sutured to the posterior endopelvic fascia and cervix and attached to the anterior longitudinal ligament of the sacrum. **B.** The mesh has been buried under the peritoneum to prevent internal intestinal hernia. (Photos courtesy of Peter L. Rosenblatt.)

lapse, once these fascial planes are reapproximated, they should be suspended using the uterosacral ligaments or other appropriate apical structures. With an abdominal or laparoscopic approach, the apical defect between the pubocervical fascia and the posterior endopelvic fascia most easily can be identified using a solid vaginal probe, and the fascial defect may be closed with or without excision of the redundant vaginal epithelium. The vaginal apex is then attached to the proximal uterosacral ligaments (26).

POSTERIOR COMPARTMENT

Posterior wall defects are most easily repaired using a transvaginal approach, either with plication of the endopelvic fascia or with a site-specific fascial defect repair. There is still a controversy in the literature as to which approach results in better success rates and fewer complications (49–51). The concept of site-specific defects has led to the rapid acceptance of the site-specific posterior repair and a general movement away from traditional levatorplasty, which may lead to postoperative dyspareunia and should probably be abandoned in sexually active women (52). Identification of discrete fascial defects can be facilitated by the surgeon placing his or her finger in the rectum after posterior vaginal dissection. These fascial breaks are then reapproximated over the surgeon's finger with delayed-absorbable sutures. Commonly, a transverse defect may be noted distally between the rectovaginal septum and the perineal body. Lateral and midline defects may be detected and repaired at the same time. Symptomatic improvement, including reductions in constipation, splinting, and tenesmus, has been demonstrated with the discrete defect rectocele repair (50). Natural and synthetic grafts have been used to augment posterior repair procedures (Fig. 39) (53), although the routine use of graft augmentation remains controversial. Apical and lateral attachment sites include the sacrospinous ligament and the lateral pelvic sidewall (levator ani fascia or arcus tendinous fascia pelvis). Distally, surgeons have described graft attachment to the perineal body or directly to the rectovaginal septum.

OBLITERATIVE PROCEDURES

Obliterative procedures may be a viable alternative to more extensive reconstructive surgery in some women who are poor surgical candidates and do not wish to preserve their sexual function. The LeFort procedure can be used to treat uterine procidentia by stripping the anterior and posterior vaginal epithelium and obliterating the vaginal canal by suturing these two denuded layers together, maintaining lateral tunnels for uterine drainage (eg, postmenopausal bleeding)

(Fig. 40). For women with posthysterectomy vaginal vault prolapse, complete colpectomy can be performed by stripping all the vaginal epithelium and suturing the vault closed with consecutive, concentric purse-string sutures, because there is no need to provide an egress for drainage. Obliterative procedures can be performed under local anesthesia, with or without intravenous sedation, which makes these procedures attractive for medically compromised patients. Careful preoperative screening is the most important determinant of patient satisfaction and lack of regret after colpocleisis. The patient must understand that vaginal intercourse is not possible after colpectomy.

PERINEORRHAPHY

For women who are satisfied with pessary use, but are unable to retain a pessary because of a lack of perineal support, a simple, extended perineorrhaphy should be considered. This procedure may be performed under local anesthesia. For some women with uterine prolapse, such a procedure may obviate the need for any pessary postoperatively, whereas for most women with vaginal vault prolapse, a pessary is required to prevent the vaginal wall from prolapsing through the introitus.

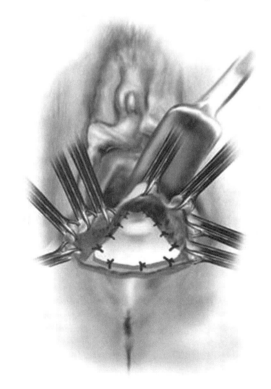

Figure 39. Posterior repair with graft augmentation. (Kohli N, Miklos JR. Dermal graft-augmented rectocele repair. Int Urogynecol J Pelvic Floor Dysfunct 2003;14:146–9. Fig. 3. © International Urogynecological Association 2003. With kind permission of Springer Science and Business Media.)

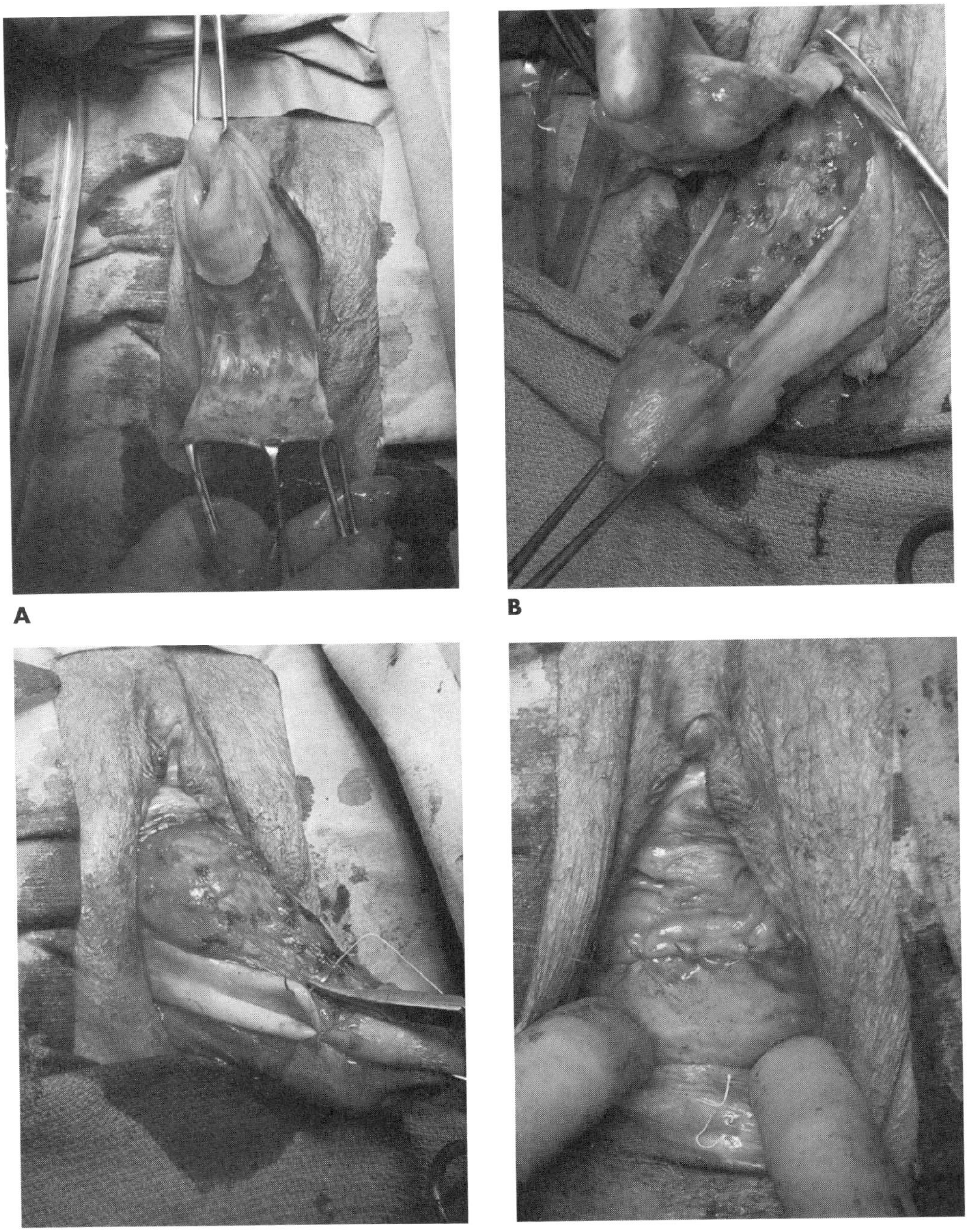

Figure 40. LeFort procedure. **A.** The posterior vaginal wall has been de-epithelialized. **B.** The epithelium has been removed from both the anterior and posterior vaginal walls. **C.** Lateral tunnels are created to allow postoperative drainage for the uterus. **D.** Completed procedure. (Photos courtesy of Peter L. Rosenblatt.)

References

1. Nygaard I, Barber MD, Burgio KL, Kenton K, Meikle S, Schaffer J, et al. Prevalence of symptomatic pelvic floor disorders in US women. JAMA 2008;300:1311–6.

2. Wu JM, Hundley AF, Fulton RG, Myers ER. Forecasting the prevalence of pelvic floor disorders in U.S. women: 2010 to 2050. Obstet Gynecol 2009;114:1278–83.

3. Handa VL, Pannu HK, Siddique S, Gutman R, VanRooyen J, Cundiff G. Architectural differences in the bony pelvis of women with and without pelvic floor disorders. Obstet Gynecol 2003;102:1283–90.

4. DeLancey JO. Anatomic aspects of vaginal eversion after hysterectomy. Am J Obstet Gynecol 1992;166;1717–24; discussion 1724–8.

5. Moalli PA, Jones Ivy S, Meyn LA, Zyczynski HM. Risk factors associated with pelvic floor disorders in women undergoing surgical repair. Obstet Gynecol 2003;101:869–74.

6. Weber AM, Richter HE. Pelvic organ prolapse. Obstet Gynecol 2005;106:615–34.

7. Thakar R, Sultan AH. Hysterectomy and pelvic organ dysfunction. Best Pract Res Clin Obstet Gynaecol 2005;19: 403–18.

8. Altman D, Falconer C, Cnattingius S, Granath F. Pelvic organ prolapse surgery following hysterectomy on benign indications. Am J Obstet Gynecol 2008;198:572.e1–572.e6.

9. Blandon RE, Bharucha AE, Melton LJ 3rd, Schleck CD, Zinsmeister AR, Gebhart JB. Risk factors for pelvic floor repair after hysterectomy. Obstet Gynecol 2009;113:601–8.

10. Dallenbach P, Kaelin-Gambirasio I, Dubuisson JB, Boulvain M. Risk factors for pelvic organ prolapse repair after hysterectomy. Obstet Gynecol 2007;110:625–32.

11. Swift SE, Tate SB, Nicholas J. Correlation of symptoms with degree of pelvic organ support in a general population of women: what is pelvic organ prolapse? Am J Obstet Gynecol 2003;189:372–7; discussion 377–9.

12. Ellerkmann RM, Cundiff GW, Melick CF, Nihira MA, Leffler K, Bent AE. Correlation of symptoms with location and severity of pelvic organ prolapse. Am J Obstet Gynecol 2001;185:1332–7; discussion 1337–8.

13. Tan JS, Lukacz ES, Menefee SA, Powell CR, Nager CW. Predictive value of prolapse symptoms: a large database study. San Diego Pelvic Floor Consortium. Int Urogynecol J Pelvic Floor Dysfunct 2005;16:203–9; discussion 209.

14. Kenton K, Shott S, Brubaker L. Vaginal topography does not correlate well with visceral position in women with pelvic organ prolapse. Int Urogynecol J Pelvic Floor Dysfunct 1997;8:336–9.

15. Kudish BI, Iglesia CB, Sokol RJ, Cochrane B, Richter HE, Larson J, et al. Effect of weight change on natural history of pelvic organ prolapse. Obstet Gynecol 2009;113:81–8.

16. Clemons JL, Aguilar VC, Tillinghast TA, Jackson ND, Myers DL. Risk factors associated with an unsuccessful pessary fitting trial in women with pelvic organ prolapse. Am J Obstet Gynecol 2004;190:345–50.

17. Clemons JL, Aguilar VC, Tillinghast TA, Jackson ND, Myers DL. Patient satisfaction and changes in prolapse and urinary symptoms in women who were fitted successfully with a pessary for pelvic organ prolapse. Am J Obstet Gynecol 2004;190:1025–9.

18. Brincat C, Kenton K, Fitzgerald M, Brubaker L. Sexual activity predicts continued pessary use. Am J Obstet Gynecol 2004;191:198–200.

19. Jones KA, Shepard JP, Oliphant SS, Wang L, Bunker CH, Lowder JL. Trends in inpatient prolapse procedures in the United States, 1979–2006. Am J Obstet Gynecol 2010; 202:501.e1–501.e7.

20. Olsen AL, Smith VJ, Bergstrom JO, Colling JS, Clark AL. Epidemiology of surgically managed pelvic organ prolapse and urinary incontinence. Obstet Gynecol 1997;89:501–6.

21. Marchionni M, Bracco GL, Checcucci V, Carabaneau A, Coccia EM, Mecacci F, et al. True incidence of vaginal vault prolapse. Thirteen years of experience. J Reprod Med 1999;44:679–84.

22. Clark AL, Gregory T, Smith VJ, Edwards R. Epidemiologic evaluation of reoperation for surgically treated pelvic organ prolapse and urinary incontinence. Am J Obstet Gynecol 2003;189:1261–7.

23. Brubaker L, Cundiff GW, Fine P, Nygaard I, Richter HE, Visco AG, et al. Abdominal sacrocolpopexy with Burch colposuspension to reduce urinary stress incontinence. Pelvic Floor Disorders Network. N Engl J Med 2006; 354:1557–66.

24. Maher C, Feiner B, Baessler K, Glazener CM. Surgical management of pelvic organ prolapse in women. Cochrane Database of Systematic Reviews 2010, Issue 4. Art. No.: CD004014. DOI: 10.1002/14651858.CD004014.pub4.

25. Weber AM, Walters MD, Piedmonte MR, Ballard LA. Anterior colporrhaphy: a randomized trial of three surgical techniques. Am J Obstet Gynecol 2001;185:1299–304; discussion 1304–6.

26. Paraiso MF, Falcone T, Walters MD. Laparoscopic surgery for enterocele, vaginal apex prolapse and rectocele. Int Urogynecol J Pelvic Floor Dysfunct 1999;10:223–9.

27. Geller EJ, Siddiqui NY, Wu JM, Visco AG. Short-term outcomes of robotic sacrocolpopexy compared with abdominal sacrocolpopexy. Obstet Gynecol 2008;112:1201–6.

28. Elliott DS, Krambeck AE, Chow GK. Long-term results of robotic assisted laparoscopic sacrocolpopexy for the treatment of high grade vaginal vault prolapse. J Urol 2006;176:655–9.

29. Pelvic organ prolapse. ACOG Practice Bulletin No. 85. American College of Obstetricians and Gynecologists. Obstet Gynecol 2007;110:717–29.

30. Iglesia CB, Fenner DE, Brubaker L. The use of mesh in gynecologic surgery. Int Urogynecol J Pelvic Floor Dysfunct 1997;8:105–15.

31. Sung VW, Rogers RG, Schaffer JI, Balk EM, Uhlig K, Lau J, et al. Graft use in transvaginal pelvic organ prolapse repair: a systematic review. Society of Gynecologic Surgeons Systematic Review Group. Obstet Gynecol 2008; 112:1131–42.

32. Richardson AC, Lyon JB, Williams NL. A new look at pelvic relaxation. Am J Obstet Gynecol 1976;126:568–73.

33. Seman EI, Cook JR, O'Shea RT. Two–year experience with laparoscopic pelvic floor repair. J Am Assoc Gynecol Laparosc 2003;10:38–45.

34. Young SB, Daman JJ, Bony LG. Vaginal paravaginal repair: one-year outcomes. Am J Obstet Gynecol 2001;185:1360–6; discussion 1366–7.

35. Hiltunen R, Nieminen K, Takala T, Heiskanen E, Merikari M, Niemi K, et al. Low-weight polypropylene mesh for anterior vaginal wall prolapse: a randomized controlled trial. Obstet Gynecol 2007;110:455–62.

36. Hinoul P, Ombelet WU, Burger MP, Roovers JP. A prospective study to evaluate the anatomic and functional outcome of a transobturator mesh kit (prolift anterior) for symptomatic cystocele repair. J Minim Invasive Gynecol 2008;15:615–20.

37. Letouzey V, de Tayrac R, Deffieux X. Long-term results after trans-vaginal cystocele repair using tension-free polypropylene mesh [abstract]. J Minim Invasive Gynecol 2008; 15:S28.

38. Maher CF, Qatawneh AM, Dwyer PL, Carey MP, Cornish A, Schluter PJ. Abdominal sacral colpopexy or vaginal sacrospinous colpopexy for vaginal vault prolapse: a prospective randomized study. Am J Obstet Gynecol 2004; 190:20–6.

39. Nygaard IE, McCreery R, Brubaker L, Connolly A, Cundiff G, Weber AM, et al. Abdominal sacrocolpopexy: a comprehensive review. Pelvic Floor Disorders Network. Obstet Gynecol 2004;104:805–23.

40. Cosson M, Rajabally R, Bogaert E, Querleu D, Crepin G. Laparoscopic sacrocolpopexy, hysterectomy, and burch colposuspension: feasibility and short-term complications of 77 procedures. JSLS 2002;6:115–9.

41. Drent D. Laparoscopic sacrocolpopexy for vaginal vault prolapse: personal experience [Letter]. N Z Med J 2001; 114:505.

42. Farnsworth BN. Posterior intravaginal slingplasty (infracoccygeal sacropexy) for severe posthysterectomy vaginal vault prolapse--a preliminary report on efficacy and safety. Int Urogynecol J Pelvic Floor Dysfunct 2002;13:4–8.

43. Karp D, Apostolis C, Lefevre R, Davila GW. Atypical graft infection presenting as a remote draining sinus. Obstet Gynecol 2009;114:443–5.

44. Luck AM, Steele AC, Leong FC, McLennan MT. Short-term efficacy and complications of posterior intravaginal slingplasty. Int Urogynecol J Pelvic Floor Dysfunct 2008;19:795–9.

45. Diwan A, Rardin CR, Kohli N. Uterine preservation during surgery for uterovaginal prolapse: a review. Int Urogynecol J Pelvic Floor Dysfunct 2004;15:286–92.

46. Maher CF, Cary MP, Slack MS, Murray CJ, Milligan M, Schluter P. Uterine preservation or hysterectomy at sacrospinous colpopexy for uterovaginal prolapse? Int Urogynecol J Pelvic Floor Dysfunct 2001;12:381–4; discussion 384–5.

47. Rosenblatt PL, Chelmow D, Ferzandi TR. Laparoscopic sacrocervicopexy for the treatment of uterine prolapse: a retrospective case series report. J Min Invasive Gynecol 2008;15:268–72.

48. Yen CF, Wang CJ, Lin SL, Lee CL, Soong YK. Combined laparoscopic uterosacral and round ligament procedures for treatment of symptomatic uterine retroversion and mild uterine descensus. J Am Assoc Gynecol Laparosc 2002;9:359–66.

49. Paraiso MF, Weber A, Walters M, Ballard L, Piedmonte MR, Skibinski C. Anatomic and functional outcome after posterior colporrhaphy. J Pelvic Surg 2001;7:335–9.

50. Cundiff GW, Weidner AS, Visco AG, Addison WA, Bump RC. An anatomic and functional assessment of the discrete defect rectocele repair. Am J Obstet Gynecol 1998;179: 1451–6; discussion 1456–7.

51. Abramov Y, Gandhi S, Goldberg RP, Botros SM, Kwon C, Sand PK. Site-specific rectocele repair compared with standard posterior colporrhaphy. Obstet Gynecol 2005; 105:314–8.

52. Lukacz ES, Luber KM. Rectocele repair: when and how? Curr Urol Rep 2002;3:418–22.

53. Kohli N, Miklos JR. Dermal graft-augmented rectocele repair. Int Urogynecol J Pelvic Floor Dysfunct 2003;14: 146–9.

Surgical Management of Incontinence

Cheryl B. Iglesia

Management of incontinence usually involves conservative measures, such as lifestyle and diet alterations, pelvic floor exercises, use of incontinence devices, and medications as a first-line therapy. When these measures fail or a patient desires a more permanent solution, surgical treatment of incontinence is indicated as the next step in therapy.

Surgery for Stress Urinary Incontinence

The two surgical treatments that have withstood the test of time and have the most evidence for long-term efficacy are the retropubic colposuspension procedure and the suburethral sling procedure. Over the past decade, significant technologic improvements for the latter have resulted in the advent of tension-free synthetic suburethral sling procedures, specifically the retropubic tension-free suburethral sling, which was developed in 1996, and the transobturator sling, which was developed in 2001.

Retropubic Colposuspension

The goal of retropubic urethropexy or colposuspension procedures is to support the bladder neck and urethra in a retropubic position, thus preventing the descent of the anterior vaginal wall during episodes of increased intraabdominal pressure (eg, coughing). Developed in

the late 1940s by Drs. Marshall, Marchetti, and Krantz and modified in the 1960s by Dr. John Burch, this urethrovaginal fixation procedure uses two or three nonabsorbable or delayed absorbable sutures placed at the level of the bladder neck and at the level of the midurethra and secures the sutures directly into the retropubic periosteum (the Marshall–Marchetti–Krantz approach) or in the Cooper (or pectineal) ligament on each side of the pubic symphysis (Burch procedure) as depicted in Figure 41. The Marshall–Marchetti–Krantz procedure is associated with the serious complication of osteitis pubis, a painful inflammatory condition of the periosteum and cartilage; therefore, the Burch procedure is the more commonly performed retropubic suspension.

With follow-up from several months to 10–20 years, the long-term success of the Burch colposuspension ranges from 69–90% (1). Conditions that may negatively affect cure rates from Burch procedures include prior antiincontinence operations and intrinsic urethral sphincter deficiency (low urethral closure or leak-point pressures on urodynamic testing). Most complications from the procedure relate to voiding dysfunction, urge incontinence, and development of vaginal vault or posterior wall prolapse.

A multicenter randomized trial found no difference between Burch colposuspension and tension-free vaginal tape procedures, with objective cure rates for urodynamic stress incontinence of 57% and 66%,

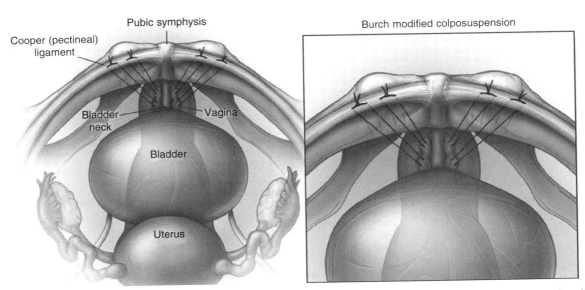

Figure 41. Burch colposuspension. (Albo ME, Richter HE, Brubaker L, Norton P, Kraus SR, Zimmern PE, et al. Burch colposuspension versus fascial sling to reduce urinary stress incontinence. Urinary Incontinence Treatment Network. N Engl J Med 2007; 356:2143–55. Copyright © 2007 Massachusets Medical Society. All rights reserved.)

respectively. Cystotomy was more common during the tension-free vaginal tape procedure than during colposuspension. Delayed voiding, operative time, and return to normal activity all lasted longer after colposuspension compared with the tension-free vaginal tape procedure (2). Five-year follow-up did not detect a significant difference between tension-free vaginal tape procedure and colposuspension for the cure of stress incontinence or for improvement in quality of life. The effect of both procedures on cure of incontinence at 5 years based on a negative 1-hour pad test was 81% in the tension-free vaginal tape group and 90% in the colposuspension group. There was an increase in enterocoele and rectocele formation postoperatively in the colposuspension group; three late tape erosions were seen in the tension-free vaginal tape group (3). Long-term follow-up rates of patients undergoing tension-free vaginal tape and laparoscopic Burch colposuspensions were compared. Tension-free vaginal tape procedure has similar long-term efficacy to laparoscopic Burch for the treatment of stress urinary incontinence at a median follow-up of 65 months (4–8 years) with 11% in the laparoscopic Burch group and 8% in the tension-free vaginal tape group reporting bothersome stress urinary incontinence symptoms (4). Open and laparoscopic Burch procedures are occasionally reserved for patients undergoing concomitant pelviscopy, those wishing future fertility in which synthetic slings are relatively contraindicated, or those with known adverse reaction to foreign mesh materials.

The Urinary Incontinence Treatment Network and the Pelvic Floor Disorders Network have published level 1 evidence on surgical treatment for stress urinary incontinence (see Appendix A). Because these prospective, multicenter clinical trials used strict outcome criteria as well as validated quality-of-life instruments, they provide some of the most accurate data ever published about the Burch procedure. The pubovaginal (autologous) sling had a higher cure rate compared to the Burch procedure, but was associated with more complications. At 24 months, the overall success rate for women who underwent the pubovaginal sling procedure was 47% compared with 38% for those who underwent the Burch procedure. Success rates specific to stress incontinence were 66% for slings versus 49% for the Burch procedure. More women who underwent the sling procedure had urinary tract infections, difficulty voiding, and postoperative urge incontinence (5). A prophylactic Burch procedure at the time of abdominal sacrocolpopexy significantly reduced both subjective and objective stress urinary incontinence. Three months after surgery, 23.8% of the women in the Burch group and 44% of the controls met the criteria for stress incontinence with 6% of Burch patients reporting bothersome symptoms of stress incontinence versus 25% of controls. By 1 year, fewer women in the

Burch group had stress incontinence (25% versus 40% for controls) and fewer women had urge incontinence as well (14.5% versus 26.8%) (6, 7).

Suburethral Sling Procedures

Suburethral sling procedures date back to the turn of the twentieth century when autologous slings were introduced. They were further popularized in the early 1940s by Dr. Aldridge who used strips of rectus fascia and secured them beneath the urethra. The mechanism of the sling was based on using the patient's own tissue to compress and partially obstruct the urethra by placing a strap support at the bladder neck; however, there was a high incidence of voiding dysfunction and urinary retention associated with this procedure. Autologous tissues used for pubovaginal sling procedures include rectus fascia, fascia lata, vaginal wall, and various allografts (cadaver tissues) and xenografts (animal tissues) (Fig. 42).

In the 1990s, a new theory was developed for the treatment of stress incontinence based on the model that continence is maintained at the midurethra with reinforcement of the pubourethral ligament and simultaneous reinforcement of the suburethral vaginal hammock and its connection to the levator ani via the pubococcygeus muscles (8). These investigators determined that the midurethra is the preferred location for slings and provided a backboard for intermittent compression of the urethra without causing outright obstruction. The midurethral sling procedure was the tension-free vaginal tape sling, a retropubic sling using synthetic polypropylene mesh material.

TECHNIQUES

Retropubic Synthetic Tension-Free Sling. The sling material is composed of monofilament polypropylene mesh and measures approximately 1.1 cm × 45 cm. The procedure can be performed under general, regional, or local anesthesia with sedation. A single dose of intravenous antibiotics is administered before making an incision. The procedure begins with a placement of an 18-French catheter for drainage of the bladder. The suprapubic sites are marked approximately 1 cm superior to the pubic symphysis and 2–3 cm, lateral to the midline. A spinal needle is used to inject 10 mL of a local anesthetic along each retropubic site. Hydrodissection is performed along the anterior vaginal wall with an additional 10 mL of local anesthetic with epinephrine. Using a scalpel, a 1.5–2 cm vertical incision is made approximately 1 cm from the external urethral meatus and the dissection is carried out laterally until the inferior margin of the pubic rami is palpated bilaterally. In contrast with a pubovaginal sling, perforation of the urogenital diaphragm is not recommended for synthetic slings.

Autologous sling procedure

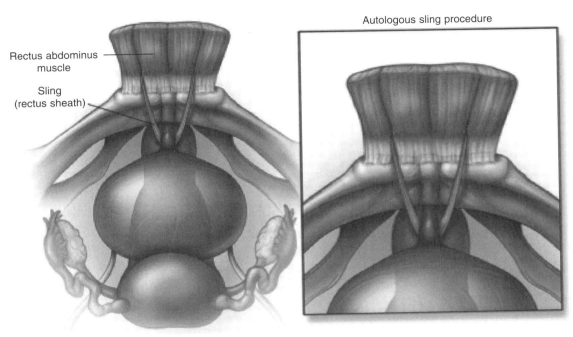

Figure 42. Autologous pubovaginal sling. (Albo ME, Richter HE, Brubaker L, Norton P, Kraus SR, Zimmern PE, et al. Burch colposuspension versus fascial sling to reduce urinary stress incontinence. Urinary Incontinence Treatment Network. N Engl J Med 2007;356:2143–55. Copyright © 2007 Massachusets Medical Society. All rights reserved.)

A rigid catheter guide is placed in the Foley catheter to move the urethra and bladder to the contralateral side as the needle is passed. Using the introducer, the needle is passed paraurethrally piercing the urogenital diaphragm in line with the patient's ipsilateral shoulder to avoid obturator and lateral pelvic sidewall structures, which are located just 3.2–3.9 cm away (Fig. 43) (9). The tip of the needle is in close contact with the pubic bone as the needle tip is directed upwards to the abdominal skin demarcations. Cystoscopy is performed after each needle passage to ensure bladder integrity. Once urethral and bladder integrity has been confirmed, the bladder is filled with approximately 300 mL and the sling is adjusted loosely without overcorrection using either a cough-stress test with the patient awake, the Credé maneuver pushing on the suprapubic region, or using an eyeball technique to judge sling tightness. Some surgeons prefer to place a right angle clamp or rigid dilator as a spacer between the inferior urethra and the mesh during sling tensioning. The plastic sheaths are removed, the excess mesh material is cut flush with the skin and skin incisions are sutured. The vaginal incision also is closed using fine absorbable suture. A transurethral catheter is placed and the patient undergoes a voiding trial after the procedure. Several modifications to the original tension-free sling have been designed to include a top-down suprapubic approach, dyed mesh, and smaller caliber needle introducers with built-in spacers at the mid-point of the mesh.

Synthetic Transobturator Sling. In 2001, the first transobturator sling that completely avoided the retropubic space was described. The path of the needle was created to avoid serious complications from bowel, vessel, and lower urinary tract injury that had all been previously associated with synthetic retropubic slings. The sling material also is composed of monofilament polypropylene mesh 1.1 cm × 50 cm and is macroporous with adequate pore size. Microporous mesh materials have been designed for use with transobturator slings in the past, but these mesh materials are less likely to incorporate into tissue and are more easily infected causing thigh abscess formation because bacteria can permeate the micropores. Specialized coatings on synthetic polypropylene mesh can also adversely affect the graft material affecting tensile strength and, thus, increase the risk for local infection and erosion as well.

The patient under general, regional, or local anesthesia with sedation is placed in the lithotomy position in adjustable stirrups. A transurethral Foley catheter is placed and the bladder is drained. With one finger in the anterior vaginal fornix and the thumb in the superior medial margin of the obturator foramen, lateral to the labium majorum, a surgeon marks the area where the skin incision should be made, which in general is in line with the clitoris. The anterior vagina is hydrodissected and a 2 cm incision is made 1 cm below the external urethral meatus. Metzenbaum scissors are used to dissect the periurethral tissue until the tip of the scissor touches the medial aspect of the inferior

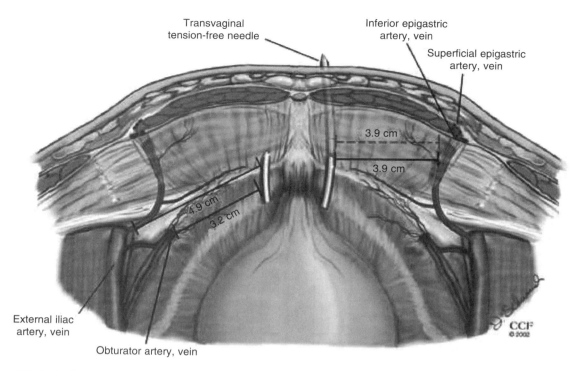

Figure 43. Path of the tension-free vaginal tape needle for synthetic retropubic slings. (Muir TW, Tulikangas PK, Fidela Paraiso MF, Walters MD. The relationship of tension-free vaginal tape insertion and the vascular anatomy. Obstet Gynecol 2003; 101:933–6.)

pubic ramus (approximately 1–1.5 cm). Fingertip dissection is performed bilaterally. Local anesthesia is used to infiltrate the transobturator region over the previously demarcated perineal skin site corresponding to the superior medical obturator foramen. Stab incisions are made and the transobturator needles are passed through the skin incision, through the obturator foramen, curving around the posterior surface of the ischiopubic ramus guiding the needle tip with the index finger into the vaginal incision as depicted in Figure 44. The needle path is around the ischiopubic ramus, penetrating the gracilis, adductor brevis, obtu-

rator externus muscles, obturator membrane, obturator internus muscle, and periurethral endopelvic fascia and exits through the vaginal incision. The transobturator sling passes on average 2.4 cm inferior–medial to the obturator canal (10). Care must be taken to avoid buttonholing or perforating the lateral vaginal sulci. The needle passage is performed bilaterally and cystoscopy should confirm urethral and bladder integrity. The mesh is attached to the needle introducer and placed without tension along the midurethra. Plastic sheaths are removed and the excess mesh is cut flush with the skin. Skin and vaginal incisions are closed with fine delayed absorbable sutures. Modifications to the transobturator slings have been made, including the use of helical and curved needle passers, as well as an inside-to-outside approach.

Trocarless Slings. This technique involves placing mini-slings as hammocks from an inside-to-outside approach via a vaginal incision with no exit points along the perineal skin or suprapubic region. Some of the slings are secured with polypropylene fixation tips directly into the obturator muscles and some are secured directly behind the pubic bone. No long-term comparative data on efficacy are available for these slings, but they may have an advantage of less vascular or visceral injury as well as less postoperative pain because they require smaller incisions compared with traditional retropubic and transobturator slings.

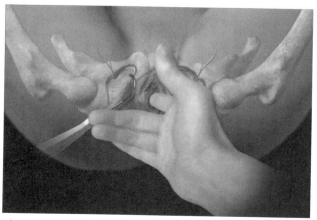

Figure 44. Path of the outside-to-inside transobturator sling. (Provided by Ethicon, Inc.)

OUTCOMES

Compared with pubovaginal slings, some of the advantages of midurethral synthetic slings are shorter operative time, ability to perform the procedure under local anesthesia on an outpatient basis, and possibly less voiding dysfunction as a result of their tension-free placement. Other complications that can occur with synthetic retropubic slings range from cystotomy (that ordinarily has no long-term sequelae) to vaginal mesh erosion. Major complications include serious synthetic mesh infection, fistula formation, as well as life-threatening bowel and vascular injuries. Despite the potential for complications, long-term data confirming durability and safety are available for synthetic mesh slings. In a review of 11 years worth of safety and efficacy data on the retropubic tension-free vaginal tape sling, the objective cure rate was 84% with a subjective cure rate of 77%. No late adverse effects of the operation were found (11).

Although the risk of complications from synthetic slings is low, surgeons should remain vigilant about searching for complications in patients undergoing synthetic sling procedures. Table 12 lists complications from a multicenter Austrian registry for tension-free vaginal tape retropubic slings and a variety of transobturator slings. Bladder injury is higher in the retropubic sling registry but the need for reoperation for loosening of the sling is similar between the two.

A few randomized comparative trials have been conducted comparing transobturator slings and retropubic slings (Table 13). In these studies, most patients in both arms had significant improvement in quality of life as well as objective cure of stress incontinence. Long-term follow-up and use of slings in patients with intrinsic sphincter deficiency, prior incontinence procedures, and concomitant prolapse surgery still need to be evaluated. The largest randomized clinical trial on retropubic versus transobturator slings by the Urinary Incontinence Treatment Network (12) showed similar objective cure rates between the two slings. In this landmark trial, there was more voiding dysfunction in the retropubic sling patients (3.4% versus 1.3%) and more early postoperative neurologic complications (numbness and weakness) in the transobturator group (9.4% versus 4%). Rates of mesh exposure in the vagina were low and did not differ between groups (1.3% retropubic and 1.0% transobturator) and new onset urge incontinence was also low (0% retropubic, 0.3% transobturator).

MANAGEMENT OF COMPLICATIONS FROM SYNTHETIC SUBURETHRAL SLINGS

Bladder injury is the most commonly reported complication after synthetic suburethral sling placement. Management entails recognition and replacement of the sling in a more lateral position. Some form of bladder drainage is recommended for a few days depending on the location and size of the injury. Voiding dysfunction and urge incontinence also are known complications after sling operations and may require sling takedown or anticholinergic medication. Timing of the sling revision is determined by the patient's symptoms and the surgeon's judgment. Although some surgeons may proceed with early sling cutting or loosening within the first 2 weeks, others may wait up to 3 months depending on the degree of bother to the patient and the comfort level with intermittent self-catheterization. Sling erosion into the urethra or bladder will require mesh excision and repair in layers as soon as the injury is recognized.

Other rare complications include vessel injury resulting in retropubic hematoma formation or significant blood loss, nerve injury, occult small bowel injury, and severe infection with necrotizing fasciitis. Case reports of each of these complications have been described. These complications may require early recognition, supportive care, vascular embolization or reoperation via exploratory laparotomy, bowel resection or repair of vascular defect. Erosion of the mesh into the vagina or thigh abscess formation will require mesh removal and appropriate antibiotic treatment and wound management.

PERIURETHRAL BULKING INJECTIONS

Urethral bulking agents may be used to increase urethral resistance at the bladder neck. Common injec-

Table 12. Complications listed in the Austrian registry for tension-free vaginal tape and transobturator sling procedures

	Retropubic synthetic slings n=2,795	Transobturator slings n=2,543
Bladder perforation	2.7%	0.4%
Urethral perforation	Not reported	0.1%
Vaginal perforation	Not reported	0.4%
Increased bleeding	2.3% (0.7% reoperation for hematoma)	3.3%
Reoperation for tape loosening or tape cutting	1.0%	0.9%
Vaginal mesh erosion	Not reported	0.4%

Data from Tamussino K, Hanzal E, Kolle D, Ralph G, Riss P. Tension-free vaginal tape operation: results of the Austrian registry. Austrian Urogynecology Working Group. Obstet Gynecol 2001;98:732–6 and Tamussino K, Hanzal E, Kolle D, Tammaa A, Preyer O, Umek W, et al. Transobturator tapes for stress urinary incontinence: Results of the Austrian registry. Austrian Urogynecology Working Group. Am J Obstet Gynecol 2007;197:634.e1–634.e5.

Table 13. Outcomes of Comparative Trials of Tension-Free Vaginal Tape Versus Transobturator Sling Procedure

Study	Follow-up	N	Cure	Complications
Ross*	12 months	105 retropubic TVT; 94 transobturator TOT	77% cure[†] TVT 81% cure[†] TOT P, not significant	More groin pain and more palpable mesh in the TOT group than in the TVT group
Barber[‡]	18 months	88 TVT 82 TOT	92% TVT 87% TOT TOT not inferior to TVT	More bladder perforations in the TVT group (7%) vs TOT group (0%)
Richter[§]	12 month	298 TVT 299 TOT	80.8% TVT 77.7% TOT equivalent objective cure[¶]	More voiding dysfunction requiring surgery or use of catheter was seen in TVT (2.7 % TVT and 0% TOT) and more neurologic symptoms (9.4% vs 4%) in TOT

Abbreviations: TOT indicates transobturator sling; TVT, tension-free vaginal tape.

*Ross S, Robert M, Swaby C, Dederer L, Lier D, Tang S, et al. Transobturator tape compared with tension-free vaginal tape for stress urinary incontinence: a randomized controlled trial. Obstet Gynecol 2009;114;1287–94.

[†]On pad test.

[‡]Barber MD, Kleeman S, Karram MM, Paraiso MF, Walters MD, Vasavada S, et al. Transobturator tape compared with tension-free vaginal tape for the treatment of stress urinary incontinence: a randomized controlled trial. Obstet Gynecol 2008;111:611–21.

[§]Richter HE, Albo ME, Zyczynski HM, Kenton K, Norton PA, Sirls LT, et al. Retropubic versus transobturator midurethral slings for stress incontinence. Urinary Incontinence Treatment Network. N Engl J Med 2010;362:2066–76.

[¶]Objective cure made by a composite of negative stress test, a negative pad test, and no retreatment.

tion agents include glutaraldehyde cross-linked bovine collagen, pyrolytic carbon coated beads, and calcium hydroxyapatite particles. These materials may be injected via transurethral or periurethral needles inserted with cystoscopic guidance at multiple sites at the bladder neck under local anesthesia or mild sedation. The periurethral injections are used in women who have medical conditions precluding them from having definitive suburethral sling or colposuspension procedures. Periurethral injections also are used for patients with intrinsic sphincter deficiency, in those who have failed prior sling or anti-incontinence operations, or in those wishing to avoid more invasive surgical options. Cure rates for urethral bulking agents are high for the first few months but most patients require repeat injections by 12 months. Few comparative trials have been published but one trial comparing calcium hydroxyapatite with collagen at 12 months showed equal efficacy with 63.4% of the patients in the calcium hydroxyapatite group and 57% of the patients in the collagen group showing improvement of one Stamey grade or more. More patients in the calcium hydroxyapatite group required only one injection with less total bulking agent during the study compared with the patients in the collagen group (13). Newer autologous and tissue-engineered urethral bulking agents are in development and these may provide more durable long-term results with less immunogenic responses and fewer complications.

Surgery for Fecal Incontinence

Fecal incontinence often coexists with urinary incontinence. Surgical treatment for fecal incontinence has much lower success rates than surgery for urinary incontinence and may relate to more significant neuromuscular impairment, especially after anal sphincter lacerations. Proper surgical repair involves identifying the separate structures involved—the bowel wall, the internal anal sphincter, the external anal sphincter, the perineal body, the bulbocavernosus muscle, and the vaginal wall. Endoanal ultrasonography and magnetic resonance imaging are useful in identifying the extent of internal and external anal sphincter defects preoperatively.

Long-term follow-up (5–10 years) from sphincteroplasty procedures shows low continence rates of 24–46% (14, 15). Improvement of anal incontinence symptoms is possible but cure is so rare that some experts advocate that prevention of anal sphincter laceration is key to maintaining fecal continence.

Muscle transposition procedures, artificial anal sphincters, and postanal repairs have also been described for fecal incontinence with mixed results. Occasionally, diverting colostomies and ileostomies are options for more refractory cases and may be most liberating to patients who have unpredictable episodes of fecal incontinence. Sacral neuromodulation, also known as direct sacral stimulation, has recently been approved by the U.S. Food and Drug Administration for treatment of fecal incontinence and involves directly stimulating nerves, primarily S3. The treatment was initially approved for refractory urge urinary incontinence as well as voiding dysfunction. Perfect continence was accomplished in 47% of patients in the sacral nerve stimulation group and a significant improvement in fecal incontinence quality of life index was noted compared to the control group undergoing optimal medical therapy (16).

Level I evidence exists for cure of stress urinary incontinence with the Burch retropubic colposuspension, tension-free vaginal midurethral slings, and pubovaginal sling procedures. Burch procedures performed prophylactically at the time of abdominal sacrocolpopexy also are beneficial. Although complications related to needle insertion and foreign mesh material do occur with retropubic and transobturator tension-free slings, both appear to have comparable subjective and objective cure rates.

Outcomes for surgery for fecal incontinence show only modest long-term cures, especially for anal sphincteroplasties. Direct sacral neuromodulation may prove to be beneficial for women with fecal incontinence.

References

1. Dainer M, Hall CD, Choe J, Bhatia NN. The Burch procedure: a comprehensive review. Obstet Gynecol Surv 1999;54:49–60.

2. Ward K, Hilton P. Prospective multicentre randomised trial of tension-free vaginal tape and colposuspension as primary treatment for stress incontinence. United Kingdom and Ireland Tension-free Vaginal Tape Trial Group. BMJ 2002;325:67–70.

3. Ward KL, Hilton P. Tension-free vaginal tape versus colposuspension for primary urodynamic stress incontinence: 5-year follow up. UK and Ireland TVT Trial Group. BJOG 2008;115:226–33.

4. Jelovsek JE, Barber MD, Karram MM, Walters MD, Paraiso MF. Randomized trial of laparoscopic Burch colposuspension versus tension-free vaginal tape:long-term follow-up. BJOG 2008;115:219–25; discussion 252.

5. Albo ME, Richter HE, Brubaker L, Norton P, Kraus SR, Zimmern PE, et al. Burch colposuspension versus fascial sling to reduce urinary stress incontinence. Urinary Incontinence Treatment Network. N Engl J Med 2007;356: 2143–55.

6. Brubaker L, Cundiff GW, Fine P, Nygaard I, Richter HE, Visco AG, et al. Abdominal sacrocolpopexy with Burch colposuspension to reduce urinary stress incontinence. Pelvic Floor Disorders Network. N Engl J Med 2006; 354:1557–66.

7. Burgio KL, Nygaard IE, Richter HE, Brubaker L, Gutman RE, Leng W, et al. Bladder symptoms 1 year after abdominal sacrocolpopexy with and without Burch colposuspension in women without preoperative stress incontinence symptoms. Pelvic Floor Disorders Network. Am J Obstet Gynecol 2007;197:647.e1–647.e6.

8. Petros PE, Ulmsten UI. An integral theory of female urinary incontinence. Experimental and clinical considerations. Acta Obstet Gynecol Scand Suppl 1990;153:7–31.

9. Muir TW, Tulikangas PK, Fidela Paraiso M, Walters MD. The relationship of tension-free vaginal tape insertion and the vascular anatomy. Obstet Gynecol 2003;101:933–6.

10. Whiteside JL, Walters MD. Anatomy of the obturator region: relations to a trans-obturator sling. Int Urogynecol J Pelvic Floor Dysfunct 2004;15:223–6.

11. Olsson I, Abrahamsson AK, Kroon UB. Long-term efficacy of the tension-free vaginal tape procedure for the treatment of urinary incontinence: A retrospective follow-up of 11.5 years post-operatively. Int Urogynecol J Pelvic Floor Dysfunct 2010;21:679–83.

12. Richter HE, Albo ME, Zyczynski HM, Kenton K, Norton PA, Sirls LT, et al. Retropubic versus transobturator midurethral slings for stress incontinence. Urinary Incontinnce Treatment Network. N Engl J Med 2010;362:2066–76.

13. Mayer RD, Dmochowski RR, Appell RA, Sand PK, Klimberg IW, Jacoby K, et al. Multicenter prospective randomized 52-week trial of calcium hydroxylapatite versus bovine dermal collagen for treatment of stress urinary incontinence. Urology 2007;69:876–80.

14. Trowbridge, ER, Morgan, D, Trowbridge MJ, Delancey JO, Fenner DE. Sexual function, quality of life, and severity of anal incontinence after anal sphincteroplasty. Am J Obstet Gynecol 2006;195:1753–7.

15. Halverson AL, Hull TL. Long-term outcome of overlapping anal sphincter repair. Dis Colon Rectum 2002;45:345–8.

16. Tjandra JJ, Chan MK, Yeh CH, Murray-Green C. Sacral nerve stimulation is more effective than optimal medical therapy for severe fecal incontinence: a randomized, controlled study. Dis Colon Rectum 2008;51:494–502.

Management of Uterine Leiomyomas

Deborah S. Lyon

Etiology and Epidemiology

Leiomyomas are known by many other names, the most common of which are "fibroids". All nomenclature reflects the nature of this tumor as part muscle, part connective tissue, and altogether benign. Leiomyomas remain the most commonly occurring solid pelvic tumors among women (1) and the most common indication for benign hysterectomy (2). Although a great deal has been learned in the past century about the nature and behavior of these tumors, much about them remains shrouded in mystery and confusion.

Prevalence of leiomyomas in the U.S. population has been reported in the 20–50% range by the time of menopause, with higher numbers quoted for African American women. However, these numbers often are based on self-reports or hysterectomy data underestimating the frequency of asymptomatic leiomyomas. A study using universal ultrasound screening showed prevalences of uterine leiomyomas of nearly 70% for white women and more than 80% for black women by age 50 years (3).

Incidence of identification of leiomyomas increases with increasing age, with a peak in the 40s and a sharp decrease after menopause. This trend is consistent with the estrogen-sensitivity of these tumors. Some experts have also reported a correlation with increasing body mass index, but this finding is variable. There is a clear increase in prevalence among African American women compared with Caucasians, which does not appear to be explained by other potentially confounding variables and which strongly suggests a genetic component to the condition (4). Of note is the fact that leiomyomas often are identified when a woman is evaluated ultrasonographically for menstrual difficulties. The latter are more prevalent as women age, thus explaining why leiomyomas are diagnosed more often with an increased age.

Genetics

Because of the racial disparity associated with occurrence of leiomyomas, there has long been suspected to be a genetic component to the pathology. Studies of families and particularly of monozygotic twins further support this connection. Studies at the histologic and molecular levels have not been very revealing, however. Most leiomyomas are chromosomally normal, and the remainder exhibit a wide variety of trisomies, translocations, deletions, and rearrangements. There is,

however, a small group of patients exhibiting a strong predisposition to both leiomyomatosis (widely disseminated leiomyomas) and renal cell carcinoma, collectively labeled as *hereditary leiomyomatosis and renal cell carcinoma syndrome*. This well-defined and highly symptomatic patient population has enabled much more detailed genetic study, including the discovery of mutations in the fumarate hydratase gene that lead to diminished suppressor function in relation to leiomyoma formation (5). This is an autosomal dominant disease, whereas most common leiomyomas appear to be inherited in a multifactorial fashion. Nonetheless, specific mutations appear likely as possible promoters or initiators of leiomyoma growth, and further research in this area may lead to refined methods of identifying risks, intervening with prevention, and providing more specific and appropriate treatments based on specific genetic findings.

Anatomic Classification

Traditionally, leiomyomas have been described based on their location relative to the myometrium (Box 16). These distinctions are of value primarily in helping to predict or explain associated symptoms. Intracavitary leiomyomas are likely to be associated with menstrual irregularities, whereas pedunculated leiomyomas are at increased risk of torsion and necrosis. Intramural and subserosal leiomyomas may be completely asymptomatic even at very large sizes.

A second classification system has been developed by the European Society of Hysteroscopy since the advent of hysteroscopic resection. This classification relates to leiomyomas that protrude into the endometrial cavity and helps predict the success and risks of hysteroscopic resection (Box 17).

Box 16

Traditional Classification of Leiomyomas

- Submucosal—leiomyomas protruding into the uterine cavity; also called intracavitary
- Intramural—leiomyomas buried within the myometrium
- Subserosal—leiomyomas bulging from the serosa
- Pedunculated—leiomyomas located on a pedicle extending from the serosa

---

Signs and Symptoms

As discussed earlier, most leiomyomas are asymptomatic. In the absence of symptoms, this diagnosis should not be sought except as a research question because treatment is based on symptoms.

Many women request imaging based on pelvic pain symptoms, and if leiomyomas are found, the patient may logically attribute the pain to these findings. In fact, pain is a relatively uncommon symptom of leiomyomas, occurring only in the setting of torsion, degeneration, or compression of other pelvic anatomy.

The most common symptoms associated with leiomyomas are bleeding abnormalities. The bleeding pattern often is described as maintaining its cyclical predictability, but worsening in intensity, duration, and associated dysmenorrhea. Caution should be used in attributing bleeding dysfunction to leiomyomas because endocrine dysfunction also is common in this population. Therefore, a hormonal management option, such as oral contraceptives or progestins, should always be considered before focusing treatment on the leiomyomas.

Other symptoms relate to compression of pelvic anatomy by enlarging leiomyomas. Patients may report urinary frequency or urgency, defecatory difficulties with a large posterior leiomyoma, or a sense of bloating and expanding abdominal girth as the uterus becomes an abdominal organ.

Infertility, like bleeding, often is associated with leiomyomas, but probably uncommonly caused by them. Most likely scenarios for leiomyoma-associated infertility are periosteal leiomyomas that occlude the tubes, or a severely distorted endometrial cavity with concomitant endometrial dyssynchrony and endometritis. Leiomyomas that do not appear to be associated with any of these mechanisms should not be considered causative.

Leiomyomas are sometimes diagnosed during pregnancy and can occasionally create pregnancy-related concerns, such as preterm labor, growth restriction, and arrest of dilation, descent, or both. They can also obstruct the surgical path at a cesarean delivery and lead to an unusual uterine incision. Such case should always be carefully noted in the operative report because it suggests a higher risk of uterine rupture in a subsequent pregnancy.

Patients frequently express concern regarding the malignant potential of leiomyomas. However, there is no clear evidence for such claims and there is some evidence for leiomyosarcomas being a completely unrelated pathology. The finding of associated malignancy occurs in less than 1 in 1,000 patients who undergo hysterectomy for leiomyomas, which is in itself an extremely small subset of the women with leiomyomas. In the setting of this low an association, causality is extremely unlikely (1).

Diagnosis

Before the widespread application of ultrasound technology to obstetrics and gynecology, most diagnoses of leiomyomas were established clinically. Ultrasonography has allowed much earlier and more precise diagnosis, although, as noted earlier, this may not be of a strong clinical benefit. Ultrasonography allows mapping the location and size of a leiomyoma to aid in selecting and deploying treatment options. However, caution should be exercised when using this modality to rule out a leiomyoma because small submucosal leiomyomas that cause most bleeding abnormalities may not be easily identified on unenhanced ultrasonography. In the case of menstrual irregularities not responsive to conventional endocrine management, a saline infusion sonohysterography or diagnostic hysteroscopy should be performed to explore the possibility of a submucosal leiomyoma.

Leiomyomas may be identified by any other pelvic imaging as well. Patients often are referred to obstetrician–gynecologists by internists or family physicians for leiomyomas discovered incidentally on imaging for other reasons. The obstetrician–gynecologist should serve as an educator to both the patient and referring clinician and should not be misled into addressing incidental findings not germane to the patient's presenting symptom.

Treatment

Although most leiomyomas do not require treatment, patients always require education and reinforcement of sound preventive health surveillance recommendations. Many experts still recommend short-interval surveillance for leiomyomas after initial identification, with at least one 3-month interval reassessment to ensure stability of the findings. This protocol has not been researched rigorously and may not be necessary in a patient who is able to self-report changing symptoms and has ready access to medical care should these occur.

Treatment is indicated in the presence of any of the following symptoms or conditions:

- Abnormal uterine bleeding not responsive to medical management
- Pain or pressure symptoms that interfere with quality of life
- Urinary tract symptoms (urgency, frequency, and obstruction)
- Infertility or recurrent pregnancy loss

Size alone has been listed as an indication because of the presumption that at least some degree of discomfort or pelvic organ crowding is likely with large leiomyomas. However, there is good evidence that conservative noninterference is acceptable even with very large leiomyomas if the patient prefers this approach (6).

If treatment is indicated by virtue of any of the listed symptoms or signs, the decision of what treatment to use is complex and should be undertaken in partnership with the patient. Nowhere has the field of gynecology changed so rapidly and dramatically as in the array of options for treatment of uterine pathology. It is incumbent upon the practicing clinician to be familiar with the possible treatments, their local availability as well as success rates and potential complications, and referral options for patients who might choose a treatment with which the clinician is not himself or herself comfortable.

Medical treatment consists largely of oral contraceptives and oral or injectable progestins. Both work by controlling the hormonal milieu (thus correcting any concomitant ovarian dysfunction that may have been present) and minimizing unopposed estrogen stimulation of the endometrium. Neither treatment significantly diminishes the size of a leiomyoma, so if bulk symptoms predominate, these therapies are unlikely to be efficacious. In contrast, gonadotropin-releasing hormone agonists may reduce uterine bulk by up to 50% within 3 months of treatment, but regrowth is almost immediate after discontinuation of the medication. Furthermore, the expense and very serious long-term consequences of therapy with gonadotropin-releasing hormone agonists have significantly limited the usefulness of this treatment regimen. Other agents currently under investigation include aromatase inhibitors and progestin receptor modulators. Both groups of therapy have showed some promise in early trials, but are not yet considered mainstays of therapy.

Minimally invasive options would include use of a progestin-bearing intrauterine device and endometrial ablation. Both of these options would be useful only for the symptom of abnormal bleeding, and both have some restrictions that make them not universally applicable. In particular, cavity size is of significant concern in the use of an intrauterine device and with the application of most currently available forms of global ablation. A third minimally invasive option is hysteroscopic resection of a small intracavitary leiomyoma. This modality is highly successful in controlling abnormal bleeding and allows for pathologic inspection of the specimen, characteristics that the other choices lack.

Hysterectomy remains the most commonly used option, with more procedures performed for leiomyomas than for all other benign indications combined (2). Hysterectomy maintains several distinct advantages over the other options. Most importantly, it remains the only definitive therapeutic option, with virtually no chance of recurrence. It also is the technique most familiar to gynecologists and most widely available in comparison with the other invasive options. Furthermore, most women undergoing intervention for leiomyomas are in their late 30s and 40s, not desiring future fertility, yet somewhat concerned about the potential for abnormal bleeding in the perimenopause. Thus, hysterectomy is an option for treatment in this population.

Uterine artery embolization has become much more widely available in the past 30 years, and high-quality research has begun to elucidate its role in the armamentarium of therapeutic options. There is a temptation to think of this as less invasive because an abdominal incision is not required, but, in terms of outcomes, uterine artery embolization has approximately the same rate of major morbidity as hysterectomy. Because of necrosis or degeneration of leiomyomas uterine artery embolization requires approximately the same amount of pain management as hysterectomy. However, hospital stays are shorter for uterine artery embolization. Minor complications, such as vaginal discharge and hematoma, are higher in women undergoing the uterine artery embolization (6). Nonetheless, embolization is a particularly attractive option for patients who are at high surgical or anesthetic risk or who wish to retain the uterus. It should not be used in those wishing to preserve fertility because limited data suggest an increased risk of implantation-related complications in pregnancies after uterine artery embolization. Therefore, secure contraception should be one of the prerequisites for undertaking this procedure.

Myomectomy is the only viable option for women wishing to retain fertility while decreasing myoma bulk. Some investigators report higher blood loss with this procedure than with hysterectomy because of the inability to definitively control blood supply, and a small percentage of cases (less than 1%) end in emergency hysterectomy. Additionally, depending on the amount of resection required, subsequent pregnancy may create a high risk of uterine rupture. These issues should be carefully explained to the patient before a myomectomy. The route of the procedure may be open or laparoscopic, depending on the size and location of the leiomyomas and the skill and interest of the surgeon. There is no clear evidence favoring one technique over the other.

Myodestructive options include magnetic resonance imaging-guided focused ultrasound surgery as well as laparoscopic myolysis and cryomyolysis. A surgical practice that mimics uterine artery embolization has also been attempted, which involves ligation of the uterine arteries laparoscopically. All of these techniques remain investigational, although they show some promise for offering the benefits of myomectomy in debulking without the disruption of the uterine integrity posed by myomectomy (2).

References

1. Wallach EE, Vlahos NF. Uterine myomas: an overview of development, clinical features, and management. Obstet Gynecol 2004;104:393–406.

2. Jacobson GF, Shaber RE, Armstrong MA, Hung YY. Hysterectomy rates for benign indications. Obstet Gynecol 2006;107:1278–83.

3. Day Baird D, Dunson DB, Hill MC, Cousins D, Schectman JM. High cumulative incidence of uterine leiomyoma in black and white women: ultrasound evidence. Am J Obstet Gynecol 2003;188:100–7.

4. Marshall LM, Spiegelman D, Barbieri RL, Goldman MB, Manson JE, Colditz GA, et al. Variation in the incidence of uterine leiomyoma among premenopausal women by age and race. Obstet Gynecol 1997;90:967–73.

5. Stewart EA, Morton CC. The Genetics of uterine leiomyomata: what clinicians need to know. Obstet Gynecol 2006;107:917–21.

6. Alternatives to hysterectomy in the management of leiomyomas. ACOG Practice Bulletin No. 96. American College of Obstetricians and Gynecologists. Obstet Gynecol 2008; 112:387–400.

First-Trimester Management
of Nonviable Pregnancy

Charles Ascher-Walsh and Terri-Ann Samuels

Nonviable pregnancies in the first trimester can be either intrauterine or extrauterine. Approximately 15% of women with a clinically diagnosed intrauterine pregnancy will have a spontaneous miscarriage during the first trimester. Approximately one half of first trimester pregnancy losses result from chromosomal abnormalities, primarily trisomies. Maternal age and reproductive history are the strongest predictors of pregnancy outcome. Extrauterine nonviable pregnancies or ectopic pregnancies account for approximately 2% of all pregnancies (1, 2). Currently, modes of management have evolved beyond suction dilation and curettage (D&C) or an exploratory laparotomy, depending on the

clinical circumstances and the patient's desires. Basic symptoms, diagnostic methods, and general management guidelines for major types of first-trimester pregnancy loss are given in Table 14. The specific details are discussed in the text.

Spontaneous Abortion

A spontaneous abortion is the umbrella label of which missed, inevitable, and threatened abortions are considered subcategories. Patients affected by any of these conditions are treated according to their presentations and their diagnoses.

Table 14. Symptoms, Evaluation, and Management of First-Trimester Pregnancy Complications

	Type of Abortion					
	Threatened	Inevitable	Incomplete	Complete	Missed	Ectopic
Signs and Symptoms						
Presence of abdominal cramping	Usually	Usually	Usually	Sometimes	Rarely	Usually
Presence of vaginal bleeding	Usually	Sometimes	Usually	Sometimes	Rarely	Sometimes
Physical Findings						
Condition of cervix	Closed	Open	Open	Closed	Closed	Closed
Size of uterus relative to pregnancy dating	Consistent	Consistent	Small	Small	Consistent or small	Consistent or small
Amount of blood in vagina	Spotting	Spotting	Bleeding	Varies	None	Scant amount
Diagnostic Testing						
Levels of β-hCG relative to gestational age	Normal	Normal	Normal or low	Low	Low or negative	Varies
Ultrasound findings	Viable intrauterine pregnancy	Viable intrauterine pregnancy	Nonviable intrauterine pregnancy	No intrauterine pregnancy	Nonviable intrauterine pregnancy	No intrauterine pregnancy and presence of adnexal mass
Management						
Medical	None and bedrest recommended	None, mifepristone, methotrexate, or misoprostol	None, mifepristone, methotrexate, or misoprostol	None, mifepristone, methotrexate, or misoprostol	N/A	Methotrexate
Surgical	N/A	N/A	Dilation and curettage	N/A	Dilation and curettage	Laparoscopy or laparotomy

Missed Abortion (Nonviable Intrauterine Pregnancy)

The term "missed abortion" is used to describe a nonviable pregnancy retained in the uterus without spontaneous passage behind a closed cervical os. The introduction of this diagnosis predated the introduction of ultrasonography and resulted from a discrepancy between the size of the uterus and duration of amenorrhea. With advent of ultrasonography, the diagnosis has extended to encompass an intrauterine pregnancy where the development of embryo and uterus lag behind reliable dating in concordance with decreasing β-hCG levels. The nonviable products of conception can be retained in a uterus behind a closed os without signs of impending expulsion for days or weeks (see Table 15). This entity is referred to as a missed abortion because generally there are no signs and just a few symptoms. Patients may report some symptoms of pregnancy, such as breast tenderness, nausea, and amen-orrhea. Eventually as progesterone levels decrease, the patient will have vaginal bleeding.

Currently, a missed abortion is most often diagnosed as an incidental finding on routine first-trimester ultrasound examination. A pregnancy is likely to be nonviable if there is no fetal cardiac activity at 6–7 weeks of gestation and the fetal pole is greater than 5 mm.

The term missed abortion often is extended to include an anembryonic pregnancy in which the embryonic disc does not develop but the trophoblast continues to implant and progress. It often is diagnosed by the visualization of an intact gestational sac of greater than 20 mm with no internal structures (3). Therefore, the ultrasound findings will be incongruent with dating and further confirmed with repeat measurements of blood β-hCG levels demonstrating abnormal increase of less than 53% over 2 days or lack of further gestational development over 7 days (Table 15).

Expectant management of a missed abortion will result in eventual expulsion of the products of con-

Table 15. Sequential First-Trimester Ultrasound Detection of Embryonic Development

Dating Reference Point	Ultrasound Feature	Comments
4.5–5 weeks from first day of last menstrual period	Gestational sac often can be seen; diameter may be 2–3 mm.	Interpret absent gestational sac with caution. False-negative findings due to early gestational age.
5.5 weeks (38 days) from last menstrual period	Gestational sac almost always seen.	Interpret absent gestational sac with caution. False-negative findings due to inaccurate recall of last menstrual period or delayed ovulation can occur.
25–26 days after hCG administration for ovulation induction or oocyte retrieval—24 days after conception	Gestational sac almost always seen.	Absent intrauterine sac indicates abnormal gestation with high degree of certainty.
25 days after home urine ovulation detection—24 days after conception	Gestational sac almost always seen.	Interpret absent gestational sac with caution. Positive urine ovulation detection may be false in 9% of cycles.
24 days after oocyte retrieval for in vitro fertilization	Gestational sac almost always seen.	Absent intrauterine sac indicates abnormal gestation with high degree of certainty.
1 week after gestational sac appears—gestational sac diameter 8–10 mm—5.5–6.5 weeks	Yolk sac appears.	Gestational sac grows 1 mm/d at this stage.
5.5–6 weeks	Embryonic heartbeat sometimes imaged.	Interpret absent embryonic heartbeat with caution. False-negative findings due to early gestational age.
6.5 weeks (46 days)—gestational sac diameter 16 mm	Embryonic heartbeat should be imaged in almost all viable gestations.	
9 weeks	Handheld Doppler ultrasonography sometimes detects fetal heart.	
10 weeks	Handheld Doppler ultrasonography detects fetal heart in 70–80% of ongoing pregnancies.	

Abbreviation: hCG indicates human chorionic gonadotropin.

ception in most patients. An observational study of outcomes of expectant management of first trimester spontaneous miscarriages showed that 70% of women (478 of 686 women) with first-trimester nonviable pregnancies opted for expectant management. The authors demonstrated that a rate of spontaneous completion (no transvaginal bleeding and endometrial thickness of less than 15 mm) in the 138 missed abortions was 76% (105 of 138 pregnancies). A total of 59% pregnancies ended in expulsion of the products of conception at 14 days; the remainder, by 46 days. Six patients had complications, details of which were not stated except that one patient underwent emergency surgery and had a blood transfusion (4).

A number of regimens have been successfully used for the medical termination of pregnancy in the first trimester, including mifepristone, methotrexate, and misoprostol (Box 18). These same agents have subse-

---

Box 18

Protocol for Intravaginal Misoprostol to Treat Nonviable First-Trimester Intrauterine Gestations

Contraindications to misoprostol: severe asthma

Caution: severe anemia, hemorrhagic disorders, and anticoagulant therapy

Protocol:

1. Obtain temperature, blood pressure, pulse, and respiratory rate.
2. Obtain complete blood count; type and screen.
3. Organize Rh immune globulin if Rh negative, antibody screen negative.
4. Obtain ultrasound confirmation of nonviable status.
5. Obtain β-hCG unless documented within previous 24 hours.
6. Administer misoprostol, 600 micrograms, intravaginally in afternoon or evening. Patient may self-administer.
7. Provide prescription for analgesia.
8. Advise patient to report to the emergency room if she is soaking two or more maxi pads per hour for 2 consecutive hours.
9. Advise patient to take her temperature every 6 hours for 24 hours after every misoprostol insertion, and call if temperature exceeds 38°C.
10. Insert misoprostol, 600 micrograms, intravaginally 18–24 hours after initial dose if products of conception have not been passed.
11. Schedule ultrasonography and test for β-hCG if products of conception have passed.
12. Monitor β-hCG level to 0.

---

quently been studied for use in terminating nonviable pregnancies.

Potential alternatives to performing medical termination in a first-trimester nonviable pregnancy were applied in a randomized clinical trial of 652 women conducted for the National Institute of Child Health and Human Development (NICHD) (5). Of these women, 491 were assigned to medical management of nonviable first-trimester pregnancy with 800 micrograms of vaginal misoprostol and 161 women underwent vacuum aspiration. Successful management was defined as complete uterine evacuation without the need for vacuum aspiration in the medical group and no repeat aspiration before 30 days in the surgical group. A success rate of 77% by day 3 increased to 84% on day 8 after the second dose of misoprostol compared with a success rate of 90% in the surgical vacuum aspiration group by day 15, which increased to 97% by day 30. The risks of pelvic infection and hemorrhage were low and the side effects were tolerable. As a result, vaginal misoprostol should be considered as a safe alternative to traditional surgical management.

Bleeding after medical management was addressed in a secondary analysis of a randomized controlled trial studying the difference in outcomes in medical management of first-trimester nonviable pregnancies using (6). The authors monitored patients treated with dry versus moistened misoprostol that were randomized with 14-day diaries to look at bleeding patterns; no difference in outcome was noted. A total of 77 patients completed their diaries. Heavy bleeding was experienced for an average of 3 days, but the median number of days of bleeding or spotting was 12 days. The median number of pads used daily was three to four in the first 7 days; however, the average change in hemoglobin was clinically insignificant 2 weeks after treatment.

Traditionally, missed abortions have been primarily managed by dilation and sharp curettage, vacuum aspiration, or a combination of the two modalities. Such surgical approach is being challenged by both expectant and medical management. Although it is the most reliable procedure in terms of success rate (defined as *complete abortion*), bleeding time, and infection rates, it is considered an invasive procedure with classic risks, such as uterine perforation, intraoperative bleeding, cervical laceration infection, and complications of anesthesia. In contrast, the benefits of a surgical procedure include completion in a predictable time period and in one step with very little follow-up necessary.

Manual vacuum aspiration is a safe and effective alternative to the traditional surgical approach. It is performed with the use of a handheld 60 mL syringe with a self-locking plunger to create the vacuum facilitating the aspiration of products of conception. It usually is an office procedure and is performed using local anesthetic, thus avoiding the use of general anesthesia and cost associated with using an operating room. The risks are the same as those of a traditional D&C. In a retrospective study of 245 patients who underwent a manual vacuum aspiration for first trimester pregnancy failure (75.5%) or incomplete abortion (24.5%), no prophylactic antibiotics were used, and cervical ripening with 400 micrograms of misoprostol was performed as per protocol (7). With a primary outcome of complete uterine evacuation without the need for further treatment, the overall efficacy of the procedure was 94.7%. No major complications (blood transfusion or uterine perforation) were reported in this group. Four patients had subsequent endometritis and the mean postprocedure hospital stay was 3.72 hours.

Although good data are lacking to support the use of prophylactic antibiotics in the operative management of a missed abortion, in view of evidence that supports the use with surgical elective abortion, the American College of Obstetricians and Gynecologists recommends that prophylactic antibiotics be considered for these procedures (8).

The Miscarriage Treatment Trial (9) was a randomized controlled trial in which nonviable gestations of less than 13 weeks were managed expectantly, surgically, or medically. The 306 women assigned to the expectant management group were discharged without a prescription for prophylactic antibiotics. There was no difference in infectious morbidity comparing expectant management group with surgical management group when using specific clinical criteria for diagnosis. Incidence of gynecologic infection was slightly lower in the expectant group than in the surgical group when comparing antibiotic use for presumed infection (5% versus 8% at 14 days; 9% versus 11% at 8 weeks). The number of unplanned D&C procedures for bleeding, retained products of conception, and on patient request (if retained products of conception were still present after 14 days) was significantly higher in the expectant management group than in the medical management group (50% versus 38%). The number of blood transfusions in the expectant management group did not significantly differ from that in the medical management group (2% versus 1%). Therefore, as opposed to what is traditionally taught, even when there are no prophylactic antibiotics used, there is no significant increase in infectious morbidity when patients are managed expectantly. RhoD immune globulin should be administered in all first-trimester abortions in Rh-negative women.

After an early pregnancy loss, many women are concerned about future fertility. A questionnaire-based retrospective study of the 762 participants of the Miscarriage Treatment Trial showed no differences in fertility rate between women who underwent medical, surgical, or expectant management (9). In fact, 80% of participants had successful pregnancies within 5 years of the index miscarriage. Time to subsequent birth was

statistically related to maternal age (age greater than 40 years was related to the least number of live births) and a history of previous miscarriage (a number greater than three miscarriages was related to the least number of live births).

A planned secondary analysis of patients in the NICHD trial (5) compared the quality of life and treatment acceptability between a group of patients treated with misoprostol and that treated with vacuum aspiration. No differences were found between the two groups in the quality of life and wellbeing; the rating of treatment acceptability, its adverse effects, and duration; or measures determining if participants would recommend or accept their treatment again in the future. These factors were significantly worse only in the group that failed medical therapy with misoprostol.

Adequate time for discussion should be allowed. A referral to a counselor also may be helpful. A follow-up examination should be scheduled and contact number should be given to the patient in the case of an emergency.

Inevitable Abortion

The term "inevitable abortion" describes a nonviable intrauterine pregnancy condition in which a cervical os has been dilated, but the products of conception have not yet been expelled. This expulsion, however, is imminent. Patients will present with vaginal bleeding, abdominal cramping, or both. On examination, the cervical os will be open with or without pregnancy tissue present. The diagnosis is made clinically on digital examination. Nonviability is confirmed by the dilatation of the cervical os that will lead to the expulsion of the products of conception.

Expectant management is an option in a patient without evidence of an infection. The approach would be similar to that in a patient with a missed abortion.

With regard to medical management, a subanalysis of the NICHD randomized controlled trial resulted in 28 out of 30 patients with inevitable or incomplete abortions who received misoprostol experiencing complete expulsion with minimal complications (5). In addition, the authors reported that women with inevitable or incomplete abortion diagnoses were more likely to have completed expulsions after one dose of misoprostol than those with the missed abortion diagnoses.

Traditionally, patients with inevitable abortion diagnoses were primarily treated with a suction D&C. This procedure is facilitated by the cervical os being already dilated, which also decreases the risk of cervical trauma.

Threatened Abortion

A threatened abortion is a condition characterized by vaginal bleeding, cramping, or both, indicating the possibility of a miscarriage. Transvaginal ultrasonography shows signs of a normal gestation, such as normal appearing gestational sac or fetal pole with cardiac activity.

The diagnosis is made clinically on examination revealing vaginal bleeding from a closed cervical os and transvaginal ultrasonography often revealing a normal viable gestation. It is most important to ascertain the source of the bleeding because, as in a normal pregnancy, bleeding can originate from a cervical laceration, vaginal lesion, or extragenital source. A thorough physical examination is essential to establish the proper diagnosis.

Expectant management is the treatment of choice for threatened abortions with a viable gestation. In one randomized trial (10), 61 women with viable pregnancies of less than 8 weeks experiencing vaginal bleeding were assigned to receive injections with β-hCG, injections with placebo, or bed rest. The abortion rates were 30%, 48%, and 75%, respectively. There was no significant difference between the treatment with a placebo and β-hCG, but there were significant differences between bed rest and β-hCG and bed rest and placebo, respectively. Although bed rest and β-hCG may be beneficial in threatened abortion, this treatment also carries the risk of ovarian hyperstimulation syndrome. Given the etiology of first trimester losses, this treatment has never become widely accepted.

Progesterone has been shown to be of no benefit in preventing the abortion of a threatened miscarriage (11). As with inevitable abortion, patients with threatened miscarriage who are experiencing vaginal bleeding and are Rh negative should receive RhoD immune globulin.

Unless gestation has been diagnosed as nonviable, there is no room for surgical intervention for a threatened abortion. If the gestation is nonviable then surgical options, such as suction D&C or manual vacuum aspiration, can be discussed as an option for termination.

Adverse prognostic factors that have been identified in patients with a threatened abortion are maternal age older than 34 years, increased number of previous miscarriages, fetal bradycardia, discrepancy between gestational age and crown–rump length, empty gestational sac, and low β-hCG levels. Favorable prognostic factors include advancing gestational age, fetal cardiac activity on presentation, and normal serum β-hCG level.

Individual counseling is based on the patient's prognostic factors on presentation. If the pregnancy appears viable, cautious optimism is appropriate, but the patient should be counseled regarding the increased risk of miscarriage. Bed rest has not been proved to be beneficial, but can be recommended as a relaxation technique.

Ectopic Pregnancy

The presentation of ectopic pregnancy varies from an asymptomatic incidental finding on early prenatal ultrasonography to an emergency room visit with signs of shock, such as hypotension, tachycardia, and rebound tenderness. Most patients will report abdominal pain secondary to peritoneal irritation by the ruptured or rupturing pregnancy, vaginal bleeding, or both. The abdominal pain can be one-sided or diffuse and vague to debilitating. The vaginal bleeding is very rarely heavy; usually it ranges from red to dark brown spotting, but rarely heavier than a normal period.

If a patient presents with abdominal pain, vaginal bleeding, or both and has a positive β-hCG level but no intrauterine gestation, she should be considered to have an ectopic pregnancy until proven otherwise. The appropriate action should be taken as per later discussion of management. However, with the advent of routine transvaginal ultrasonography and early prenatal care, the treatment quandary now exists, because with the diagnosis of an ectopic pregnancy before rupture, medical management becomes an option.

An accurate gestational age is the most helpful factor in determining appropriate pregnancy characteristics on transvaginal ultrasonography. In gestations longer than 5.5 weeks, an intrauterine pregnancy can be demonstrated with an almost 100% accuracy. An early intrauterine pregnancy can be diagnosed when transvaginal ultrasonography reveals an early gestational sac (12), which can be seen as early as 4.5 weeks of gestation. It is a small fluid-filled sac surrounded by an echogenic ring. It is located within the endometrium just beneath the endometrial stripe. To confirm its presence, the intradecidual sign should be visualized in two planes and remain the same in both (13). Sensitivities and specificities of the intradecidual sign were reported to be 60–68% and 97–100%, respectively. A true gestational sac should be differentiated from a pseudogestational sac or decidual cyst that is centrally located, with no surrounding echogenic ring, is asymmetric, and associated with septations. Of limited value is the subsequent visualization of the double decidual sac sign. It is caused by an inner rim of chronic villi surrounded by a thin crescent of fluid in the endometrial cavity, then surrounded by the outer rim of decidua vera. This sign appears only in the short window between the intradecidual sign and the appearance of a yolk sac at 5.5 weeks of gestation, which is a definitive sign of an intrauterine gestation.

If no gestational sac has been identified or if there appears to be a pseudogestational sac, then one must look elsewhere for the gestation. The most common location for an ectopic pregnancy is within the fallopian tube. Other sites that have been reported are the ovary, abdomen, cornua of a rudimentary uterine horn, cervix, and prior abdominal scar. The common findings include a complex adnexal mass separate from the ovary. If color Doppler ultrasonography is available, a physician should search for a "ring of fire" surrounding the ectopic pregnancy. A complex cyst within the ovary is more likely to be a corpus luteum, which generally has a more hypoechoic wall than an ectopic pregnancy.

Heterotopic pregnancy was an extremely rare entity with a reported incidence of 1 in 4,000 women in the general population. But with the advent of assisted reproductive technology, its incidence has increased to 1 case per 100 women who undergo vitro fertilization (14). One should be diligent in looking for an ectopic pregnancy even though a gestational sac is seen in utero.

In contrast to patients who underwent ovulation induction or embryo transfer, accuracy in pregnancy dating is not as reliable in patients who conceived spontaneously. Unless a clear gestational sac is seen on ultrasonography, these women will require further evaluation with serum β-hCG levels. The "discriminatory zone" is the cutoff created for the appearance of a normal intrauterine gestation on ultrasonography. It is generally 1,500–2,000 milli-international units per milliliter. Therefore, if the transvaginal ultrasound result is nondiagnostic and the β-hCG level is higher than the discriminatory zone, an ectopic pregnancy is probable. Other possibilities that confuse the diagnosis are the possibility of multiple gestations where the β-hCG level is higher than 2,000 milli-international units per milliliter before the gestation would be identifiable by ultrasonography and the possibility that the women completed a spontaneous abortion before presentation.

Serial β-hCG measurements are useful if the ultrasound result is nondiagnostic and the β-hCG level on presentation is below the discriminatory zone. They may help to make the distinction between a viable intrauterine pregnancy, ectopic pregnancy, and spontaneous abortion. The β-hCG levels will be increased by 53% in 48 hours in 99% of viable pregnancies (15). Approximately 50% of women with an ectopic pregnancy have increasing β-hCG levels and 50% have decreasing β-hCG levels (16). When the β-hCG level reaches the discriminatory zone, repeat ultrasound examination should be performed to confirm or exclude intrauterine pregnancy. β-hCG levels should be monitored until cardiac activity is seen; then the pregnancy can be determined as viable. Asymptomatic patients whose β-hCG levels are decreasing should be monitored until the levels reach those in nonpregnant patients. Serial β-hCG levels will continue to decrease but the rate will depend on the initial β-hCG level—lower initial values have a slower decrease (15). As with spontaneous abortion, an ectopic pregnancy can also resolve without intervention. The concern is that during the delay, an ectopic pregnancy may rupture.

Although the mortality from ectopic pregnancies has decreased over the years to 0.5 deaths per 1,000 pregnancies (17), it is still responsible for 6% of all maternal deaths. There is little room for expectant management with respect to ectopic pregnancies. If the initial β-hCG level is low and continues to decrease, only a small number of ectopic pregnancies can and will regress expectantly, but they still require vigilance and extensive counseling and a high degree of suspicion with regard to potential rupture. If the β-hCG level is increasing, the ectopic pregnancy is more likely to rupture. But if the β-hCG is decreasing, there is no correlation between the β-hCG level and likelihood of rupture. A report on expectant management of ectopic pregnancies showed that if the β-hCG level is greater than 1,500 milli-international units per milliliter, such management is more likely to fail. The authors report a 67% success rate of expectant management if β-hCG levels are between 175 milli-international units per milliliter and 1,500 milli-international units per milliliter and 95% success rate for the same if initial values of β-hCG were less than 175 milli-international units per milliliter. There have been reports of rupture of ectopic pregnancy when β-hCG levels were undetectable (18).

Medical management with methotrexate is the conservative noninvasive alternative to surgical management. Methotrexate is a folic acid antagonist that acts by inactivating the enzyme dihydrofolate reductase that is required for DNA and RNA synthesis. Therefore, it affects rapidly dividing, tissues such as bone marrow, buccal and intestinal mucosa, respiratory epithelium, malignant cells, and trophoblastic tissue. Before initiating methotrexate treatment, patients should have baseline hematologic, renal, and liver function tests (see Box 19). The reported success rate for the treat-

---

Box 19

Contraindication to Medical Therapy

Absolute Contraindications

- Breastfeeding
- Overt or laboratory evidence of immunodeficiency
- Alcoholism, alcoholic liver disease, or other chronic liver disease
- Preexisting blood dyscrasias, such as bone marrow hypoplasia, leukopenia, thrombocytopenia, or significant anemia
- Known sensitivity to methotrexate
- Active pulmonary disease
- Peptic ulcer disease
- Hepatic, renal, or hematologic dysfunction

Relative Contraindications

- Gestational sac larger than 3.5 cm
- Embryonic cardiac motion

Medical management of ectopic pregnancy. ACOG Practice Bulletin No. 94. American College of Obstetricians and Gynecologists. Obstet Gynecol 2008;111:1479–85.

ment of ectopic pregnancies and the preservation of tubal patency is more than 90% (19). Methotrexate is an option for ectopic pregnancies that present in more unusual sites, such as the cervix, tubal isthmus, or abdomen. It can be administered intramuscularly or directly injected into the site of the ectopic pregnancy.

There are three published regimens for the administration of methotrexate: 1) a single dose regimen, 2) a more recent two-dose regimen, or 3) a multiple-dose regimen (Box 20). In the single dose regimen (20), the dose is calculated by body surface area. A 15% decrease in β-hCG levels between posttreatment day 4 and day 7 is expected. The β-hCG levels should then be checked weekly until undetectable. It has been reported that 15% of patients (19) will not have an adequate decrease in the β-hCG level on day 7 and require a

---

Box 20

Methotrexate Treatment Protocols

Single-dose regimen:*

- Administer a single dose of methotrexate 50 mg/m² intramuscularly day 1.
- Measure human chorionic gonadotropin (hCG) level on posttreatment days 4 and 7.
- Check for 15% hCG decrease between days 4 and 7.
- Then measure hCG level weekly until reaching the nonpregnant level.
- If results are less than the expected 15% decrease, re-administer methotrexate 50 mg/m² and repeat hCG measurement on days 4 and 7 after second dose. This can be repeated as necessary.
- If, during follow-up, hCG levels plateau or increase, consider repeating methotrexate administration.

Two-dose regimen:†

- Administer 50 mg/m² intramuscularly on day 0.
- Repeat 50 mg/m² intramuscularly on day 4.
- Measure hCG levels on days 4 and 7, and expect a 15% decrease between days 4 and 7.
- If the decrease is greater than 15%, measure hCG levels weekly until reaching nonpregnant level.
- If less than a 15% decrease in hCG levels, re-administer methotrexate 50 mg/m² on days 7 and 11, measuring hCG levels.
- If hCG levels decrease 15% between days 7 and 11, continue to monitor weekly until nonpregnant hCG levels are reached.
- If the decrease is less than 15% between days 7 and 11, consider surgical treatment.

Fixed multiple-dose regimen:‡

- Administer methotrexate 1 mg/kg intramuscularly (on days 1, 3, 5, 7), alternate daily with folinic acid 0.1 mg/kg intramuscularly (on days 2, 4, 6, 8).
- Measure hCG levels on methotrexate-dose days and continue until hCG level has decreased by 15% from its previous measurement.
- The hCG level may increase initially above pretreatment value, but after 15% decrease, monitor hCG levels weekly until reaching the nonpregnant level.
- If the hCG level plateaus or increases, consider repeating methotrexate using the regimen described.

*Stovall TG, Ling FW. Single-dose methotrexate: an expanded clinical trial. Am J Obstet Gynecol 1993;168:1759–62; discussion 1762–5.

†Barnhart K, Hummel AC, Sammel MD, Menon S, Jain J, Chakhtoura N. Use of "2-dose" regimen of methotrexate to treat ectopic pregnancy. Fertil Steril 2007;87:250–6.

‡Rodi IA, Sauer MV, Gorrill MJ, Bustillo M, Gunning JE, Marshall JR, et al. The medical treatment of unruptured ectopic pregnancy with methotrexate and citrovorum rescue: preliminary experience. Fertil Steril 1986;46:811–3.

Medical management of ectopic pregnancy. ACOG Practice Bulletin No. 94. American College of Obstetricians and Gynecologists. Obstet Gynecol 2008;111:1479–85.

second dose of methotrexate. The multiple-dose regimen is administrated by mg/kg. Methotrexate is given every other day interspersed with leucovorin "rescue" injections. Levels of β-hCG levels are measured daily and if there is a decrease of greater than 15% or more between 2 consecutive days, the patient should be monitored with serial measurements of β-hCG levels until undetectable. A failure of the multiple dose regimen is defined as less than 15% decrease in β-hCG levels after four doses of methotrexate. The multiple-dose protocol (93% success rate) has been found to be superior to the single-dose protocol (88% success rate) in two systematic meta-analyses (19, 21). It was demonstrated that the success rate was higher for the multiple-dose regimens with higher β-hCG levels and cardiac activity present. The single-dose regimen is easier to administer with fewer side effects but the multiple dose regimen may be more appropriate for ectopic pregnancies with a higher β-hCG level and cardiac activity.

In a subsequent prospective trial, a third regimen was proposed where women with an ectopic pregnancy were given their first dose of methotrexate on day 0 and a second dose on day 4 (22). If by day 7 β-hCG levels decreased by at least 15%, the patient was monitored with weekly β-hCG measurements until the result was negative. If the decrease was insufficient between day 4 and day 7, the patient received a third dose on day 7. The participant returned on day 11 and if the 15% decrease in the β-hCG levels was not attained, a fourth dose was given. On day 14 if the 15% decrease did not occur, the patient was referred for surgical treatment. The authors reported a success rate of 87% with this new regimen. The regimen itself was reported to be well tolerated by the patients.

For patients who are Rh negative, there have been reports of Rh isoimmunization even with ectopic pregnancies (23, 24). Therefore, RhoD immune globulin should be administered to these patients as prophylaxis.

An ectopic pregnancy also can be approached surgically, by laparoscopy or laparotomy. Laparoscopy is more cost effective with shorter hospital stays and easier recovery for patients and is the preferred approach. Laparotomy is indicated for patients with extensive hemoperitoneum, intravascular compromise, poor visualization of the pelvic structures at the time of laparoscopy, or simply if the surgeon is not able to complete the surgery laparoscopically.

Three observational studies have examined salpingostomy versus salpingectomy. They reported higher rates of subsequent pregnancy in the salpingostomy group (73% versus 57%), but rates of subsequent ectopic were also higher in the salpingostomy group (15% versus 10%) (25). The decision depends on the extent of the damage to the affected and contralateral tube, the patient's reproductive history, and the skill of the surgeon and usually is made intraoperatively.

Risk factors for ectopic pregnancies (history of sexually transmitted infections, previous tubal surgery, previous ectopic pregnancy, in vitro fertilization, smoking, and age older than 35 years) especially those pertaining to the patient's lifestyle should be discussed in an attempt to increase awareness and minimize them in the future. If the patient is hemodynamically stable without abdominal pain secondary to rupture, then she may be able to participate in her management.

For medical management to be safe, a careful medical history has to be taken and a subjective and objective assessment of the patient's ability to adhere to the chosen regimen must be attained. It is unsafe to commence methotrexate without adequate follow-up. If the patient is eligible, she should be informed of the potential side effects of the methotrexate treatment and the failure rate of the chosen protocol. If the methotrexate treatment is unsuccessful or the patient develops symptoms of tubal rupture, she should be prepared for surgical management, if necessary.

If there is time for discussion, the risks and benefits of surgical management should be addressed and the approach taken justified. Patients who desire future fertility should be counseled fertility is unchanged or decreased with one fallopian tube if they undergo salpingectomy. Salpingostomy has less of a negative effect on fertility compared with salpingostomy, but increases the risk of recurrent ectopic pregnancies. The risk of recurrence is approximately 10% among women with one previous ectopic pregnancy and at least 25% among women with two or more previous ectopic pregnancies (25).

Sepsis Associated With Abortion

Sepsis with abortion is more frequent in regions where illegal abortions are performed than in areas with legalized abortions. Since the legalization of abortion, rates have decreased significantly. Symptoms and signs include fever, abdominal pain, purulent discharge, general malaise, and high white cell count.

For nonviable pregnancy management, none of the studies reviewed recommended prophylactic antibiotics for expectant, medical, or surgical management strategies, and the gynecologic infection rates were low. In order to prevent sepsis one must have a high index of clinical suspicion. The management of septic abortion needs an early recognition and aggressive removal of the products of conception generally by surgical intervention with the administration of the appropriate antibiotic therapy.

Resident Education

Education of residents in the management of first-trimester pregnancy loss should emphasize attention to detail and high index of suspicion for ectopic pregnancies and resulting infection. Early diagnosis requires proficiency in endovaginal scanning. Residents also need education and training in manual vacuum extraction and conscious sedation to most efficiently, safely, and economically treat this challenging group of women. In addition, residents will need to be prepared to cope with the emotional and psychologic aspects of these diagnoses.

References

1. Ectopic Pregnancy--United States, 1990–1992 Center for Disease Control and Prevention. MMWR Morb Mortal Wkly Rep 1995;44:46–8.

2. Van Den Eeden SK, Shan J, Bruce C, Glasser M. Ectopic pregnancy rate and treatment utilization in a large managed care organization. Obstet Gynecol 2005;105:1052–7.

3. Trinder J, Brocklehurst P, Porter R, Read M, Vyas S, Smith L. Management of miscarriage: expectant, medical, or surgical? Results of randomised controlled trial (miscarriage treatment (MIST) trial). BMJ 2006;332:1235–40.

4. Luise C, Jermy K, May C, Costello G, Collins WP, Bourne TH. Outcome of expectant management of spontaneous first trimester miscarriage: observational study. BMJ 2002;324: 873–5.

5. Zhang J, Gilles JM, Barnhart K, Creinin MD, Westhoff C, Frederick MM. A comparison of medical management with misoprostol and surgical management for early pregnancy failure. National Institute of Child Health and Human Development (NICHD) Management of Early Pregnancy Failure Trial. N Engl J Med 2005;353:761–9.

6. Davis AR, Robilotto CM, Westoff CL, Forman S, Zhang J. Bleeding patterns after vaginal misoprostol for the treatment of early pregnancy failure. NICHD Management of Early Pregnancy Failure Trial group. Hum Reprod 2004;19:1655–8.

7. Milingos DS, Mathur M, Smith NC, Ashok PW. Manual vacuum aspiration: a safe alternative for the surgical management of early pregnancy loss. BJOG 2009;116:1268–71.

8. Antibiotic prophylaxis for gynecologic procedures. ACOG Practice Bulletin No. 104. American College of Obstetricians and Gynecologists. Obstet Gynecol 2009;113:1180–9.

9. Smith LF, Ewings PD, Quinlan C. Incidence of pregnancy after expectant, medical, or surgical management of spontaneous first trimester miscarriage: long term follow–up of miscarriage treatment (MIST) randomised controlled trial. BMJ 2009;339:b3827.

10. Harrison RF. A comparative study of human chorionic gonadotrophin, placebo, and bed rest in women with early threatened abortion. Int J Fertil Menopausal Stud 1993;38:160–5.

11. Haas DM, Ramsey PS. Progestogen for preventing miscarriage. Cochrane Database of Systematic Reviews 2008, Issue 2. Art. No.: CD003511. DOI:10.1002/14651858. CD003511.pub2.

12. Levine D. Ectopic pregnancy. Radiology 2007;245:385–97.

13. Chiang G, Levine D, Swire M, McNamara A, Mehta T. The intradecidual sign: is it reliable for diagnosis of early intrauterine pregnancy? AJR Am J Roentgenol 2004;183:725–31.

14. Maymon R, Shulman A. Controversies and problems in the current management of tubal pregnancy. Hum Reprod Update 1996;2:541–51.

15. Barnhart K, Sammel MD, Chung K, Zhou L, Hummel AC, Guo W. Decline of serum human chorionic gonadotrophin and spontaneous complete abortion: defining the normal curve. Obstet Gynecol 2004;104:975–81.

16. Silva C, Sammel MD, Zhou L, Gracia C, Hummel AC, Barnhart K. Human chorionic gonadotrophin profile for women with ectopic pregnancy. Obstet Gynecol 2006;107: 605–10.

17. Chang J, Elam-Evans LD, Berg CJ, Herndon J, Flowers L, Seed KA, et al. Pregnancy related mortality surveillance--United States, 1991--1999. MMWR Surveill Summ 2003;52:1–8.

18. Montgomery Irvine L, Padwick ML. Case report: serial serum HCG measurements in a patient with an ectopic pregnancy: a case for caution. Hum Reprod 2000;15: 1646–7.

19. Barnhart KT, Gosman G, Ashby R, Sammel M. The medical management of ectopic pregnancy: a meta analysis comparing "single dose" and "multidose" regimens. Obstet Gynecol 2003;101:778–84.

20. Stovall TG, Ling FW. Single-dose methotrexate: an expanded clinical trial. Am J Obstet Gynecol 1993;168: 1759–62; discussion 1762–5.

21. Hajenius PJ, Mol F, Mol BW, Bossuyt PM, Ankum WM, van der Veen F. Interventions for tubal pregnancy. Cochrane Database of Sytematic Reviews 2007, Issue 1. Art. No.: CD000324. DOI: 10.1002/14651858.CD000324.pub2.

22. Barnhart K, Hummel AC, Sammel MD, Menon S, Jain J, Chakhtoura N. Use of "2-dose" regimen of methotrexate to treat ectopic pregnancy. Fertil Steril 2007;87:250–6.

23. Von Stein GA, Munsick RA, Stiver K, Ryder K. Fetomaternal hemorrhage in threatened abortion. Obstet Gynecol 1992; 79:383–6.

24. Dayton VD, Anderson DS, Crossno JT, Cruikshank SH. A case of Rh isoimmunization: should threatened first trimester abortion be an indication for Rh immune globulin prophylaxis? Am J Obstet Gynecol 1990;163:63–4.

25. Seeber BE, Barnhart KT. Suspected ectopic pregnancy [published erratum appears in Obstet Gynecol 2006;107:955]. Obstet Gynecol 2006;107:399–413.

Management of Ovarian Cysts and Adnexal Masses

Richard G. Moore and Shannon MacLaughlan

Each year in the United States more than 380,000 women are hospitalized with benign adnexal masses and ovarian cysts. It is estimated that approximately 200,000 women will undergo surgery for this indication (1). Most women undergoing surgery will have a benign tumor, and a small percentage of women ultimately will receive a diagnosis of an ovarian malignancy. The challenge in the diagnosis and management of women presenting with an ovarian cyst or pelvic mass is the ability to differentiate between benign and malignant tumors. The incidence of ovarian malignancy increases with age; therefore, the risk assessment of a pelvic mass must take into consideration different factors for adolescent, premenopausal, and postmenopausal women.

Premenarchal and Adolescent Females

Ovarian malignancies are rare in premenarchal and adolescent females, representing only 1% of all childhood malignancies. However, the incidence of malignancy among young females with adnexal masses is approximately 10% (2). In an age group in which ovarian conservation is important, identification of characteristics predictive of malignancy is crucial.

In the premenarchal and adolescent population, ovarian masses are most commonly diagnosed in women who present with pain, ovarian torsion, palpable mass, or precocious puberty or are discovered as an incidental finding at the time of surgery for another indication. Acute pain or suspicion of torsion is an indication for surgical intervention. However, the extent and approach of surgery for this indication are somewhat controversial. Ovaries that have undergone torsion are discolored, edematous, and enlarged and assessment for malignancy can be difficult. Surgeons often perform an oophorectomy out of concern for missing an underlying malignancy. However, most ovaries removed from females aged 19 years or younger because of torsion will have either benign cysts or neoplasms or no pathology at all, with a malignancy rate of only 1–3.5% (3). Accordingly, a reasonable and more conservative approach in premenarchal and adolescent females with evidence of torsion would be a diagnostic laparoscopy with detorsion of the affected ovary. In the absence of signs of malignancy, such as metastatic disease, solid mass on the affected ovary, or bilateral masses, the procedure can be concluded, and the patients monitored by pelvic ultrasonography postoperatively.

Among females who present with masses on imaging or physical examination who are asymptomatic, most will require surgery for further characterization. Pubertal females will have follicles of various stages of development and simple cysts of less than 8 cm in size can be observed. If small simple cysts are causing pain, they can be aspirated or fenestrated with little risk of recurrence (4). Ovarian masses that are heterogeneous or solid should be removed for risk of malignancy or torsion. The most common ovarian neoplasm in this age group is the mature teratoma or dermoid. The most common malignant ovarian tumors in this age group are germ cell tumors, representing 50% of all ovarian malignancies in females younger than 20 years (2). Characteristics most concerning for malignancy in young females with ovarian masses include solid tumors, elevated tumor markers, tumor size of 8 cm or greater, and age 1–8 years (2). Also, children presenting with precocious puberty and an adnexal mass are at high risk of sex cord stromal tumors, the second most common ovarian malignancy in this age group (2).

Females younger than 19 years with complex or solid adnexal masses should undergo preoperative testing for tumor markers, including CA 125, HE4, inhibin A, inhibin B, total inhibin, L-lactate dehydrogenase, alpha fetoprotein, and β-hCG level measurements. Although limited in specificity in this population, the CA 125 level is a marker for epithelial ovarian cancer, as is the serum biomarker HE4 level. An elevated inhibin level may indicate a juvenile granulosa cell tumor. Germ cell tumors, such as dysgerminomas and embryonal tumors, are the most common ovarian malignancies in this population, and may be marked by elevated L-lactate dehydrogenase levels, alpha-fetoprotein levels, or both. Finally, β-hCG levels can be elevated among patients with germ cell tumors and can be crucial in ruling out ectopic pregnancy as a diagnosis. Patients with elevated tumor markers, masses greater than 8 cm, or signs of precocious puberty should be counseled regarding the indication for laparotomy and likely staging, although fertility-sparing surgical procedures are appropriate even in the setting of malignancy. Females in this age group with solid or heterogeneous masses without characteristics concerning for malignancy should undergo conservative surgery for evaluation and prevention of torsion. Young women with evidence of ovarian torsion should have ovarian-sparing procedures in the absence of obvious malignancy.

Premenopausal Women

Ovarian cysts and adnexal masses are a common problem in women during their reproductive years. Most commonly, these cysts represent functional or corpus luteal cysts that will resolve on their own. However, the differential diagnosis in this age group includes ectopic pregnancy and tubo–ovarian abscesses; therefore, evaluation of the adnexal mass must include assessment for pregnancy and risk factors for sexually transmitted diseases. The most common benign ovarian neoplasms seen in the premenopausal age group include teratomas and serous and mucinous cystadenomas. The incidence of malignancies is lower in the premenopausal women than in postmenopausal women; however, invasive epithelial ovarian cancer should be included in the differential diagnosis. Tumors of low malignant potential are more commonly found in premenopausal women compared with postmenopausal women. Equally important, premenopausal women are at higher risk of germ cell tumors than postmenopausal women and should have the appropriate tumor marker test as part of their initial evaluation and risk assessment. The considerations for management of an adnexal mass are given in Box 21.

Patient Symptomatology

The adnexal mass in premenopausal women is likely to be discovered because of an evaluation for abdominal or pelvic pain. Emergent surgical intervention is required

---

Box 21

Considerations for the Management of Adnexal Masses

- Patient symptomatology
- Preoperative risk assessment for malignancy (American College of Obstetricians and Gynecologists guidelines, Society of Gynecologic Oncologists guidelines, Risk of Ovarian Malignancy Algorithm, and Risk of Malignancy Index)
- Indications for expectant management with imaging surveillance
- Indications for laparotomy versus a minimally invasive surgical approach
- Oophorectomy versus cystectomy with ovarian preservation
- Indications for fertility preservation
- Risk of surgery versus observation

---

for clinical suspicion of ovarian torsion in order to preserve the ovary in a reproductive-aged woman. Ruptured hemorrhagic cysts also can cause hemodynamic instability and require emergent surgery.

Preoperative Risk Assessment

There are multiple tools available to the obstetrician–gynecologist to evaluate adnexal masses in premenopausal women, including clinical history and examination, imaging modalities, serum tumor marker technologies, and decision-making algorithms that combine multiple components to maximize the sensitivity and specificity of individual tests.

The most useful imaging modality for evaluating the architectural features of an ovarian cyst or pelvic mass is transvaginal ultrasonography. The following features are characteristic of a malignant adnexal mass (5):

- Thick septations
- Papillary projections into the lumen of cyst
- Intramural nodule
- Cystic and solid component
- Increased overall volume of ovary
- Increased Doppler flow measurement

Serum tumor markers also play a role in the evaluation of adnexal masses in premenopausal women. However, the commonly used serum biomarker CA 125 measurement has a decreased specificity in premenopausal patients because its level often is elevated in many benign obstetric–gynecologic conditions, such as endometriosis, leiomyomas, pelvic inflammatory disease, and pregnancy. For this reason, the American College of Obstetricians and Gynecologists (the College) recommends a higher threshold for referral to a gynecologic oncologist based on serum CA 125 levels. The novel serum biomarker HE4 measurement has improved specificity over CA 125 measurement in this population (6); the level of HE4 is not elevated in patients with endometriosis and other benign gynecologic conditions. The combination of serum HE4 and CA 125 levels has been demonstrated to differentiate between endometriomas and ovarian malignancies effectively (7, 8), and the Risk of Ovarian Malignancy Algorithm (or predictive probability algorithm) (Box 22) has a sensitivity of 95% at a specificity of 75% in this population.

The combination of multiple parameters improves the gynecologist's ability to differentiate between benign masses and malignant masses preoperatively. Both the College (Box 23) and the Society of Gynecologic Oncologists (SGO) (Box 24) have published recommendations for evaluation of adnexal masses and guidelines for referral to gynecologic oncologists. Various algorithms combine history, clinical examination, serum tumor

Box 22

Risk of Ovarian Malignancy Algorithm

Risk of ovarian malignancy algorithm is a formula that calculates a predictive probability of ovarian cancer using the results of serum CA 125 and HE4 measurements and a menopausal status. First, the predictive index is determined using the coefficient for the natural logarithm (ln) of HE4 value and that for the CA 125 value*:

- For premenopausal women:

$$\text{Predictive index} = -12.0 + 2.38*\ln(HE4) + 0.0626*\ln(CA\ 125)$$

- For postmenopausal women:

$$\text{Predictive index} = -8.09 + 1.04*\ln(HE4) + 0.732*\ln(CA\ 125)$$

The risk of ovarian malignancy algorithm is then used to calculate the predictive probability of ovarian malignancy:

$$\text{Predictive probability} = \exp(\text{predictive index})/[1+\exp(\text{predictive index})]$$

Preoperative referral to a gynecologic oncologist is recommended if

- predictive probability is greater than 27.7% for premenopausal women

- predictive probability is greater than 13.1% for postmenopausal women

CA 125 values are for the Abbott Architect platform. Other CA 125 platforms will have different cutoff values.

*Moore RG, McMeekin DS, Brown AK, Di Silvestro P, Miller MC, Allard WJ, et al. A novel multiple marker bioassay utilizing HE4 and CA125 for the prediction of ovarian cancer in patients with a pelvic mass. Gynecol Oncol 2009;112:40–6.

Box 23

Guidelines of the American College of Obstetricians and Gynecologists for Referral to a Gynecologic Oncologist

Women with a pelvic mass and at least one of the following clinical characteristics should be referred to a gynecologic oncologist:

- Elevated CA 125 level
  - Greater than 35 units/mL in postmenopausal women
  - Greater than 200 units/mL in premenopausal women
- Ascites
- Nodular or fixed pelvic mass
- Evidence of abdominal or distant metastases
- Family history of one or more first-degree relative with ovarian cancer or breast cancer

The role of the generalist obstetrician–gynecologist in the early detection of ovarian cancer. ACOG Comittee Opinion No. 280. American College of Obstetricians and Gynecologists. Obstet Gynecol 2002;100:1413–6.

Indications for Expectant Management

Premenopausal women with cystic ovarian masses and minimal symptoms can be treated expectantly with repeat ultrasonography in 6–12 weeks to document resolution or stability (9). Historically, patients in this category have been treated with oral contraceptives to decrease a risk of persistence or recurrence of functional ovarian cysts. However, research has shown no benefit to this approach over observation alone (10). Cysts that are completely simple and less than 5 cm do not require further follow-up. Simple cysts in this age group that are greater than 5 cm can undergo repeat ultrasound in one year (11).

Ovarian masses that persist on imaging often represent benign neoplasms, such as cystadenomas, endometriomas, or mature teratomas (10). Both endometriomas and teratomas have distinctive characteristics on ultrasound and magnetic resonance imaging and can be diagnosed accurately with these modalities. Surgical intervention in these cases rests on the patient's symptoms and the stability of the mass over time. If conservative management is selected, repeat ultrasound should be obtained yearly (11). If there is any concern for malignancy, surgical intervention should be pursued for diagnostic purposes.

Postmenopausal Women

The prevalence of an adnexal mass in postmenopausal women is as high as 15.4% (12). The differential diag-

marker measurements, and imaging characteristics in an objective fashion. When reasonable concern exists for malignancy in a woman with an adnexal mass, the patient should be referred to a gynecologic oncologist.

Other ovarian malignancies, such as malignant germ cell and sex cord stromal tumors, although rare, must be considered. Accordingly, evaluation of an adnexal mass with malignant characteristics on imaging should include serum measurements of L-lactate dehydrogenase, alpha-fetoprotein, inhibin, and β-hCG. Women with elevated values of one or more of these tumor markers should be referred to a gynecologic oncologist. Many premenopausal women desire future fertility and multidisciplinary teams, including gynecologic oncologists and reproductive endocrinologists, should be used. Fertility-sparing surgery for some malignancies and tumors of low malignant potential often is appropriate.

nosis is broad and can include benign and malignant ovarian neoplasms, tubo–ovarian or diverticular abscesses, and metastatic implants (Table 16). The risk of malignancy is increased in postmenopausal women compared with their premenopausal counterparts, and historically, the presence of an adnexal mass in a postmenopausal woman has been an indication for surgical intervention. However, postmenopausal ovaries continue to produce functional cysts, and most adnexal masses in this population are benign. In a population of 48,230 asymptomatic postmenopausal women screened with ultrasonography alone, 92.4% of the 845 women who underwent surgery for adnexal masses had either benign neoplasms or normal ovaries (13). When multimodality screening with both CA 125 level measurement and ultrasonography was performed on 50,078 women, 97 women eventually underwent surgery for a high-risk finding. Therefore, when caring for

postmenopausal women with adnexal masses, a clinician must consider the risk of unnecessary surgery for asymptomatic benign lesions versus the possibility of delayed diagnosis of an early ovarian or fallopian tube malignancy. Important features to consider are listed in Box 21.

Patient Symptomatology

Patients with symptomatic pelvic masses should undergo surgical intervention to alleviate discomfort and rule out malignancy. Ovarian cancer is associated with the following symptoms (14):

- Pelvic or abdominal pain
- Urinary urgency or frequency
- Increased abdominal size or bloating
- Difficulty eating or feeling full (particularly when present for less than 1 year and more than 12 days per month)

Preoperative Risk Assessment

The same tools available to evaluate the malignant potential of adnexal masses in reproductive-aged women should be applied to postmenopausal women, considering the differences between the two populations. Malignant ovarian neoplasms have the same characteristics on imaging in postmenopausal and premenopausal women. It is important to keep in mind that the incidence of epithelial ovarian cancer is higher in postmenopausal women than in other populations, so masses must be evaluated with a higher index of suspicion of malignancy.

The risk of malignancy index uses ultrasound imaging features, menopausal status, and serum CA 125 levels to calculate a preoperative risk (Box 25)(15). This algorithm has been validated in multiple studies and is commonly used in the United Kingdom for referral guidelines (16). However, ultrasound imaging is subjective in nature with variations in results between operators, centers, and geographic regions. Furthermore, an accurate risk of malignancy index cannot be calculated if the architectural features of the mass are inadequately described.

The most commonly used serum tumor marker in the evaluation of women with a pelvic mass is CA 125 measurement. Its level is elevated in up to 80% of women with advanced stage epithelial ovarian cancer but in only one half of women with early-stage disease. The novel tumor marker HE4 measurement is evolving as a useful tool in evaluating adnexal masses, and has increased sensitivity and specificity over that of CA 125 testing alone (6). As in premenopausal women, the dual marker combination of CA 125 and HE4 measurement has higher sensitivity and specificity for

Table 16. Differential Diagnosis of the Adnexal Mass in Women According to Age

Type of Mass	Postmenopausal Women	Premenopausal Women	Premenarchal and Adolescent Females
Benign	Cystadenoma Follicular cyst Corpus luteal cyst Hydrosalpinx Endometrioma Teratoma Tubo-ovarian abscess Leiomyoma Fibroma Thecoma Brenner tumor	Follicular cyst Corpus luteal cyst Hemorrhagic cyst Ectopic pregnancy Cystadenoma Hydrosalpinx Tubo-ovarian abscess Endometrioma Teratoma Leiomyoma	Teratoma Functional cyst Cystadenoma Torsion without pathology Endometrioma Paraovarian cyst
Malignant	Epithelial ovarian cancer Low malignant potential tumor of the ovary Nonepithelial ovarian cancer Primary peritoneal cancer Fallopian tube cancer Metastatic implant (breast, gastrointestinal, and uterine cancer)	Low malignant potential tumor of the ovary Nonepithelial ovarian cancer Epithelial ovarian cancer Primary peritoneal cancer Fallopian tube cancer Metastatic implant (breast, gastrointestinal, and uterine cancer)	Germ cell tumor Sex cord stromal tumor Low malignant potential tumor of the ovary Epithelial ovarian cancer
Nongynecologic	Diverticular abscess Lymphadenopathy	Lymphadenopathy	Lymphadenopathy Lymphoma or leukemia

detecting malignancy in patients with ovarian masses than either tumor marker measurement alone (7, 8). The combinations of the two markers used in the Risk of Ovarian Malignancy Algorithm can accurately discriminate between benign adnexal masses and malignant adnexal masses (Box 22) (7). A postmenopausal woman with normal CA 125 and HE4 levels in the setting of an adnexal mass has minimal risk of malignancy. Consideration of these two biomarkers in the context of a patient's constellation of symptoms improves the preoperative risk evaluation for malignancy (17). The use of algorithms using quantitative measures, such as serum tumor markers, and menopausal status allow for reproducible results without regards to operators or geographic location.

Expectant Management

The natural history of unilocular ovarian cysts less than 10 cm in diameter in postmenopausal women has been well described. The malignant potential of these masses is essentially zero in the setting of a normal CA 125 level and HE4 level. The most common diagnosis after surgery for excision of an ovarian cyst is a serous cystadenoma. Nearly one half of simple cysts in this population will resolve without intervention, especially among women who are less than 10 years from men-

strual cessation (18). Completely solid masses are most often benign and may represent fibromas or thecomas. These tumors will not resolve over time and most often will require surgical intervention. A dermoid cyst or teratoma has distinct imaging features, including fat and calcifications that can be characterized accurately with magnetic resonance imaging.

It is reasonable to offer expectant management to postmenopausal women with benign-appearing ovarian cysts of less than 10 cm in diameter with normal tumor markers. For simple cysts less than 7 cm, surveillance should include repeat ultrasonography annually. Larger cysts may need further imaging for characterization. Cystic masses that are complex in nature but still benign in appearance may also be observed in the setting of normal tumor markers. Surveillance for these masses should include repeat ultrasound examination in 6–12 weeks to document stability, followed by annual follow-up (11). Increase in size, development of complex characteristics, such as papillations or solid components, development of symptoms, or rising serial tumor marker levels should prompt surgical intervention.

Surgical Intervention

Postmenopausal women with symptomatic adnexal masses or imaging findings that raise concerns for

Box 25

Risk of Malignancy Index

Risk of malignancy index is calculated based on the following formula*:

Risk of Malignancy Index = ultrasound score[†] × menopausal score[‡] × serum CA 125 level

A risk of malignancy index of 200 warrants a preoperative referral to a gynecologic oncologist.

*Jacobs I, Oram D, Fairbanks J, Turner J, Frost C, Grudzinskas JG. A risk of malignancy index incorporating CA 125, ultrasound and menopausal status for the accurate preoperative diagnosis of ovarian cancer. Br J Obstet Gynaecol 1990;97:922–9.

[†]Ultrasound score is determined by assigning the value of 1 for each of the following characteristics of an adnexal mass on ultrasonography (a score of 3 is assigned for the presence of two to five features):

- Multiloculated ovarian cyst
- Solid component in ovarian mass
- Bilateral adnexal masses
- Ascites
- Evidence of intraabdominal metastases

[‡]Menopausal score of 1 is assigned if a woman is premenopausal and menopausal score of 3 is assigned if a woman is postmenopausal.

malignancy should undergo surgical evaluation for both diagnostic and therapeutic purposes. The standard approach for postmenopausal patients with adnexal masses, elevated levels of tumor markers, and evidence of ascites or other metastatic disease has been laparotomy. However, most women with adnexal masses will have benign disease and minimally invasive surgery is appropriate. Minimally invasive surgery has the benefits of decreased pain and morbidity, shorter hospital stay, and faster recovery times for patients. However, the decision regarding a surgical approach will depend on a number of factors, including the following:

- Level of surgeon's experience with laparoscopic surgery
- Size of the adnexal mass
- Ability to determine malignancy intraoperatively

Algorithms, such as those based on the College or SGO guidelines, along with tumor marker measurements (HE4 and CA 125) using ROMA can be used to assess the risk of malignancy and the choice of surgical approach. Tumors larger than 10 cm can be technically difficult to remove laparoscopically because of challenges in visualization and ability to remove the mass intact, although there may be a role for experienced surgeons in appropriate circumstances. In a series of 186 women who underwent laparoscopy for ovarian masses 10 cm or larger, the surgery was completed laparoscopically in 174 women. Laparoscopic procedures were converted to laparotomy for technical difficulties (n=7) or incidental malignancies requiring staging (n=5). However, tumor spillage occurred in 121 cases (19). The implications of a ruptured benign cyst are negligible, but rupture of a stage IA or stage IB ovarian malignancy may result in a decreased disease-free survival and also subject a patient to chemotherapy that might not have otherwise been needed (20). Therefore, the goal of any surgery for an adnexal mass should be the intact removal of the mass or placement of the cyst into an endoscopic bag with a controlled rupture and drainage for removal.

Patients undergoing surgery for an adnexal mass should be counseled regarding the risk of a malignancy, and the discussion should address the potential need for a staging procedure. Availability of a subspecialist to perform appropriate surgical staging should be taken into account, and preoperative referral to a gynecologic oncologist should be considered based on the risk assessment as discussed previously. The procedure should begin with an inspection of the mass, pelvis, and abdomen to determine the likelihood of malignancy. Gross inspection of a mass intraoperatively by the surgeon is a reliable way to determine the need for frozen section, which has good sensitivity and specificity for determining malignancy and the need for more extensive surgery (21, 22).

References

1. DeFrances CJ, Cullen KA, Kozak LJ. National Hospital Discharge Survey: 2005 annual summary with detailed diagnosis and procedure data. Vital Health Stat 13 2007; 165:1–209.

2. Oltmann SC, Garcia N, Barber R, Huang R, Hicks B, Fischer A. Can we preoperatively risk stratify ovarian masses for malignancy? J Pediatr Surg 2010;45:130–4.

3. Oltmann SC, Fischer A, Barber R, Huang R, Hicks B, Garcia N. Pediatric ovarian malignancy presenting as ovarian torsion: incidence and relevance. J Pediatr Surg 2010;45:135–9.

4. Hayes-Jordan A. Surgical management of the incidentally identified ovarian mass. Semin Pediatr Surg 2005;14: 106–10.

5. van Nagell J Jr, DePriest PD, Ueland FR, DeSimone CP, Cooper AL, McDonald JM, et al. Ovarian cancer screening with annual transvaginal sonography: findings of 25,000 women screened. Cancer 2007;109:1887–96.

6. Moore RG, Brown AK, Miller MC, Skates S, Allard WJ, Verch T, et al. The use of multiple novel tumor biomarkers for the detection of ovarian carcinoma in patients with a pelvic mass. Gynecol Oncol 2008;108:402–8.

7. Moore RG, McMeekin DS, Brown AK, DiSilvestro P, Miller MC, Allard WJ, et al. A novel multiple marker bioassay

utilizing HE4 and CA125 for the prediction of ovarian cancer in patients with a pelvic mass. Gynecol Oncol 2009; 112:40–6.

8. Huhtinen K, Suvitie P, Hiissa J, Junnila J, Huvila J, Kujari H, et al. Serum HE4 concentration differentiates malignant ovarian tumours from ovarian endometriotic cysts. Br J Cancer 2009;100:1315–9.

9. Alcazar JL, Castillo G, Jurado M, Garcia GL. Is expectant management of sonographically benign adnexal cysts an option in selected asymptomatic premenopausal women? Hum Reprod 2005;20:3231–4.

10. Grimes DA, Jones LB, Lopez LM, Schulz KF. Oral contraceptives for functional ovarian cysts. Cochrane Database of Systematic Reviews 2009, Issue 2. Art. No.: CD006134. DOI: 10.1002/14651858.CD006134.pub3.

11. Levine D, Brown DL, Andreotti RF, Benacerraf B, Benson CB, Brewster WR, et al. Management of asymptomatic ovarian and other adnexal cysts imaged at US: Society of Radiologists in Ultrasound Consensus Conference Statement. Radiology 2010;256:943–54.

12. Dorum A, Blom GP, Ekerhovd E, Granberg S. Prevalence and histologic diagnosis of adnexal cysts in postmenopausal women: an autopsy study. Am J Obstet Gynecol 2005;192:48–54.

13. Menon U, Gentry-Maharaj A, Hallett R, Ryan A, Burnell M, Sharma A, et al. Sensitivity and specificity of multimodal and ultrasound screening for ovarian cancer, and stage distribution of detected cancers: results of the prevalence screen of the UK Collaborative Trial of Ovarian Cancer Screening (UKCTOCS). Lancet Oncol 2009;10:327–40.

14. Goff BA, Mandel LS, Drescher CW, Urban N, Gough S, Schurman KM, et al. Development of an ovarian cancer symptom index: possibilities for earlier detection. Cancer 2007;109:221–7.

15. Jacobs I, Oram D, Fairbanks J, Turner J, Frost C, Grudzinskas JG. A risk of malignancy index incorporating CA 125, ultrasound and menopausal status for the accurate preoperative diagnosis of ovarian cancer. Br J Obstet Gynaecol 1990;97:922–9.

16. Bailey J, Tailor A, Naik R, Lopes A, Godfrey K, Hatem HM, et al. Risk of malignancy index for referral of ovarian cancer cases to a tertiary center: does it identify the correct cases? Int J Gynecol Cancer 2006;16 Suppl 1:30–4.

17. Andersen MR, Goff BA, Lowe KA, Scholler N, Bergan L, Drescher CW, et al. Use of a Symptom Index, CA125, and HE4 to predict ovarian cancer. Gynecol Oncol 2010;116:378–83.

18. Castillo G, Alcazar JL, Jurado M. Natural history of sonographically detected simple unilocular adnexal cysts in asymptomatic postmenopausal women. Gynecol Oncol 2004;92:965–9.

19. Ghezzi F, Cromi A, Bergamini V, Uccella S, Siesto G, Franchi M, et al. Should adnexal mass size influence surgical approach? A series of 186 laparoscopically managed large adnexal masses. BJOG 2008;115:1020–7.

20. Bakkum-Gamez JN, Richardson DL, Seamon LG, Aletti GD, Powless CA, Keeney GL, et al. Influence of intraoperative capsule rupture on outcomes in stage I epithelial ovarian cancer. Obstet Gynecol 2009;113:11–7.

21. Ghaemmaghami F, Fakour F, Karimi ZM, Behtash N, Modares Gilani M, Mousavi, A et al. Clinical assessment, gross examination, frozen section of ovarian masses: do patients benefit? Arch Gynecol Obstet 2008;278:209–13.

22. Geomini P, Bremer G, Kruitwagen R, Mol BW. Diagnostic accuracy of frozen section diagnosis of the adnexal mass: a metaanalysis. Gynecol Oncol 2005;96:1–9.

Recognition and Management
of Surgical Injuries

Fidel A. Valea

With the advances in videolaparoscopy, electrosurgical equipment, and mechanical devices, minimally invasive surgical techniques are now used to perform operations that were exclusively performed, just a few years ago, through a laparotomy. Despite all the technologic advances, injuries to other organs still occur during gynecologic surgery because of the close proximity of the other pelvic organs to the female reproductive tract. The types and frequency of injuries that can occur are dependent on the experience of the surgeon, the type of surgery performed (with the more radical surgery having greater risks), and the condition of the patient.

Urinary Tract

The incidence of urinary tract injury during gynecologic surgery is between 0.33% and 4.8% depending on the type of surgery and the surgical approach (1). Laparoscopic surgery has the highest incidence, although in the United States, most injuries occur during an abdominal hysterectomy for benign indications because it is the most common type of hysterectomy performed (2). Injury to the bladder represents approximately 80% of all urinary tract injuries. Risk factors for urinary tract injury include previous pelvic surgery with adhesion formation, the presence of cancer, previous history of radiation, and any entity that distorts normal anatomy, such as a large mass. Because urinary tract injuries can lead to significant morbidity and increased costs, it is important to identify these injuries at the time they occur. The universal use of cystoscopy after hysterectomy was evaluated in one prospective study in which an overall 4.8% rate of urinary injury at the time of hysterectomy was detected in 471 patients (2). Bladder injury occurred 3.6% of the time and ureteral injury was detected in 1.7% of the patients. However, only 12.5% of ureteral injuries and 35.3% of bladder injuries were identified before cystoscopy. This was confirmed in a multiinstitutional trial in the United States (3). As a result, one may consider cystoscopy after hysterectomy, especially if there is any question of urinary injury, hematuria, or both, so that repair can be immediate and morbidity to the patient reduced.

Ureters

Seventy five percent of all ureteral injuries are associated with gynecologic surgery. Of all injuries to the urinary tract, those involving the ureter are the most difficult to recognize and may produce the most serious complications. Although ureteral injury during hysterectomy is relatively uncommon, occurring in approximately 0.3–0.5% of all cases, it is more common in laparoscopic hysterectomies than in other types of hysterectomy.

Understanding the anatomy of the ureter is essential to avoid injury. The ureter enters the pelvis by crossing over the lower common iliac artery and beneath the infundibulopelvic ligament containing the ovarian vessels. As the ureter dips into the pelvis, it can be seen beneath the thin transparent peritoneum along the lateral pelvic sidewall, where it lies between the uterosacral ligament and the hypogastric artery. The ureter then turns anteriorly 1.5 cm lateral to the cervix and continues beneath the uterine artery. Between the uterine artery and its entrance into the bladder, the ureter crosses a tunnel in the cardinal ligament. It turns anteriorly and medially over the anterior vaginal fornix to join the bladder approximately 1.5 cm below the cervix. The relationship between the lower ureter and the cervix may vary on each side. A periurethral pseudosheath protects a rich anastomosis of vessels that run along the ureter. In mobilizing the ureter, these vessels will not be injured as long as the sheath is not damaged.

In its course through the pelvis, the ureter is susceptible to involvement, distortion, or compression by a variety of normal and pathologic conditions, including pregnancy, pelvic tumors, gynecologic malignancies, endometriosis, pelvic infection, retroperitoneal tumors, uterine procidentia, pelvic hematomas, ovarian remnants, and a variety of other problems. Almost all major gynecologic operations, including abdominal, vaginal, and laparoscopic hysterectomies, have been implicated in ureteral injury. Specifically, laparoscopic hysterectomy, radical hysterectomy, surgery for endometriosis, and concurrent prolapse surgery carry the highest risk. It should be noted that high uterosacral ligament vaginal vault suspension has been associated with a high ureteral injury rate of 11% (4). Subtotal (supracervical) hysterectomy was rarely associated with ureteral injury, suggesting that removal of the cervix places the ureter at greatest risk of injury. Recent randomized trials failed to show a difference in operative complications between supracervical and total abdominal hysterectomy (5).

There are several measures one could take to prevent ureteral injury. The first step should be to identify the patient at risk, so she can be counseled appropriately. Adequate exposure so the ureter can be identified, visualized or palpated, dissected, mobilized, and retracted out of harm's way also is helpful in preventing ureteral injuries. When performing a laparoscopic hysterectomy, the use of a Koh ring on the uterine manipulator allows for the easier identification of the cervix and serves to push the ureters laterally away from the cervix when the manipulator is pushing the cervix and uterus cephalad.

The treatment of ureteral injuries depends on the location and type (Boxes 26 and 27). Ureteral injuries are less common during hysterectomy when dissection

---

Box 26

Locations of Ureteral Injuries

- At or above the infundibulopelvic ligament and near the pelvic brim—during infundibulopelvic ligament ligation or during an aortic lymphadenectomy

- In the base of the broad ligament where the ureter passes beneath the uterine vessels—during the dissection out of the cardinal ligament during a radical hysterectomy

- Along the lateral pelvic sidewall just above the uterosacral ligaments—during a pelvic lymphadenectomy or when the rectovaginal septum is developed during a radical hysterectomy or during desperate measures to control pelvic sidewall bleeding

- As the ureter leaves the cardinal ligament and enters the bladder—with both an extrafascial and radical hysterectomy; however, the ureter is most vulnerable to injury in the lowest 3 cm of dissection during the removal of the cervix.

Box 27

Types of Ureteral Injuries in Pelvic Surgery

- Crushing injury from misapplication of surgical instruments
- Ligation with suture
- Thermal injury from surgical energy devices
- Ischemia due to the stripping of the ureteral adventitia and subsequent devascularization
- Transection (either partial or complete)
- Kinked with secondary, partial, or complete obstruction
- Resection of a segment of ureter as part of radical pelvic surgery for cancer

---

is accomplished immediately adjacent to the cervix, medial to the ureter. If the ureteral sheath is traumatized by a misplaced clamp or thermal injury, the placement of a semipermanent ureteral catheter for a few weeks should be considered while revascularization of the ureter takes place if the injury is small and identified immediately. Perioperative, retroperitoneal, closed suction drains can be used when ureteral damage is suspected, not only to identify but also to prevent urinoma formation. Similarly, if the ureter is kinked by a suture, the suture should be removed and a ureteral stent should be placed to allow it to heal as detailed earlier. When the ureter has been partially or completely divided or is so devitalized by suture or clamping that necrosis is likely to occur, more aggressive management is indicated. The appropriate repair for a severely injured ureter depends on the level of the ureteral injury in the pelvis, the length of the segment traumatized or removed, the mobility of the ureter and bladder, the quality of the pelvic tissues, the condition for which the operation is being performed, and the general condition and anticipated lifetime of the patient. When possible, direct reimplantation of the ureter, an ureteroneocystostomy, is the preferred method because the blood supply to the bladder is excellent and promotes healing. When injury to the pelvic ureter is so extensive that the proximal ureter cannot be brought to the bladder without tension, several techniques are available to reduce the ureteral–vesical gap. These modalities include the Boari bladder flap tube technique and the psoas muscle hitch (Fig. 45 and Fig. 46). If the ureter is transected above the pelvic brim, the preferred method is either an ureteroureterostomy or the interposition of an intestinal segment between the injured ureter and the bladder. If a stent is placed in the management of a ureteral injury, it should be left in place for a few weeks to allow the injured area to heal.

Controversy exists as to the management of ureteral obstruction secondary to ureteral ligation discovered in the immediate postoperative period. Early repair (48–72 hours after surgery usually involving ureteroneocystostomy) is favored by many clinicians because it may be accomplished before inflammation and scarring occur. Certainly, surgery should be delayed in the patient with significant pelvic infection or in any patient whose medical status is compromised and in whom surgery for ureteral obstruction might pose a significant threat.

Bladder

In the United States, bladder injuries most commonly occur during an abdominal hysterectomy for benign indications because this is the most common type of hysterectomy performed in the United States. However,

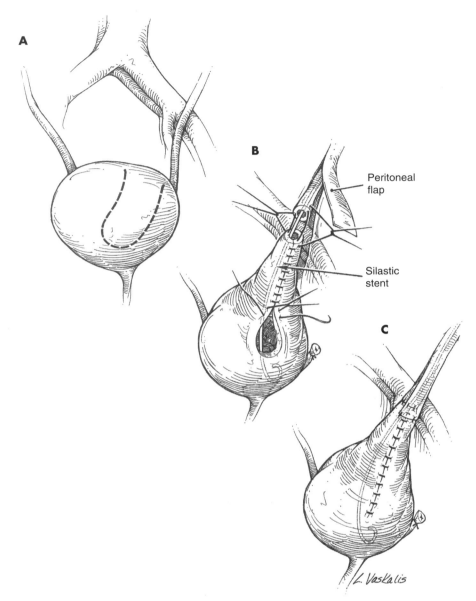

Figure 45. A–C. Boari–Ockerblad bladder flap. (This figure was published in Nichols DH, Clarke-Pearson DL, eds. Gynecologic, obstetric, and related surgery. 2nd ed. Mosby: St. Louis (MO); 2000. p. 861, Copyright Elsevier [2000].)

on a case-by-case basis, bladder injuries are more common with the vaginal approach. Bladder injury complicates up to 1–2% of all hysterectomies and 5% of all retropubic midurethral sling operations making them more common than ureteral injuries. Risk factors for bladder injury include prior cesarean delivery because of the scarring that forms between the bladder base and the pubocervical fascia (but this is not a contraindication to vaginal surgery). Any anatomic distortion of the lower uterine segment, such as by a leiomyoma also can make it difficult to find the proper plane and increase the risk of a bladder injury. Similarly, when performing a trachelectomy, the dissection of the bladder away from the top of the cervix after a previous subtotal (supracervical) hysterectomy can be difficult. Finally, radical pelvic surgery also is associated with an increased risk of bladder injury especially if the patient has previously undergone radiation therapy.

During an abdominal hysterectomy, the bladder is at risk of injury during the creation of the bladder flap, when the bladder dome is dissected from the lower uterine segment. During a vaginal hysterectomy, the injury usually occurs during the dissection of the bladder from the vaginal wall and can involve the trigone. As such, it is imperative that the surgeon identify the ureteral orifices when this injury does occur.

Prevention of bladder injury begins with the thorough familiarity with the anatomy of the bladder, especially

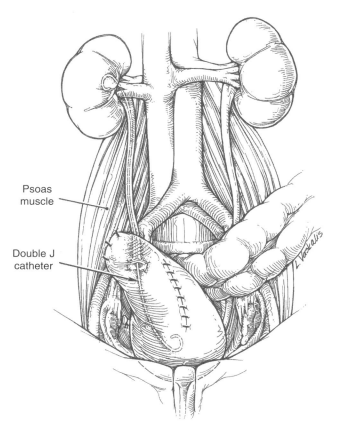

Psoas
muscle

Double J
catheter

Figure 46. Vesicopsoas hitch. (This figure was published in Nichols DH, Clarke-Pearson DL, eds. Gynecologic, obstetric, and related surgery. 2nd ed. Mosby: St. Louis (MO); 2000, Copyright Elsevier [2000].)

Box 28

Prevention of Bladder Injuries

- Empty the bladder completely before making an incision in the lower abdomen.
- Use sharp rather than blunt dissection to mobilize the bladder away from the cervix in all directions when initially creating a bladder flap.
- Develop the pubovesicocervical fascia anterior to the cervix.
- When difficulty is anticipated or encountered, place 5 mL of diluted indigo carmine or methylene blue solution in the bladder to help identify an inadvertent opening in the bladder. Sterile milk also may be used for this purpose because it stains the tissues less.
- Place an instrument in the bladder through the urethra to identify the proper plane for dissection.
- Use an omental pedicle graft to bring new vascularity to the bladder base when hysterectomy is done after pelvic irradiation.
- Use sharp dissection to separate the bladder away from the base of the cervix and upper part of the vagina before excising the uterus and cervix at hysterectomy.

---

its boundaries in relation to the lower uterine isthmus, the cervix, and the upper third of the anterior vaginal wall. Some injuries to the bladder are caused by vigorous blunt dissection in the wrong plane. Injury also may result from inadequate mobilization of the bladder away from the cervix in all directions in either total abdominal or vaginal hysterectomy—the bladder may accidentally be caught in clamps or sutures that are placed in the cardinal ligaments or anterior vaginal cuff. Finding a proper plane for dissection may be especially difficult in patients who have had a previous low-cervical cesarean delivery. Practical measures to help prevent bladder injuries from gynecologic and obstetric surgery are listed in Box 28.

If an injury to the bladder is discovered, it should be carefully assessed to determine the extent and proximity to the ureteral orifices. The hysterectomy should be completed before the repair to optimize exposure and simplify the identification of the proper planes. The closure is in layers, with the first layer consisting of a running horizontal mattress suture of 3-0 or 4-0 delayed-absorbable suture that carefully approximates and inverts the bladder mucosa. The surgeon must ensure that the closure goes beyond the limits of the

defect. By instilling approximately 200 mL of a dilute methylene blue solution or sterile milk into the bladder the surgeon can confirm the security of the closure. Any point of leakage should be reinforced with sutures. A second and possibly even a third layer of mattress sutures approximate the muscle layer without tension and reinforces the closure. Some authors even advocate the closure of the peritoneum to interpose yet another layer between the bladder and the vaginal apex. At the completion, cystoscopy with intravenous indigo carmine should be performed to confirm ureteral integrity. A catheter should be placed in the bladder should be catheterized for 5–7 days to allow for healing. If the injury is at the dome of the bladder, some experts have even recommended not using prolonged catheterization if the repair was simple.

Gastrointestinal Injuries

The incidence of bowel injury during gynecologic surgery is low, approximately 0.3%. Clearly, there are conditions that can increase this risk significantly, such as adhesions from prior surgery, endometriosis, inflammatory bowel disease, the presence of cancer, and previous history of radiation. In addition, there is a higher rate of bowel injury with abdominal hysterectomy than with vaginal hysterectomy. The management of each specific injury is variable and depends on a variety of factors, including the location and extent of the injury, the skill of the surgeon, and the overall condition of the patient. Paramount to the management of bowel injury is the prevention.

Prevention includes identifying the patients at risk, so that they can be appropriately counseled and prepared, as well as the use of meticulous surgical technique to avoid injuries. Alternative routes of surgery, such as a vaginal hysterectomy instead of an abdominal hysterectomy also should be considered. If the patient is having laparoscopic surgery one could use an open entry technique to insert the trocar, use a micro-laparoscope to evaluate the state of the adhesions, and perform the initial entry in the left hypochondrium, Palmer's point, to avoid the most likely location of adhesions and still evaluate the pelvis. Nasogastric decompression has also been recommended to minimize the risk of perforating a viscus.

The use of bowel preparation to prevent complications is not supported by the literature. A Cochrane Database review could not find any benefit to the routine use of a mechanical bowel preparation before abdominal surgery and also questioned the potential for complications (6). However, a subsequent meta-analysis looking specifically at the incidence of complications failed to show any clinical difference in complications whether a mechanical bowel preparation was used or not (7).

Small Bowel

Small bowel injuries during gynecologic surgery usually are a result of blunt or sharp dissection to release adhesions and restore normal anatomy. The small bowel is injured much more commonly than the large bowel. Although the technique of adhesiolysis varies depending on the type of adhesions and the surgeon's skill, in general, sharp dissection is preferred but at times blunt dissection or even electrocautery may be required to restore normal anatomy.

With the increasing use of laparoscopic surgery, more attention has been paid to the incidence of small bowel injury. However, it remains low ranging from 0.13% to 0.3%. In one large population study, the trocar or Veress needle were responsible for approximately 42% of the injuries, followed by the injuries caused by laser or coagulator (26%), those caused by grasping forceps and scissors (1%), and those caused by scissors (less than 1%). Approximately 32% of the time, the injury was caused by some other factor (8). Although the small Veress needle punctures of the small bowel may not require any special care other than careful follow-up, some experts advocate oversewing the area with a 3-0 delayed absorbable suture to limit the potential injury; other injuries will require more extensive repair or possibly even resection of the damaged segment of the bowel (Fig. 47).

Unrecognized thermal bowel injuries can have serious consequences and can be difficult to recognize. In fact, 15% of all laparoscopic bowel injuries are not recognized at the primary surgery. The tissue necrosis and subsequent perforation that occur with thermal injuries does so 72–96 hours after surgery when the patient is already home. A high index of suspicion is necessary to diagnose this injury early because delay in diagnosis is usually associated with increased morbidity and mortality.

When the serosa of the small bowel is torn exposing the underlying muscularis layer, it usually is repaired immediately because it can be difficult to find later. The repair involves oversewing the seromuscular layer of the bowel with a few interrupted sutures of a 3-0 delayed absorbable suture placed transversely through the longitudinal axis of the bowel to limit the narrowing of the lumen. This technique can be performed in several areas of the bowel if necessary. However, if the defect is large, there are numerous defects within a small section of the bowel, or if the defect involves the mesentery of the bowel, it is usually best to resect and reanastomose that segment of small bowel. Such repair usually is performed in a side-to-side fashion with two layers of interrupted delayed absorbable sutures or a surgical stapling device.

If the defect actually enters the lumen of the bowel, care should be taken to limit gross soilage with the use of laparotomy packs. Occasionally, bowel clamps can be used to limit the efflux from the enterotomy. The injury should be isolated, inspected, débrided, if necessary, and assessed for a primary repair or resection. Usually, if the injury involves less than 50% of the circumference of the bowel, a primary repair may be performed. If not, that area of small bowel will need to be resected and reanastomosed as described earlier.

At times, usually during an extensive adhesiolysis, one may encounter numerous areas of the bowel with a variety of injuries. The decision to resect or repair should be made judiciously because numerous resections of multiple segments of bowel are not recommended. In that setting, consultation with a surgeon experienced in bowel surgery would be helpful to assist in the decision of which injuries to repair and which to resect.

For crush injuries that are recognized early and are not necrotic, the area can be inspected and, if intact, the area of injury should be oversewn with interrupted 3-0 delayed absorbable seromuscular sutures taking care not to compromise the lumen of the bowel. It is not always necessary to excise the injured site.

Thermal injuries, such as the ones that occur most commonly with the use of electrosurgery especially during laparoscopy, are more difficult to assess. One must try to decide whether the injury is superficial, such as a small, 2 mm, surface cautery burn to control

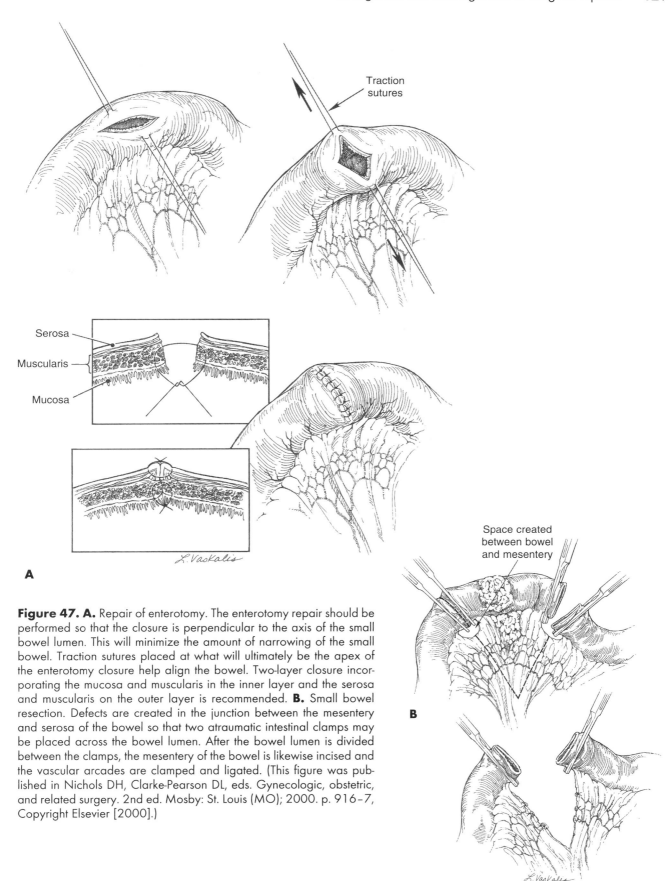

Traction
sutures

Serosa

Muscularis

Mucosa

L. Vaskalis

A

Space created
between bowel
and mesentery

B

Figure 47. A. Repair of enterotomy. The enterotomy repair should be performed so that the closure is perpendicular to the axis of the small bowel lumen. This will minimize the amount of narrowing of the small bowel. Traction sutures placed at what will ultimately be the apex of the enterotomy closure help align the bowel. Two-layer closure incorporating the mucosa and muscularis in the inner layer and the serosa and muscularis on the outer layer is recommended. **B.** Small bowel resection. Defects are created in the junction between the mesentery and serosa of the bowel so that two atraumatic intestinal clamps may be placed across the bowel lumen. After the bowel lumen is divided between the clamps, the mesentery of the bowel is likewise incised and the vascular arcades are clamped and ligated. (This figure was published in Nichols DH, Clarke-Pearson DL, eds. Gynecologic, obstetric, and related surgery. 2nd ed. Mosby: St. Louis (MO); 2000. p. 916–7, Copyright Elsevier [2000].)

L. Vaskalis

a small bleeding vessel, or extensive, which would require surgical repair. There is no steadfast rule to evaluate the injury and it is usually at the discretion of the surgeon and based on clinical experience. If there is any question, the area should be repaired either by oversewing (if the injury is small with no resection) or resection (if the area is larger) and repair as detailed earlier. One must remember that the extent of thermal injury usually exceeds the visual findings. With rare exceptions, there is no need for the routine use of closed suction drains after a small bowel repair.

Large Bowel

Injuries to the large bowel at the time of gynecologic surgery are even less common than injuries to the small bowel making up 41% of all bowel injuries in one laparoscopic series (9). In this series, 77% of the small bowel injuries were entry related and 41% of the large bowel injuries were entry related. The rest of the injuries were attributable to dissection injuries. Up to 70% of the small bowel and 51% of the large bowel injuries were not diagnosed at the initial surgery.

Risk factors for large bowel injury are similar to those of small bowel injuries and include adhesions, cancer, endometriosis, inflammatory bowel disease, and history of radiation. Prevention also is similar with meticulous dissection and a high index of suspicion. On occasion, in cases with extensive pelvic adhesive disease, a subtotal (supracervical) hysterectomy can be performed to limit the extent of dissection and potential

injury to the rectosigmoid colon. However, the current literature does not substantiate this benefit.

Injuries to the rectosigmoid colon can be managed similarly to the small intestine. Even in the presence of unprepared bowel, a Cochrane Database review supported the primary repair rather than fecal diversion with colostomy, especially if there is no gross fecal soilage in the peritoneal cavity (10). A diverting colostomy can be considered if rectosigmoid colon cannot be repair adequately or if the patient's health is compromised. A "bubble test" may be performed intraoperatively after the repair to see if there is an air leak. The pelvis is filled with a saline solution and the proctoscope is introduced through the anus and air is pushed across the anastomosis (Fig. 48). If an air leak is detected and bowel is repaired and made airtight, a colostomy can be avoided. However, if there is a persistent air leak, it is prudent to perform a diverting colostomy to allow the anastomosis to heal on its own. Most such injuries do not require any further surgery other than the reversal of the colostomy because they heal on their own if the fecal stream is diverted and they were not irradiated. Prophylactic drains have not shown any benefit in reducing the incidence of postoperative infections or anastomotic breakdown (11). If the large bowel is entered, coverage also should include better anaerobic and Gram-negative prophylaxis for 24 hours.

If a rectal injury is encountered at the time of vaginal surgery or at the time of an obstetric delivery, the management includes identification, inspection, débride-

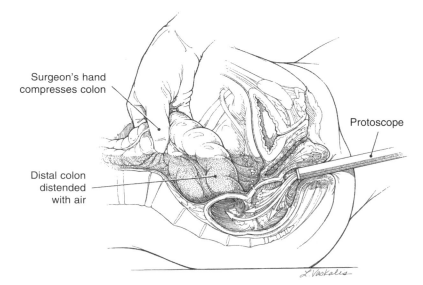

Figure 48. "Bubble test." To evaluate the possibility of an occult rectal injury, the pelvis is filled with a saline solution, and a proctoscope is introduced through the anus. The sigmoid colon at the pelvic brim is compressed between the surgeon's fingers and the rectosigmoid colon is insufflated with air. The appearance of bubbles coming from the rectum indicates rectal injury, which needs to be immediately repaired. (This figure was published in Nichols DH, Clarke-Pearson DL, eds. Gynecologic, obstetric, and related surgery. 2nd ed. Mosby: St. Louis (MO); 2000. p. 519, Copyright Elsevier [2000].)

ment, and closure in layers (at least two) with delayed absorbable 3-0 sutures. The surgeon should ensure that the sphincter is intact or properly repaired. A diverting colostomy is not routinely necessary. The administration of antibiotics at the time of a third- or fourth-degree perineal laceration repair after the delivery process has been shown to significantly decrease the perineal breakdown rate at 2 weeks. Of the patients seen at 2 weeks postpartum, 4 of 49 patients (8.2%) who received antibiotics and 14 of 58 patients (24.1%) who received placebo developed a perineal wound complication (P=0.037) (12).

Any patient with a rectosigmoid repair should avoid placing anything in the rectum and be placed on a low residue diet with stool softeners for a few weeks postoperatively. Enemas should be avoided during this time period to allow the anastomosis to heal.

References

1. Stany MP, Farley JH. Complications of gynecologic surgery. Surg Clin North Am 2008;88:343–59, vii.

2. Vakili B, Chesson RR, Kyle BL, Shobeiri SA, Echols KT, Gist R, et al. The incidence of urinary tract injury during hysterectomy: a prospective analysis based on universal cystoscopy. Am J Obstet Gynecol 2005;192:1599–604.

3. Ibeanu OA, Chesson RR, Echols KT, Nieves M, Busangu F, Nolan TE. Urinary tract injury during hysterectomy based on universal cystoscopy. Obstet Gynecol 2009;113:6–10.

4. Aronson MP, Aronson PK, Howard AE, Morse AN, Baker SP, Young SB. Low risk of ureteral obstruction with "deep" (dorsal/posterior) uterosacral ligament suture placement for transvaginal apical suspension. Am J Obstet Gynecol 2005;192:1530–6.

5. Learman LA, Summitt RL Jr, Varner RE, McNeeley SG, Goodman-Gruen D, Richter HE, et al. A randomized comparison of total or supracervical hysterectomy: surgical complications and clinical outcomes. Total or Supracervical Hysterectomy (TOSH) Research Group. Obstet Gynecol 2003;102:453–62.

6. Guenaga KK, Matos DD, Wille-Jorgensen P. Mechanical bowel preparation for elective colorectal surgery. Cochrane Database of Systematic Reviews 2009, Issue 1. Art. No.: CD001544. DOI: 10.1002/14651858.CD001544.pub3.

7. Contant CM, Hop WC, van't Sant HP, Oostvogel HJ, Smeets HJ, Stassen LP, et al. Mechanical bowel preparation for elective colorectal surgery: a multicentre randomised trial [published erratum appears in Lancet 2008;371:1664]. Lancet 2007;370:2112–7.

8. van der Voort M, Heijnsdijk EA, Gouma DJ. Bowel injury as a complication of laparoscopy. Br J Surg 2004;91:1253–8.

9. Baggish MS. One-hundred and thirty small- and large-bowel injuries associated with gynecologic laparoscopic operations. J Gynecol Surg 2007;23:83–96.

10. Nelson RL, Singer M. Primary repair for penetrating colon injuries. Cochrane Database of Systematic Reviews 2003, Issue 3. Art. No.: CD002247. DOI: 10.1002/14651858.CD002247.

11. de Jesus EC, Karliczek A, Matos D, Castro AA, Atallah AN. Prophylactic anastomotic drainage for colorectal surgery. Cochrane Database of Systematic Reviews 2004, Issue 2. Art. No.: CD002100. DOI: 10.1002/14651858.CD002100.pub2.

12. Duggal N, Mercado C, Daniels K, Bujor A, Caughey AB, El-Sayed YY. Antibiotic prophylaxis for prevention of postpartum perineal wound complications: a randomized controlled trial. Obstet Gynecol 2008;111:1268–73.

Postoperative Complications

Daniel L. Clarke-Pearson

Gynecologic surgery infrequently results in significant surgical complications. However, the gynecologic surgeon must be prepared to recognize and manage complications in an expeditious fashion, in order to obtain the best surgical outcomes. Complications are more likely to occur in women with gynecologic cancer who undergo radical surgery and in older women and those who have medical comorbidities. Minimizing these problems often is accomplished by the astute clinician who is aware of potential complications and is proactive in prevention and early intervention.

Postoperative Hemorrhage

The early recognition and correction of postoperative hemorrhage is critical in order to prevent shock, multiorgan failure, and death. Early signs of postoperative bleeding may be low urine output, tachycardia, or hypotension. Intraabdominal or retroperitoneal bleeding is more difficult to recognize when compared with vaginal bleeding. A few basic principles are very important in the control of hemorrhage after gynecologic surgery. First, the patient's blood volume and coagulation factors must be maintained at all times. Loss of coagulation factors during intraoperative and postoperative hemorrhage results in continued bleeding that cannot be controlled by surgical means. In all cases, it should be emphasized that prompt replacement of clotting factors provided by transfusion of fresh frozen plasma and platelets is critical to achieve hemostasis in the face of hemorrhage.

Replacement of platelets and clotting factors in patients with massive transfusion is dependent on clinical and surgical assessments. According to the published guidelines from the American Society of Anesthesiologists platelet transfusion rarely is indicated for platelet counts greater than 100,000 per microliter and usually indicated for counts of less than 50,000 per microliter (with intermediate platelet counts of 50,000 per microliter to 100,000 per microliter, transfusion should be based on the risk of bleeding) (1). Fresh frozen plasma therapy is indicated in massively transfused patients if the prothrombin or activated partial thromboplastin time values exceed 1.5 times the normal values. In cases of massive postoperative blood loss, it may be prudent to administer fresh frozen plasma empirically (after four units of packed red blood cells). This strategy is aimed at preventing the patient from becoming hypocoagulable while awaiting the laboratory results (prothrombin time and partial thromboplastin time), which may take nearly an hour and another hour to thaw the fresh frozen plasma before it is available to be administered. Cryoprecipitate transfusions are recommended for correction of bleeding in massively transfused patients with fibrinogen concentrations of less than 80–100 mg/dL.

Hemorrhaging patients should receive blood products, crystalloids, and colloids to attain hemodynamic and metabolic balance. In gynecologic patients, the most common causes of postoperative life-threatening hemorrhage are bleeding from the angle of the vaginal cuff, retraction of ovarian or uterine vessels during hysterectomy, and retroperitoneal venous bleeding associated with radical cancer operations. Whatever the cause, immediate control of bleeding and reoperation as soon as the patient's condition is stable are essential for the treatment of shock from blood loss. Under any conditions, reoperation for postoperative hemorrhage is difficult, and a highly experienced gynecologic surgeon should be present or standing by. Expert administration of anesthesia, constant monitoring, and blood and fluid replacement are vital in continued emergency care.

Vaginal Bleeding

If the patient has continued vaginal bleeding after hysterectomy and is soaking several pads an hour, there is little to be gained by blind vaginal packing. After the patient is properly stabilized and prepared, reoperation should be undertaken. Careful vaginal examination with anterior and posterior exposure usually reveals a vaginal angle arterial "pumper." A single suture or two usually controls the bleeding. Small, oozing vessels on the cut surface of the vaginal wall may be cauterized with care to avoid bladder or rectal wall injury. Compression packs in the vagina may help slow venous ooze from the vaginal wall.

Uterine or Ovarian Vessel Bleeding

Bleeding from a uterine or ovarian vessel usually is the result of a slipped ligature or retraction of an artery. Compression should be applied to control bleeding, then the ureter must be identified before ligation or clipping of the bleeding vessel. When the bleeding is retroperitoneal, usually it is from the uterine artery or its branches. Hypogastric artery ligation may be required but, occasionally, does not control bleeding because of the rich collateral supply. In this case, radiographically controlled arterial embolization can be used.

Retroperitoneal Bleeding

Venous bleeding after retroperitoneal procedures is a more difficult problem than uterine or ovarian vessel bleeding. The blood loss may appear as a boggy mass that fills the broad ligament area or as a massive hematoma that extends into the iliac fossa and dissects to the renal area. Frequently, the source of the continuous oozing is difficult to locate. Expanding hematomas should be evacuated, bleeding vessels clamped and tied off or clipped, and the field dried. When the veins are in the presacral or terminal hypogastric areas, sutures often tear into another vein, and the bleeding becomes worse.

Under these circumstances, metal hemostatic clips may be used to halt the bleeding. Microfibrillar collagen, oxidized cellulose gauze, a hemostatic matrix, and fibrin sealant may help control hemostasis. Gauze packing, carefully placed with continuous compression, is a measure of last resort; yet, potentially lifesaving. When the area must be packed or drained, the exit for the pack may be facilitated through the vaginal cuff or by an extraperitoneal low flank incision. The pack may be removed after 24–48 hours once the patient is stabilized. Bleeding from sacral veins, such as the bleeding encountered during sacral colpopexy, may be controlled through tamponade by a sterile stainless-steel thumbtack pushed into the sacrum.

Management of Shock

During and after gynecologic surgery, blood volume deficit that results from intraoperative blood loss or postoperative hemorrhage is the most common cause of shock. This shock usually is manifested by arterial hypotension, tachycardia, a weak pulse, anxiety, skin pallor, diminished urinary output, and peripheral vasoconstriction. In addition to hemorrhage (hypovolemic shock), the differential diagnosis of shock must include other causes, such as cardiogenic (myocardial infarction) and cardiac compressive conditions (cardiac tamponade or pneumothorax), sepsis, drug overdose, and pulmonary embolus. Appropriate studies are dictated by the patient's signs and symptoms.

Consideration should be given to obtaining arterial blood gas analysis, an electrocardiogram, a chest radiograph, blood chemistry studies, and blood cultures. The patient should be prepared for blood transfusion. The degree and duration of postoperative shock determine the need for resuscitation, central venous pressure monitoring, and Swan–Ganz pulmonary artery catheterization.

Central Monitoring

Invasive cardiovascular (CV) monitoring may be lifesaving for patients with massive hemorrhage or patients who are at an additional risk because of preexisting cardiopulmonary disorders. The monitoring allows the rational use of fluids and cardioactive medications while avoiding the complications from their use. In patients with marked hemodynamic instability, peripheral artery cannulation allows continuous monitoring of systemic arterial pressure as well as ready access to obtain repeated analysis of arterial blood gases.

In patients without cardiac or pulmonary disease, monitoring of central venous pressure along with monitoring of the vital signs, urine output, and other clinical signs may be sufficient for fluid resuscitation. In addition, central venous pressure monitoring avoids several of the complications of a pulmonary artery (Swan–Ganz) catheter and may be accomplished with a simple manometer.

The usefulness of the Swan–Ganz catheter in critically ill patients (even those without heart disease) who do not respond to therapy based on an initial noninvasive assessment has been well documented. Additional diagnostic information may be obtained concerning unsuspected cardiac dysfunction, pulmonary artery embolization, or sepsis. Data available from central monitoring facilitate better management in patients without primary myocardial insult, but with hypotension and evidence of inadequate perfusion of vital organs (eg, oliguria, acidosis, and mental obtundation). Unnecessary fluid overload can be prevented and the risk of congestive failure and pulmonary edema reduced.

In patients with cardiac or pulmonary disease, cardiac output and resistance measurements allow the proper use of pressors, afterload and preload reducers, and fluids. In addition, if sepsis is part of the clinical picture, careful monitoring of pulmonary capillary wedge pressures may be necessary to prevent pulmonary edema, which is seen with even mild increases in left atrial pressure as a result of the increased permeability of the pulmonary vascular bed. This increased permeability also may be seen in patients in hypovolemic shock, again leading to pulmonary edema at relatively normal wedge pressures. Finally, invasive monitoring not only provides a direct measurement of cardiac function but also provides information within minutes about the effects of therapy. Complications of use of pulmonary artery catheters include pulmonary infarction distal to the catheter (1–2% of cases), pulmonary artery rupture (0.2% of cases), balloon rupture (3% of cases), and sepsis (2% of cases), all of which are made more likely by prolonged use of the catheter.

Venous Thromboembolic Complications

The causal factors of venous thromboembolism were first proposed by Virchow in 1858 and include a hypercoagulable state, venous stasis, and vessel endothelial injury. Preoperative evaluation of the patient should include a complete history and physical examination in order to identify the risk factors of venous thromboembolism listed in Box 4 (section "Perioperative Care").

In addition, intraoperative factors associated with postoperative venous thromboembolism included increased anesthesia time, increased blood loss, and the need for transfusion in the operating room. Prophylactic methods to reduce the risk of venous thromboembolism are discussed in the section "Perioperative Care."

Diagnosis and Treatment of Deep Vein Thrombosis

During the postoperative recovery, the early recognition of deep vein thrombosis (DVT) and pulmonary embolism and immediate treatment are critical. The signs and symptoms of DVT of the lower extremities include pain, edema, erythema, and prominent vascular pattern of the superficial veins. These signs and symptoms are relatively nonspecific; 50–80% of patients with these symptoms will not actually have DVT. Conversely, approximately 80% of patients with symptomatic pulmonary emboli have no signs or symptoms of thrombosis in the lower extremities. Because of the lack of specificity when signs and symptoms are recognized, additional diagnostic tests should be performed to establish the diagnosis of DVT.

B-mode duplex Doppler imaging is the most common technique used to diagnose symptomatic DVT. With duplex Doppler imaging, the femoral vein can be visualized and clots may be seen directly. Compression of the vein with the ultrasound probe tip allows assessment of venous collapsibility; the presence of a thrombus diminishes vein wall collapsibility. It should be recognized that ultrasound imaging is less accurate when evaluating the calf and the pelvic veins.

Magnetic resonance venography has a sensitivity and specificity comparable to venography. In addition, magnetic resonance venography may detect thrombi in pelvic veins that are not imaged by venography. The primary drawback of magnetic resonance venography is the time involved in examining the lower extremity and pelvis as well as the expense of this technology.

Although venography has been the standard technique for diagnosis of DVT, it is used only in cases where the clinical suspicion of DVT remains high after evaluation with ultrasonography and magnetic resonance venography. Venography requires the injection of a contrast dye into a vein on the dorsal surface of the foot, which may cause allergic reaction or renal injury, and may result in phlebitis in approximately 5% of patients.

Once a DVT is diagnosed, anticoagulant therapy should be instituted immediately. Treatment may be with either unfractionated heparin or low molecular weight heparin, followed by 6 months of oral anticoagulant therapy with warfarin.

Treatment with unfractionated heparin is intended to prevent proximal propagation of a thrombus and allow physiologic thrombolytic pathways to dissolve the clot. An initial bolus of 80 units of unfractionated heparin per kilogram is given intravenously, followed by a continuous infusion of 1,000–2,000 units/h (18 units/kg/h). Heparin dosage is adjusted to maintain activated partial thromboplastin time levels at a therapeutic level 1.5–2.5 times the control value. Initial activated partial thromboplastin time should be measured after 6 hours of heparin administration and the dose adjusted as necessary (2). A weight-based nomogram has proved helpful in achieving a therapeutic activated partial thromboplastin time (Table 17).

Low molecular weight heparin (enoxaparin and dalteparin) also is effective in the treatment of VTE and has a cost-effective advantage over intravenous heparin in that it may be administered in the outpatient setting (Box 29). Because low molecular weight heparin has a minimal effect on activated partial thromboplastin

Table 17. Heparin Administration for Treatment of Deep Vein Thrombosis or Pulmonary Embolism—Weight-Based Nomogram

Time of Administration	Dose
Initial dose	80-units/kg bolus, then 18 units/kg/h
APTT* less than 35 seconds (less than 1.2 × control)	80-units/kg bolus, then 4 units/kg/h
APTT* 35–45 seconds (1.2–1.5 × control)	40-units/kg bolus, then 2 units/kg/h
APTT* 46–70 seconds (1.5–2.3 × control)	No change
APTT* 71–90 seconds (2.3–3 × control)	Decrease infusion rate by 2 units/kg/h
APTT* greater than 90 seconds (greater than 3 × control)	Hold infusion for 1 h, then decrease infusion rate by 3 units/kg/h

Abbreviation: APTT indicates activated partial thromboplastin time.

*The APTT should be measured every 6 hours and the heparin dose adjusted as indicated.

Raschke RA, Reilly BM, Guidry JR, Fontana JR, Srinivas S. The weight-based heparin dosing nomogram compared with a "standard care" nomogram. A randomized controlled trial. Ann Intern Med 1993;119:874–81.

Box 29

Therapeutic Dosages of Low Molecular Weight Heparin

Enoxaparin
- 1 mg/kg subcutaneously twice daily or
- 1.5 mg/kg daily

Dalteparin
- First 30 days: 200 international units per kilogram of body weight subcutaneously once daily
- Months 2–6: 150 international units per kilogram of body weight subcutaneously once daily

The total daily dose should not exceed 18,000 international units. A pharmacist should be consulted if the patient has renal failure because the dose of dalteparin should be modified.

time, serial laboratory monitoring of partial thromboplastin time levels is not necessary. Similarly, monitoring of anti-Xa activity (except in difficult cases or those with renal impairment) has not been shown to be of significant benefit in a dose adjustment of low molecular weight heparin.

In most cases, the conversion from parenteral heparin or low molecular weight heparin to oral warfarin may start on the initial day of therapy. Once the warfarin dose is confirmed to be therapeutic (international normalized ratio [INR] of 2–3 for 2 consecutive days), heparin may be discontinued. Initially, the INR should be monitored frequently in order to appropriately adjust the warfarin dose. Once a stable warfarin dose is established, the INR may be checked less frequently. Patients should be cautioned to avoid the use of drugs and dietary products that might alter the metabolism or absorption of warfarin.

Diagnosis and Treatment of Pulmonary Embolism

Many of the signs and symptoms of pulmonary embolism are associated with other, more commonly occurring postoperative pulmonary complications. The classic findings of pleuritic chest pain, hemoptysis, shortness of breath, tachycardia, and tachypnea should alert the physician to the possibility of a pulmonary embolism. However, the signs often are much more subtle and may be suggested only by a persistent tachycardia or a slight elevation in the respiratory rate. Initial evaluation should include a chest X-ray, electrocardiography, and arterial blood gas assessment. Any evidence of abnormality should be further evaluated by ventilation–perfusion lung scan or a spiral CT scan of the chest. A high percentage of lung scan results may be

interpreted as "indeterminate." In this setting, careful clinical evaluation and judgment are required to decide whether pulmonary arteriography should be obtained. The treatment of pulmonary embolism includes the following steps:

1. Immediate anticoagulant therapy, identical to that outlined for the treatment of DVT
2. Respiratory support, including oxygen and bronchodilators—Intubation in an intensive care unit may be necessary.
3. Pulmonary embolectomy—Although massive pulmonary emboli are usually rapidly fatal, pulmonary embolectomy has been performed successfully on rare occasions.
4. Pulmonary artery catheterization with the administration of thrombolytic agents—Although it bears further evaluation, it may be important in patients with massive pulmonary embolism.
5. A vena cava filter—It may be necessary in situations in which anticoagulant therapy is ineffective in the prevention of repeated embolization.

Urinary Tract Complications

Infections

Historically, the urinary tract has been the most common site of infection in surgical patients. Recent studies indicate that the incidence of urinary tract infections after hysterectomy is 1–5% (3), but may approach 15% in patients undergoing pelvic floor operations (4). This decrease in the rates of urinary tract infections (UTIs) is most likely the result of increased perioperative use of prophylactic antibiotics. Catheterization of the urinary tract, either intermittently or continuously with the use of an indwelling catheter, has been implicated as a main cause of urinary tract contamination. Therefore, catheters should be used judiciously and in a sterile environment and discontinued as soon as possible. After most types of gynecologic surgery the catheter may be removed the day of surgery or in the morning of the first postoperative day.

Despite the high incidence of UTIs in the postoperative period, few of these infections are serious. Most are confined to the lower urinary tract, and pyelonephritis is a rare complication. The treatment of UTI includes hydration and antibiotic therapy. Commonly prescribed and effective antibiotics include sulfonamide, cephalosporins, fluoroquinolones, and nitrofurantoin. The choice of antibiotic should be based on knowledge of the susceptibility of organisms cultured at a particular institution. In some institutions, for example, more than 40% of *Escherichia coli* strains are resistant to ampicillin. For uncomplicated UTIs, an antibiotic that has good activity against *E coli* should be administered in the interim while awaiting the urine culture and sensitivity data.

Patients who have a history of recurrent UTIs, those with chronic indwelling catheters (Foley catheters or ureteral stents), and those who have urinary conduits should be treated with antibiotics that will be effective against the less common urinary pathogens, such as *Klebsiella* and *Pseudomonas* species. Chronic use of the fluoroquinolones for prophylaxis is not advised because these agents are notorious for inducing antibiotic-resistant strains of bacteria.

Injury

Unless bilateral ureteral obstruction has been caused by surgery, most patients with postoperative anuria or severe oliguria will have these findings secondary to prerenal hypovolemia that is resolved by hydration and diuresis. However, unilateral ureteral injury may not be recognized until several days postoperatively and may be manifest by flank pain, pyelonephritis, or a slight increase in the serum creatinine level. The volume of urinary output is rarely altered. When postoperative ureteral obstruction is suspected, evaluation may include the use of intravenous pyelography (IVP) or CT with contrast (in cases where serum creatinine level is normal) or with renal ultrasonography or furosemide renal scan. If ureteral obstruction is discovered, initial management should include cystoscopy with retrograde stent placement. If successful, the obstruction is likely due to tethering from nearby sutures or extrinsic compression from a mass. Leaving the stent in place for 6 weeks and then reevaluating with follow-up imaging is recommended. However, if a retrograde stent cannot be inserted, consideration should be given to reexploration to correct the obstruction. If reoperation is not reasonable, a percutaneous nephrostomy tube should be inserted.

Vaginal leakage of fluid during the first 10 weeks postoperatively is an ominous finding and requires evaluation for a urinary tract fistula. Confirming the presence of a fistula and, if present, identifying the location is the next priority. Initially, the bladder should be filled with a dyed (indigo carmine) saline solution. A vaginal examination should reveal dye draining from the upper vagina. If there is no leakage from the bladder, then intravenous indigo carmine solution should be administered. Dye draining from the vagina strongly suggests a ureteral vaginal fistula. Further investigation with IVP or CT (with intravenous contrast) and cystoscopy may further delineate the location of the fistula. A vesicovaginal fistula should be managed by decompression of the bladder by insertion of an indwelling Foley catheter to allow continuous drainage. This technique often will allow the fistula to close spontaneously. Similarly, if

an ureterovaginal fistula is discovered, a ureteral stent should be placed across the section of ureter that is fistulized. This technique usually will allow the ureteral injury to heal "over" the stent.

Gastrointestinal Complications

Ileus

After abdominal or pelvic surgery, most patients will experience some degree of intestinal ileus. The exact mechanism by which this arrest and disorganization of gastrointestinal motility occurs is unknown, but it appears to be associated with the opening of the peritoneal cavity and aggravated by manipulation of the intestinal tract and prolonged surgical procedures. Infection, peritonitis, and electrolyte disturbances also may result in ileus. For most patients undergoing gynecologic operations, the degree of ileus is minimal and gastrointestinal function returns relatively rapidly, allowing the resumption of oral intake within a few days of surgery. Patients who have persistently diminished bowel sounds, abdominal distention, and nausea and vomiting require further evaluation and more aggressive treatment.

Ileus usually is manifested by abdominal distention and should be evaluated initially by physical examination assessing the quality of bowel sounds and searching for tenderness or rebound on palpation. The possibility that the patient's signs and symptoms may be associated with a more serious intestinal obstruction or other intestinal complication must be considered. Pelvic examination should be performed to evaluate the possibility of a pelvic abscess or hematoma that may contribute to the ileus. Results of abdominal X-ray to evaluate the abdomen in the supine position as well as in the upright position usually will aid in the diagnosis of an ileus. The most common radiographic findings include dilated loops of small and large bowel as well as air-fluid levels in the upright position. In the postoperative gynecologic patient, especially in the upright position, the flat plate of the abdomen also may show evidence of free air. This is a common finding immediately after surgery and is not indicative of a perforated viscus in most patients. The remote possibility of distal colonic obstruction or pseudoobstruction (Ogilvie syndrome) suggested by a dilated cecum should be excluded by rectal examination, colonoscopy, or barium enema.

The initial management of a postoperative ileus is aimed at gastrointestinal tract decompression and maintenance of appropriate intravenous replacement fluids and electrolytes and includes the following steps:

1. A nasogastric tube should be used with discretion when gastric distention occurs.
2. Fluid and electrolyte replacement must be adequate to keep the patient well perfused. Significant

amounts of third-space fluid loss occur in the bowel wall, the bowel lumen, and the peritoneal cavity during the acute episode. Gastrointestinal fluid losses from the stomach may lead to a metabolic alkalosis and depletion of other electrolytes as well. Careful monitoring of serum chemistries and appropriate replacement are necessary.

3. Chewing gum has been shown to relieve ileus (5).

4. Most cases of severe ileus will begin to improve over a period of several days. In general, this is recognized by reduction in the abdominal distention, return of normal bowel sounds, and passage of flatus or stool. Follow-up abdominal radiographic results should be obtained as necessary for further monitoring.

5. If a patient shows no evidence of improvement during the first 48–72 hours of medical treatment, other causes of ileus should be sought. Such cases may include ureteral injury, peritonitis from pelvic infection, unrecognized gastrointestinal tract injury with peritoneal spill, or fluid and electrolyte abnormalities, such as hypokalemia. In the evaluation of persistent ileus, the use of water-soluble upper gastrointestinal contrast studies may assist in the resolution of the ileus.

Although ileus is a common complication after open abdominal–pelvic surgery, it is rare after vaginal and laparoscopic surgery. An ileus and abdominal distention or pain after these surgical procedures should raise a high degree of suspicion that a more serious complication (eg, bowel injury) has occurred.

Small Bowel Obstruction

Obstruction of the small bowel after abdominal surgery occurs in approximately 1–2% of patients, but may be more frequent after radical gynecologic oncology procedures because of the extensive dissection and sometimes extensive manipulation of the small bowel. The most common cause of small bowel obstruction is adhesions to the operative site. If the small bowel becomes adherent in a twisted position, partial or complete obstruction may result from distention, ileus, or bowel wall edema. Less common causes of postoperative small bowel obstruction include entrapment of the small bowel into an incisional hernia and an unrecognized defect in the small bowel or large bowel mesentery. Early in its clinical course, a postoperative small bowel obstruction may exhibit signs and symptoms identical to those of ileus. Initial conservative management as outlined for the treatment of ileus is appropriate. Because of the potential for mesenteric vascular occlusion and resulting ischemia or perforation, worsening symptoms of abdominal pain, progressive distention, fever, leukocytosis, or acidosis should

be evaluated carefully because immediate surgery may be required.

In most cases of postoperative small bowel obstruction, the obstruction is only partial and the symptoms usually resolve with conservative management, which may include the following steps:

1. After several days of conservative management further investigation may be necessary. Evaluation of the gastrointestinal tract with barium enema and an upper gastrointestinal series with small bowel follow-through are appropriate. Alternatively, an abdominal and pelvic CT scan with gastrointestinal contrast dye may be useful in identifying the location of obstruction (and also evaluates for the presence of an abscess, lymphocele, or ureteral injury.) In most cases, complete obstruction is not documented, although a narrowing or tethering of the segment of small bowel may indicate the site of the problem.

2. Further conservative management with nasogastric decompression and intravenous fluid replacement may allow time for bowel wall edema or torsion of the mesentery to resolve.

3. If resolution is prolonged and the patient's nutritional status is marginal, the use of total parenteral nutrition may be necessary.

4. Conservative medical management of postoperative small bowel obstruction usually results in complete resolution. However, if persistent evidence of small bowel obstruction remains after full evaluation and an adequate trial of medical management, exploratory laparotomy may be necessary to evaluate and manage the obstruction. In most cases, lysis of adhesions is all that is required, although a segment of small bowel that is badly damaged or extensively sclerosed from adhesions may require resection and reanastomosis.

Colonic Obstruction

Colonic obstruction after gynecologic surgery is exceedingly rare. Advanced ovarian carcinoma is the most common cause of colonic obstruction in the postoperative gynecologic surgery patient and is caused by extrinsic impingement on the colon by the pelvic malignancy. Occult intrinsic colonic lesions (eg, colon cancer) also may cause obstruction. When colonic obstruction is manifested by abdominal distention and abdominal radiography reveals a dilated colon and enlarging cecum, further evaluation of the large bowel is required by barium enema or colonoscopy. Dilation of the cecum to more than 10–12 cm in diameter as viewed by abdominal X-ray requires immediate evaluation and surgical decompression by performing a colectomy or colostomy. In some circumstances, an intraluminal stent may be placed endoscopically. Surgery should be performed as soon as the obstruction is documented. Conservative management of colonic obstruction is not appropriate, because the complication of colonic perforation has an exceedingly high mortality rate.

Diarrhea

Episodes of diarrhea often occur after abdominal and pelvic surgery as the gastrointestinal tract returns to its normal function and motility. However, prolonged and multiple episodes may represent a pathologic process, such as impending small bowel obstruction, colonic obstruction, or pseudomembranous enterocolitis. Excessive amounts of diarrhea should be evaluated by abdominal X-ray and stool samples tested for the presence of ova and parasites, bacterial culture, and *Clostridium difficile* toxin. Proctoscopy and colonoscopy also may be advisable in severe cases. Evidence of intestinal obstruction should be managed as outlined previously. Infectious causes of diarrhea should be managed with the appropriate antibiotics as well as fluid and electrolyte replacement. *Clostridium difficile*-associated pseudomembranous enterocolitis may result from exposure to any antibiotic. Discontinuation of these antibiotics (unless they are needed for another severe infection) is advisable, along with the institution of appropriate therapy. Because of the expense and nephrotoxicity of vancomycin, therapy with oral metronidazole may be preferred. Therapy should continue until the diarrhea abates, and several weeks of oral therapy may be required in order to obtain complete resolution of the pseudomembranous enterocolitis.

Pulmonary Complications

The respiratory tract is a relatively common site for complications after gynecologic surgery performed under general anesthesia. Risk factors include extensive or prolonged atelectasis, preexistent chronic obstructive pulmonary disease, severe or debilitating illness, central neurologic disease causing an inability to clear oropharyngeal secretions effectively, and nasogastric suction. In surgical patients, early ambulation and aggressive management of atelectasis are the most important preventive measures.

Significant proportions (40–50%) of hospital-acquired cases of pneumonia are caused by Gram-negative organisms. These organisms gain access to the respiratory tract from the oral pharynx. Gram-negative colonization of the oral pharynx has been shown to be increased in patients in acute care facilities and has been associated with the presence of nasogastric tubes, preexisting respiratory disease, mechanical ventilation, tracheal intubation, and paralytic ileus, which is associated with microbial overgrowth in the stomach.

A thorough lung examination should be included in the assessment of all febrile surgical patients. In the absence of significant lung findings, a chest X-ray should nonetheless be obtained in patients at high risk of pulmonary complications. A sputum sample also should be obtained for Gram stain and culture. The treatment should include postural drainage, aggressive pulmonary toilet, and antibiotics. The antibiotic chosen should be effective against both Gram-positive and Gram-negative organisms, and in patients who are receiving assisted ventilation, the antibiotic spectrum should include drugs that are active against *Pseudomonas* organisms.

Control of the airway is critical in the immediate postoperative period. Extubation may not be prudent or possible at the end of the case due to tracheal edema resulting from a difficult intubation. Alternatively, the patient may not have the physical capacity to adequately ventilate due to suppression of the respiratory drive from anesthetics and excess chest wall weight. Many obese patients have the obesity hypoventilation syndrome, which increases their baseline hypercarbia and also may delay extubation. It often is prudent to plan immediate postoperative admission to a surgical intensive care unit with mechanical ventilation and serial arterial blood sampling to aid in the proper timing for extubation.

After extubation, ventilation of the obese patient during sleep may be aided by the use of noninvasive positive pressure ventilation units, particularly if the patient has a history of sleep apnea and uses a continuous positive airway pressure machine at home. Respiratory therapists can be of assistance in patient instruction and management of continuous positive airway pressure equipment, in addition to other respiratory instruction. Monitoring with continuous pulse oximetry will assist the detection of impending respiratory failure.

There is a higher risk of aspiration in obese patients due to increased gastric residual volumes, a higher rate of gastroesophageal reflux disease, and increased intraabdominal pressure from mass effect. Neutralization of the stomach contents with a proton pump inhibitor can minimize the chemical burn potential of aspirated stomach contents. Gastrointestinal motility agents, such as metoclopramide, may decrease residual volume by increasing intestinal transit. It also is prudent to raise the head of the bed to prevent aspiration. Prophylaxis for postoperative venous thromboembolism and pulmonary embolism should be ordered for obese patients because they are at higher risk of these complications.

References

1. Practice guidelines for blood component therapy: a report by the American Society of Anesthesiologists Task Force

on Blood Component Therapy. Anesthesiology 1996;84: 732–47.

2. Raschke RA, Reilly BM, Guidry JR, Fontana JR, Srinivas S. The weight-based heparin dosing nomogram compared with a "standard care" nomogram. A randomized controlled trial. Ann Intern Med 1993;119:874–81.

3. Nieboer TE, Johnson N, Lethaby A, Tavender E, Curr E, Garry R, et al. Surgical approach to hysterectomy for benign gynaecological disease. Cochrane Database of Systematic Reviews 2009, Issue 3. Art. No.: CD003677. DOI: 10.1002/14651858.CD003677.pub4.

4. Falagas ME, Athanasiou S, Iavazzo C, Tokas T, Antasaklis A. Urinary tract infections after pelvic floor gynecological surgery: prevalence and effect of antimicrobial prophylaxis. A systematic review. Int Urogynecol J Pelvic Floor Dysfunct 2008;19:1165–72.

5. Purkayastha S, Tilney HS, Darzi AW, Tekkis PP. Meta-analysis of randomized studies evaluating chewing gum to enhance postoperative recovery following colectomy. Arch Surg 2008;143:788–93.

Surgical Site Infections

David A. Eschenbach

Approximately 2 million obstetric and gynecologic surgical procedures are performed annually in the United States. The large number of surgical site infections after surgery lead to national efforts to prevent postoperative infection, including the Surgical Care Improvement Project. Surgical site infections account for approximately 40% of nosocomial infections in patients who undergo surgery (1). From 2% to 5% of patients undergoing all types of surgery develop surgical site infections; however, some procedures, such as cesarean delivery have an even higher infection rate. Approximately two thirds of surgical site infections involve the surgical incision; the remaining one third involves the deep organs or spaces accessed during surgery (2).

The rate of surgical site infections depends on the degree of wound contamination (highest for contaminated or dirty wounds), the physical status of the patients (as determined by the American Society of Anesthesiologists), the duration of surgery (highest for surgery times beyond the 75th percentile of time) and body mass index (BMI) greater than 30 (expressed as weight in kilograms divided by height in meters squared). In patients with one of these risk factors, the risk of surgical site infections after abdominal hysterectomy (4.1%) is only slightly lower than those of surgical site infections after colon surgery (8.5%) and small bowel surgery (6.9%) (3).

Pathophysiology

Microbial contamination of the surgical site is necessary to produce a surgical site infection; however, microbial contamination alone does not necessarily produce infection. The risk of a surgical site infection also depends on the number of bacteria multiplied further by the virulence of those bacteria. Surgical site infections particularly increase when the number of bacteria exceeds 10^5 microbes per gram of tissue. The host's resistance to infection counters these effects to produce a surgical site infection (1). Most of this resistance to infection occurs at the local tissue level and includes normal glucose levels, temperature, and oxygen levels and limited tissue damage. The presence of antibiotics in the tissue before surgical incision reduces the risk of a surgical site infection by the local inhibition of bacterial growth in these spaces.

Bacteria most commonly arise from those present on the skin, vagina, or cervix and are carried by direct contamination of the surgical site. Breaches of the urinary or gastrointestinal systems allow direct contamination by flora in these areas. This flora usually is confined by anatomic barriers, such as skin or vagina, but surgical opening of these barriers exposes the deep tissue to microbes that exist on the skin or vaginal surface. A markedly increased contamination and subsequent surgical site infection rate occur with exposure to a high microbe concentration (in the colon), or particularly virulent microbes, such as with methicillin-resistant *Staphylococcus aureus* (MRSA), or both (active skin furuncles).

Hysterectomy presents special pathophysiologic considerations. In the case of vaginal hysterectomy or complete abdominal hysterectomy, vaginal and cervical flora not only contaminate the surgical site, but more than one third of patients undergoing complete hysterectomy accumulate ultrasound-apparent fluid collections between the vagina and the peritoneum and this collection supports microbial growth and increases the risk of a surgical site infection (4). A low rate of surgical site infections exists with subtotal hysterectomy where the cervix is left in situ and the surgical site is not contaminated by vaginal flora. Further, laparoscopic hysterectomy compared with other approaches immediately reduces the risk of postoperative nosocomial infection by more than 50% and minimizes the readmission rates for nosocomial infection (5); a similar reduction is reported after robotic hysterectomy.

Risk Factors

The skin is the source of gram-positive streptococci and staphylococci. The genital tract is the source of a wide variety of *Escherichia coli* and other gram-negative bacteria, streptococci, enterococci, and anaerobic bacteria. Occasionally, very virulent bacteria, such as group A streptococci and *Clostridium species*, are found in the vagina; infections from these bacteria often are life threatening.

Surgery is much more likely to cause infection when contamination occurs from bacterial vaginosis flora rather than from lactobacillus-dominant vaginal flora. The odds ratio of surgical site infections in women with bacterial vaginosis compared with lactobacillus-dominant flora is increased threefold to fourfold after complete hysterectomy. Normal lactobacillus-dominant vaginal flora has a low pH, hydrogen peroxide-producing bacteria, and bacteriocidins levels that all inhibit the growth of most other bacteria. Relatively avirulent *Lactobacillus* bacteria make up 90–95% of the bacterial count in this environment and limit the growth of potentially virulent bacteria.

By contrast, the vaginal flora in bacterial vaginosis has a concentration of 20–1,000 times more bacteria than lactobacillus-dominant flora. The high concentration and the potential virulence of these bacteria contribute to infection in the setting of bacterial vaginosis. In addition, the flora in bacterial vaginosis produces enzymes that increase virulence both by the inhibition of neutrophil function and the enhancement of invasion through the cervix.

Preoperative shaving increases the risk of wound infection threefold compared with hair clipping. Shaving causes small cuts of the skin that are readily colonized by bacteria, a condition that increases wound infection. Most operating rooms now use clippers and no razors. Control of distant skin and urinary tract infection also reduces the risk of a surgical site infection.

Patients with diabetes mellitus typically have confounding conditions that may independently increase the risk of a surgical site infection. However, control of diabetes before surgery as indicated by hemoglobin A_{1C} levels and low 48-hour postoperative glucose levels is associated with fewer infections (6). Furthermore, the intraoperative control of glucose levels in patients without overt diabetes may improve monocyte function and decrease wound infection. As mentioned, a BMI greater than 30 is associated with increased wound infection.

Several other patient characteristics are associated with surgical site infections, but no randomized study either has or can be done to determine if they are independent surgical site infection risk factors. Cigarette smoking, obesity, advanced age, poor nutrition, steroid use, and preoperative hospitalization all are associated with an increased rate of surgical site infections (1). In addition, it has long been suspected that surgical site infection risk is reduced by the careful handling of tissue, control of bleeding, obliteration of dead space, irrigation of dry tissue, use of fine suture, wound closure without tension, and the removal of blood clots. Close attention to these techniques prevents bacteria from being sequestered in sites not accessible to leukocytes and antibiotics.

Prevention

Distant preoperative chlorhexidine shower or intravaginal povidone–iodine application the night before surgery does not conclusively reduce surgical site infection. However, immediate preoperative chlorhexidine skin preparations and vaginal povidone–iodine cleansing reduce surgical site infection after cesarean delivery (7).

Data support the role of normal temperature, oxygen levels, and glucose levels during surgery in reducing the risk of a surgical site infection. A low core body temperature produces vasospasm, reduces oxygenation, and reduces immune responses (8). Patients undergo-

ing abdominal and prolonged procedures often develop hypothermia. Normal oxygen and glucose levels during surgery also prevent surgical site infections.

Appropriately administered perioperative antibiotics reduce the risk of surgical site infections in procedures with vaginal or colorectal contamination (Table 18) (9). A brief one- to two-dose course of antibiotics administered for prophylaxis before the surgical incision allows antibiotics to be absorbed in the tissue and the spaces where they can reduce, although not eliminate, tissue bacterial counts. A prophylactic agent should be chosen that is active against most (but not necessarily all) potential contaminating bacteria, safe and inexpensive, and not used to treat serious postoperative infection (to reduce antibiotic resistance).

The antibiotic should achieve a bactericidal concentration in serum and tissue by the time of incision (10). Cephalosporins should be administered within 1 hour before the incision (9). Infection rates increase in direct relation to a decrease in time between the antibiotic administration and the skin incision. Failure to administer prophylactic antibiotics before the incision is common; therefore, close communication between the surgeon, pharmacy, and an anesthesiologist is necessary to ensure timely and appropriate administration (11).

Antibiotic serum levels should be maintained during the procedure and for several hours after surgery. Dosages need to account for the half-life and the minimal inhibitory concentration for the expected microbes. For example, cefazolin should be administered every 3–4 hours during surgery and cefotetan every 6–8 hours of surgery (12). Antibiotics can be discontinued at the end of surgery. After that time no prophylactic benefit accrues; instead antibiotic use becomes detrimental. For existing infection, treatment with antibiotics is necessary and simple prophylaxis does not suffice. For colorectal surgery, parenteral metronidazole can be combined with cefotetan for prophylaxis.

Details of antibiotic use for gynecologic procedures have been published by the American College of Obstetricians and Gynecologists (the College) (9). Gynecologic procedures that require antibiotic prophylaxis include hysterectomy, urogynecology procedures, hysterosalpingography, and surgical abortion. Adverse reactions to antibiotics also are covered in the College document. Antibiotic prophylaxis is not recommended for laparoscopy, hysteroscopy, intrauterine device insertion, endometrial biopsy, or urodynamic procedures. Although currently not routinely recommended, the addition of a second prophylactic antibiotic to cefotetan appears to further reduce surgical site infection after cesarean section (13).

Prophylactic ciprofloxacin reduces bacteriuria from an indwelling urinary catheter. Short-term use of an indwelling urinary catheter does not require the use of antibiotic prophylaxis.

Table 18. Antibiotic Prophylactic Regimens by Procedure

Procedure	Antibiotic	Dose (single dose)
Hysterectomy	Cefazolin[†]	1 or 2[‡] gram IV
Urogynecology procedures, including those involving mesh	Clindamycin[§] plus gentamicin or quinolone[‖] or aztreonam	600 mg IV 1.5 mg/kg IV 400 mg IV 1 gram IV
	Metronidazole[§] plus gentamicin or quinolone[‖]	500 mg IV 1.5 mg/kg IV 400 mg IV
Laparoscopy Diagnostic Operative Tubal sterilization	None	
Laparotomy	None	
Hysteroscopy Diagnostic Operative Endometrial ablation Essure	None	
Hysterosalpingography or Chromotubation	Doxycycline[¶]	100 mg orally, twice daily for 5 days
IUD insertion	None	
Endometrial biopsy	None	
Induced abortion and dilation and evacuation	Doxycycline	100 mg orally 1 hour before procedure and 200 mg orally after procedure
	Metronidazole	500 mg orally twice daily for 5 days
Urodynamics	None	

Abbreviations: IUD indicates intrauterine device; IV, intravenously.

*A convenient time to administer antibiotic prophylaxis is just before induction of anesthesia.

†Acceptable alternatives include cefotetan, cefoxitin, cefuroxime, or ampicillin–sulbactam.

‡A 2-g dose is recommended in women with a body mass index greater than 35 (expressed as weight in kilograms divided by height in meters squared) or weight greater than 100 kg or 220 lb.

§Antimicrobial agents of choice in women with a history of immediate hypersensitivity to penicillin

‖Ciprofloxacin or levofloxacin or moxifloxacin

¶If patient has a history of pelvic inflammatory disease or procedure demonstrates dilated fallopian tubes. No prophylaxis is indicated for a study without dilated tubes.

Antibiotic prophylaxis for gynecologic procedures. ACOG Practice Bulletin No. 104. American College of Obstetricians and Gynecologists. Obstet Gynecol 2009;113:1180–9.

Postoperative Considerations

Initial Evaluation and Antibiotic Treatment

Postoperative infection usually is diagnosed from indirect data, such as a fever of 38.5°C or higher in the first 24 hours after surgery, in addition to other abnormalities, such as tachycardia, leukocytosis, and unusual pain and tenderness. The workup of a surgical site infection should include a careful physical examination and, if necessary, directed pelvic and abdominal, renal, or lung imaging. Infection at other sites (particularly the urinary tract and lung) should be excluded. In addition, other noninfectious causes of fever, including thrombophlebitis, also need to be excluded. The distinction of a surgical site infection from other causes of a fever is a critical step because based on the diagnosis, therapy moves in separate directions.

Direct evidence of a wound infection includes redness, swelling, and purulent wound drainage. Cultures must be obtained from wounds or postsurgical infection sites that appear life threatening to identify group A streptococci, clostridia and MRSA from wounds that do not respond to usual antibiotic treatment. Cultures are of limited use for other intraabdominal infections and blood cultures and although occasionally positive, do not generally help guide therapy (14).

Most women with postoperative infection have a polymicrobial infection that includes anaerobic bacteria. Antibiotics are effective for most pelvic infections if the antibiotic selected covers both common gram-negative and gram-positive aerobic and anaerobic bacteria. Antibiotic-resistant *S aureus* and *Pseudomonas* and *Enterobacter* species are unusual in obstetric and gynecologic care and do not require initial coverage. Antibiotic choices are similar to those used to treat intraabdominal infections (14) and include a single β-lactam or β-lactamase inhibitor combination (ampicillin–sulbactam, piperacillin–tazobactam, and ticarcillin–clavulanic acid), carbapenems (ertapenem, imipenem–cilastatin, and meropenem), extended cephalosporins (cefotetan and cefoxitin), or combination regimens (aminoglycoside plus clindamycin or metronidazole, cefuroxime plus metronidazole, ceftriaxone cefotaxime or cefepime plus metronidazole, or a quinolone combination [ciprofloxacin plus metronidazole]). For postoperative infections, all regimens are equally effective and none has superiority in randomized trials.

Clindamycin has extended anaerobic coverage and an ability to achieve high serum levels and even inhibit bacteria in sites with low oxygen tension. Clindamycin also inhibits gram-positive aerobic bacteria. Further, clindamycin has an antitumor necrosis factor effect that could reduce the overexpressed systemic inflammatory response that occurs in septic shock.

Metronidazole can be substituted for clindamycin, but it covers only anaerobes. Still, metronidazole remains effective against most anaerobic bacteria. The clinical efficacy of metronidazole and gentamicin is virtually the same as clindamycin and gentamicin in direct comparisons.

Gentamicin inhibits virtually all gram-negative aerobic bacteria associated with pelvic infections; antibiotic resistance usually is confined to hospital acquired respiratory and urinary tract gram-negative infection. However, gentamicin and other aminoglycosides are nephrotoxic. A serum level of 5 micrograms per milliliter is considered therapeutic to treat the more resistant gram-negative bacteria present in the lung or urinary tract. However, most gram-negative bacteria in female pelvic infections remain very susceptible to all of the aminoglycosides. Thus, young healthy women do not need peak and trough levels determined because the usual dose of all aminoglycosides produces antibiotic

concentrations that easily inhibit the aminoglycoside sensitive gram-negative bacteria found in pelvic infection. In pregnancy and the postpartum period, aminoglycoside peak and trough level tests also are not necessary. Although these women have the ability to rapidly excrete aminoglycosides because of their high glomerular filtration rates, even subtherapeutic aminoglycoside levels in these women are sufficient to inhibit gram-negative bacteria. By contrast, peak and trough levels of aminoglycosides should be measured in older women (particularly with cancer) or preeclamptic women who might have reduced renal function. Because of a potentially reduced renal function in these women, peak and trough levels are needed to detect unexpectedly high gentamicin levels and prevent both renal toxicity and hearing loss. The current recommended dosing of gentamicin is 4.5mg/kg daily. Although all of the aminoglycosides have similar coverage for the usual pelvic gram-negative bacteria, amikacin provides extended coverage for unusually antibiotic resistant gram-negative bacteria.

Many genital bacteria in pelvic infection produce β-lactam enzymes. The extended penicillins use a combination of penicillin with a β-lactam inhibitor, clavulanic acid, or tazobactam to inhibit β-lactam producing bacteria. Extended penicillins have good activity against both gram-positive aerobic and anaerobic bacteria. Extended cephalosporins have a similar ability to inhibit β-lactam-producing bacteria. However, cephalosporins are frequently used, particularly for prophylaxis, and there is more induced resistance with the cephalosporin that with extended penicillins.

Enterococci are frequent isolates from surgical site infections, especially when cephalosporins are used for prophylaxis. Neither cephalosporins nor penicillins inhibit enterococci, but ampicillin does. However, both intraabdominal infections and surgical site infections in which enterococci are isolated usually respond to antibiotics that do not inhibit enterococci. Still, it is appropriate to add ampicillin to regimens if enterococci are isolated and the patient does not clinically respond to a cephalosporin or a penicillin regimen.

Fluoroquinolones were originally indicated to treat urinary tract infections because of their excellent gram-negative spectrum. Ciprofloxacin and ofloxacin also have gram-positive aerobic activity as well as activity against gonorrhea and chlamydia. However, overuse of quinolones has led to bacterial resistance. Fluoroquinolones are second-line choices for surgical site infections.

Failure of Initial Treatment

A true failure of antibiotic therapy is unusual because most bacteria found in female pelvic infections are susceptible to antibiotics. Thus, continued signs of infection should prompt a search for a wound infection, urinary infection, pneumonia, and an abscess or, rarely, for toxin-producing bacteria that produce serious rapid infection and septic shock.

Postoperative cultures from transvaginal cervical, endometrial, or vaginal cuff sites usually contain contaminated or predictable bacteria. For these reasons, selection of treatment usually is made on an empirical basis because contaminated surgical site cultures are of limited benefit. Blood cultures, except in very ill or immunocompromised patients also are of limited benefit because a positive blood culture does not predict the patient who fails antibiotic therapy. Aerobic cultures suffice in most instances of wound infection, because even though anaerobes often are present, antibiotic therapy usually is chosen that appropriately covers the anaerobes; therefore, anaerobic resistance to antibiotics is unusual with pelvic-derived infection. Pelvic abscesses contain anaerobic bacteria in a polymicrobial infection and because material from an abscess is difficult to obtain, empirical coverage of both aerobic and anaerobic bacteria should be started.

However, a culture must be obtained before treatment in two cases: 1) grossly infected wound infections where MRSA is possible and 2) in the setting of a serious, rapidly developing infection, septic shock, or both where it is necessary to determine if the toxin-producing group A streptococci and clostridia are present in which case a rapid and complete surgical excision is required.

Leukocyte counts and the pulse are more sensitive indicators than the temperature to monitor a patient's response to antibiotics. Patients with no clinical improvement usually have the same or more abdominal tenderness, perhaps signs of wound infection, and usually no change in leukocytosis or tachycardia compared with patients who respond to the treatment. Patients with a slow response may continue to have a fever, but tenderness, leukocytosis, and pulse may be reduced. Patients with clinical improvement, but a slow response, should continue the antibiotic regimen for an additional day before a consideration of an antibiotic change. Patients with no clinical improvement or worsening signs need evaluation for wound infection, infection at other sites, and abscess. In rare cases of very ill patients with worsening signs, a surgical exploration should be considered to exclude a toxic-producing infection or a ruptured or injured viscus.

Grossly infected wounds should be drained and débrided. Extensive débridement requires general anesthesia to ensure patient's comfort and complete removal of devitalized tissue. Most localized infections can be débrided under a field block of local anesthesia. After adequate débridement, gentle tissue handling is advocated using only one–two daily changes of loosely applied wet gauze. Negative pressure vacuum therapy

to the wound also has improved healing. Medical grade honey is available and honey's limited but impressive value in even grossly infected wounds needs consideration (15). Rough handling of the wound should be avoided because it prevents fibroblast formation and inhibits healing. Healthy granulation tissue is associated with a low bacterial count, so once healthy granulation tissue appears, the wound can be closed safely and effectively. Secondary wound closure, as opposed to spontaneous healing of the wound reduces healing time and reduces both pain and costs (16). A field block of local anesthesia allows the placement of deep sutures; the skin can be approximated with sterile strips.

Wound or pelvic abscesses of more than 6 cm in diameter usually require surgical drainage. Abscess drainage removes enzymes and bacteria and restores leukocyte function and antibiotic levels. An abscess attached to the vagina that dissects the bladder from the rectum and is in the midline bulging into the vaginal can be safely drained vaginally. Small or unilocular abscesses along the anterior abdominal wall are most amenable to interventional radiologic drainage. Percutaneous drainage of intraabdominal abscess by interventional radiology also can be considered, but the catheter frequently plugs and up to one third of patients eventually need open abscess drainage (17). Open laparoscopy can be considered instead of open laparotomy to drain deep pelvic or multiloculated abscesses. The abscess is confirmed by aspiration of pus with a large bore needle and large drains can then be placed under laparoscopic visualization to provide continued drainage. The abscess cavity can be gently irrigated with water to improve and hasten drainage. However, patients who develop peritonitis with an abscess usually have a ruptured abscess and they need consideration for immediate laparotomy to remove intraabdominal pus and prevent septic shock.

Life-Threatening Infection

Most patients who die of obstetric or gynecologic infection in developed countries either have infection from toxin-producing bacteria (group A streptococci or clostridia) or necrotizing fasciitis. Neither of these infections responds to antibiotics alone (18). These infections must be properly distinguished from the usual surgical site infections. They manifest unusual symptoms, such as severe pain, extreme anxiety or confusion, rapidly increasing erythema around the wound despite appropriate antibiotics, respiratory distress, hemolysis, disseminated intravascular coagulation, multiorgan failure, or signs of septic shock. These infections are caused by the toxin-producing group A streptococci or clostridia. The toxins cause an overwhelming systemic inflammatory response in addition to local tissue damage that causes tissue necrosis and the sequestration of bacteria in dead tissue without a blood supply. In this setting, small toxin molecules continue to leak out of this space to cause the systemic effects while antibiotics are not able to adequately penetrate into the space because of the dead tissue, occluded blood vessels, or both. When these life-threatening infections are suspected, immediate surgical exploration is necessary to confirm and, if present, to remove the dead tissue and the source of toxin production (19). Delay of the surgical treatment of these infections and delay after septic shock that occurs in this setting markedly increases the already high 40–50% death rate with septic shock. Typically, such patients initially respond to fluid resuscitation. However, a failure to perform surgery in the small window of opportunity immediately after diagnosis and fluid resuscitation usually leads to a fetal outcome. Pressor therapy should be used as a bridge to allow surgery and not as a continued support tactic without surgery. Faced with these clinical findings, the clinician changes from a strategy of "treat with antibiotics and wait" used for the usual infection to a strategy of immediate surgical removal of infection.

The overall death rate for even previously healthy young patients in septic shock is approximately 40%. In most cases, infection so severe as to cause widespread systemic dysfunction, including disseminated intravascular coagulation or respiratory distress syndrome and especially septic shock, cannot be managed by antibiotics alone. As mentioned previously, virtually all such infections are caused by toxin-producing bacteria that need surgical removal. The one exception is surgical site infection from toxic shock syndrome, and virtually no postoperative patients should be considered to have a toxic shock syndrome without an exploratory operation.

Necrotizing fasciitis is another unusual, but potentially lethal, infection that can occur in any postoperative patient, but it is most common in patients with diabetes or impaired immunity (19). Most spontaneous infections that develop over days are caused by synergism between streptococci and staphylococci. However, a particularly lethal form of the infection can occur within a few hours of surgery; usually rapid infection results from group A streptococci. Necrotizing fasciitis usually involves only the superficial fascia and the subcutaneous tissue. Because the skin is not infected, little skin change occurs in early stages. Typically, excessive fluid collects and this produces significant local swelling and extreme pain. Fever is variable as is leukocytosis, but leukocyte counts higher than 30,000 per microliter are not unusual. Low serum calcium levels result from the combining of calcium with digested fat to form soap. Wound discharge typically is watery and lacks pus or a foul odor. The presence of gas in the wound also indicates necrotizing fasciitis. Late findings are continued spread of obvious cellulitis despite appropriate antibiotics and the development of septic shock in a patient with cellulitis.

Treatment with antibiotics alone does not control the infection. The baseline death rate of patients with necrotizing fasciitis is 50% and this rate increases to nearly 100% without surgical débridement. The necrotic area typically looks like cellulitis on inspection. However, tissue manipulation by gentle suction or débridement produces sloughing without bleeding. The area should be débrided back to the point where bleeding ensues. Extensive débridement of the entire abdominal wall or perineum is sometimes necessary in advanced cases. In such instances, the skin can be undermined and laid over the lower tissue level as a skin graft; however, with extensive devascularization, even the skin will eventually slough.

References

1. Mangram AJ, Horan TC, Pearson ML, Silver LC, Jarvis WR. Guideline for the prevention of surgical site infection, 1999. The Hospital Infection Control Practices Advisory Committee. Infect Control Hosp Epidemiol 1999;20:250–78; quiz 279–80.

2. National Nosocomial Infections Surveillance (NNIS) System Report, data summary from January 1992 to June 2002, issued August 2002. National Nosocomial Infections Surveillance System. Am J Infect Control 2002;30:458–75.

3. Culver DH, Horan TC, Gaynes RP, Martone WJ, Jarvis WR, Emori TG, et al. Surgical wound infection rates by wound class, operative procedure, and patient risk index. National Nosocomial Infections Surveillance System. Am J Med 1991;91:152S–7S.

4. Toglia MR, Pearlman MD. Pelvic fluid collections folowing hysterectomy and their relation to febrile morbidity. Obstet Gynecol 1994;83:766–70.

5. Soper DE, Bump RC, Hurt WG. Wound infection after abdominal hysterectomy: effect of the depth of subcutaneous tissue. Am J Obstet Gynecol 1995;173:465–9; discussion 469–71.

6. Estrada CA, Young JA, Nifong LW, Chitwood WR Jr. Outcomes and perioperative hyperglycemia in patients with or without diabetes mellitus undergoing coronary artery bypass grafting. Ann Thorac Surg 2003;75:1392–9.

7. Hass DM, Morgan AL, Darei S, Contreras K. Vaginal preparation with antiseptic solutions before cesarean section for preventing postoperative infection. Cochrane Database of Systematic Reviews 2010, Issue 3. Art. No.: CD007892. DOI: 10.1002/14651858.CD007892.pub2.

8. Melling AC, Ali B, Scott EM, Leaper DJ. Effects of preoperative warming on the incidence of wound infection after clean surgery: a randomized controlled trial [published erratum appears in Lancet 2002;359:896]. Lancet 2001; 358:876–80.

9. Antibiotic prophylaxis for gynecologic procedures. ACOG Practice Bulletin No 104. American College of Obstetricians and Gynecologists. Obstet Gynecol 2009;113:1180–9.

10. Owens SM, Brozanski BS, Meyn LA, Wiesenfeld HC. Antimicrobial prophylaxis for cesarean section before skin incision. Obstet Gynecol 2009;114:573–9.

11. Bratzler DW, Houck PM, Richards C, Steele L, Dellinger EP, Fry DE, et al. Use of antimicrobial prophylaxis for major surgery: baseline results from the National Surgical Infection Prevention Project. Arch Surg 2005;140:174–82.

12. Bratzler DW, Houck PM. Antimicrobial prophylaxis for surgery: an advisory statement from the National Surgical Infection Prevention Project. Surgical Infection Prevention Guidelines Writers Workgroup; American Academy of Orthopaedic Surgeons; American Association of Critical Care Nurses; American Association of Nurse Anesthetists; American College of Surgeons; American College of Osteopathic Surgeons; American Geriatrics Society; American College of Anesthesiologists; American Society of Colon and Rectal Surgeons; American Society of Health-System Pharmacists; American Society of PeriAnesthesia Nurses; Ascension Health; Association of periOperative Registered Nurses; Association for Professionals in Infection Control and Epidemiology; Infectious Diseases Society of America; Medical Letter; Premier; Society for Healthcare Epidemiology of America; Society of Thoracic Surgeons; Surgical Infection Society. Clin Infect Dis 2004;38:1706–15.

13. Tita AT, Hauth JC, Grimes A, Owen J, Stamm AM, Andrews WW. Decreasing incidence of postcesarean endo-metritis with extended-spectrum antibiotic prophylaxis. Obstet Gynecol 2008;111:51–6.

14. Solomkin JS, Mazuski JE, Baron EJ, Sawyer RG, Nathens AB, DiPiro JT, et al. Guidelines for the selection of anti-infective agents for complicated intraabdominal infections. Infectious Diseases Society of America. Clinical Infect Dis 2003;37:997–1005.

15. Al-Waili NS, Saloom KY. Effects of topical honey on post-operative wound infections due to gram positive and gram negative bacteria following caesarean sections and hyster-ectomies. Eur J Med Res 1999;4:126–30.

16. Walters MD, Dombroski RA, Davidson SA, Mandel PC, Gibbs RS. Reclosure of disrupted abdominal incisions. Obstet Gynecol 1990;76:597–602.

17. Shuler FW, Newman CN, Angood PB, Tucker JG, Lucas GW. Nonoperative management for intraabdominal abscesses. Am Surg 1996;62:218–22.

18. Eschenbach DA. Preventing and managaing incisional sur-gical site infections. Contemp Ob Gyn 1998;43(9):69–85.

19. Gallup DG, Freedman MA, Meguiar RV, Freedman SN, Nolan TE. Necrotizing faciitis in gynecologic and obstet-ric patients: a surgical emergency. Am J Obstet Gynecol 2002;187:305–10; discussion 310–1.

Sterilization

Amy J. Voedisch and Paul D. Blumenthal

Sterilization procedures are safe and effective methods of permanent contraception that are used by more than 220 million couples globally. In the United States, tubal sterilization (used by approximately 10.3 million women annually) is the second most common form of contraception overall and the most common form of contraception in women older than 35 years. Tubal sterilization combined with vasectomy is the leading method of birth control in the United States (1).

Patient Selection and Counseling

Sterilization procedures result in permanent, lifelong contraception. Although reversal techniques for both men and women are available, they may not be successful. Therefore, counseling should emphasize the permanence of these methods and only patients who are interested in a permanent, nonreversible method of birth control are realistic candidates for sterilization.

Such counseling should involve a thorough review of all contraceptive methods, including forms of long-acting reversible contraception that have similar efficacies as sterilization. Patients should also be informed of the various methods of sterilization, including the multiple tubal ligation and vasectomy techniques. Risks of the procedures should be reviewed in detail, including surgical risks, failure rates, and long-term effects. Physicians also need to comply with any regulatory requirements regarding the informed consent process and timing of the procedure.

Tubal Occlusion Methods

There are multiple approaches to tubal sterilization and method selection often is determined by the timing of the surgery in relation to pregnancy. Procedures can be performed postpartum, postabortion, or as interval procedures remote from pregnancy.

Postpartum Methods

Tubal sterilizations can be performed at the time of a cesarean delivery or in the postpartum period after a vaginal delivery through an infraumbilical minilaparotomy incision. Postpartum sterilization is most expeditiously performed either immediately after delivery or within 24–48 hours. Such postpartum tubal ligation procedures usually are partial salpingectomies or tubal resections. Several techniques have been described, including Pomeroy and Parkland methods, which are the most commonly used (Fig. 49 and Fig. 50). These and other techniques are compared in Table 19. Laparoscopic, suprapubic minilaparotomy, and transvaginal partial salpingectomies also can be performed outside of the postpartum period. Postpartum tubal ligation procedures account for approximately 50% of procedures performed in the United States (2). These techniques have one of the lowest failure rates with a 0.3–1% 10-year probability of pregnancy (3).

One of the challenges of postpartum sterilization is providing the desired procedure in a timely fashion. Only 50–60% of women who consent to postpartum

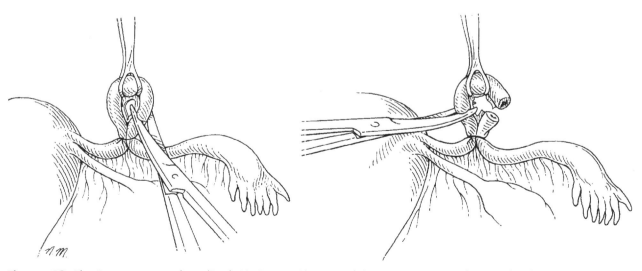

Figure 49. The Pomeroy procedure. (Rock JA, Jones HW. Te Linde's operative gynecology 10th edition. Philadelphia [PA]: Wolters Kluwer/Lippincott Williams & Wilkins; 2008.)

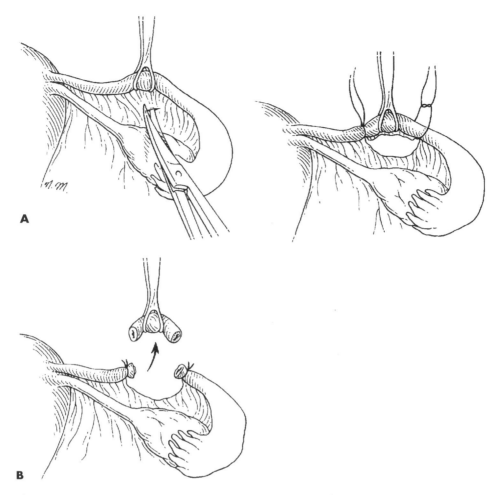

Figure 50. The Parkland procedure. (Rock JA, Jones HW. Te Linde's operative gynecology 10th edition. Philadelphia [PA]: Wolters Kluwer/Lippincott Williams & Wilkins; 2008.)

sterilization undergo the surgery during the obstetric hospital stay. Identified barriers to the procedure include maternal medical complications and contraindications to surgery, lack of hospital resources and personnel to perform the surgery, insufficient anesthesia services, last-minute maternal misgivings, and lack of a valid Medicaid consent form (4). Young women (younger than 25 years) who have had vaginal deliveries also are less likely to have the surgery than older women or those who have had a cesarean delivery (5). One study reported that 18% of women who did not receive their desired postpartum sterilization procedures had subsequent pregnancies with the mean time between deliveries of 19.8 months (6).

Interval Methods

Interval sterilizations can be performed laparoscopically, transcervically, transvaginally, or by suprapubic minilaparotomy. In recent years, these procedures are typically performed laparoscopically with a 10-year failure rate ranging from 0.1% to 5% depending on the method

used and age at time of sterilization. New transcervical approaches have recently been described and are safe and equally effective alternatives.

Laparoscopic Techniques

Electrocoagulation and methods using various mechanical devices (the silicone rubber band [Falope ring], spring-loaded [Hulka–Clemens] clip, and titanium clip lined with silicone rubber [Filshie clip]) (Fig. 51 and Fig. 52) comprise the most common forms of laparoscopic tubal sterilizations and are reviewed in Table 19. Although these methods typically are used as interval laparoscopic procedures, they can also be employed postpartum, at the time of cesarean delivery or through a suprapubic interval minilaparotomy.

Transcervical Techniques

Transcervical approaches to tubal sterilization are cost-effective and offer the advantage of avoiding a transabdominal procedure. A variety of techniques have

Table 19. Postpartum and Interval Sterilization Methods

Sterilization Method	Surgical Technique	Efficacy	Comments
Postpartum			
Pomeroy*	Partial salpingectomy Ligation of tube in a loop with plain catgut Excision of ligated tissue	3.8 pregnancies per 1,000 cases	Most common method Delayed absorbable suture increases failure due to fistula formation, recanalization, or both
Parkland*	Partial salpingectomy Segment excised after ends individually ligated	3.8 pregnancies per 1,000 cases	
Irving[†]	Partial salpingectomy similar to Parkland Proximal portion buried into uterine myometrium	Less than 1 pregnancy per 1,000 cases	Typically performed with cesarean deliveries Increase risk of intraoperative blood loss Decreased risk of fistula
Uchida[‡]	Partial salpingectomy Proximal portion buried by closure of mesosalpinx	No pregnancies in 20,000 cases	Uncommon method
Fimbriectomy[§]	Distal one third of tube and fimbriae excised	24 pregnancies per 1,000 cases	Rarely used due to higher failure rates from incomplete fimbriae excisions
Interval–Laparoscopic			
Unipolar coagulation*	Unipolar coagulation with hook or forceps	1.8 pregnancies per 1,000 cases	First laparoscopic method Risk of thermal injury
Bipolar coagulation*	Bipolar coagulation with forceps of 3 cm tubal segment with 25W of current	6.3 pregnancies per 1,000 cases	Lower thermal injury risk Replaced unipolar method Optical flow meter decreases failure rate
Falope ring*	Silicone rubber band placed over loop of tube	4.5 pregnancies per 1,000 cases	Tubal pathology relative contra-indication
Spring clip*	Clip placed perpendicular to tube Cannot be repositioned	18.2 pregnancies per 1,000 cases	Tubal pathology relative contra-indication
Filshie clip[‖]	Similar application to spring clip	2.3 pregnancies per 1,000 cases	Easier to apply than spring clip Tubal pathology relative contra-indication

*Peterson HB, Xia Z, Hughes JM, Wilcox LS, Tylor LR, Trussell JP. The risk of pregnancy after tubal sterilization: findings from the U.S. Collaborative Review of Sterilization. Am J Obstet Gynecol 1996;174:1161–8; discussion 1168–70.
[†]Milad M, Le L. Laparoscopic Irving tubal sterilization. A case report. J Reprod Med 1998;43:215–8.
[‡]Uchida H. Uchida tubal sterilization. Am J Obstet Gynecol 1975;121:153–8.
[§]Oskowitz S, Haverkamp AD, Freedman WL. Experience in a series of fimbriectomies. Fertil Steril 1980;34:320–3.
[‖]Penfield J. The Filshie clip for female sterilization: a review of world experience. Am J Obstet Gynecol 2000;182:485–9.

been researched over the years, most of them using hysteroscopic guidance, including thermal, mechanical, and sclerosing methods. Thermal-only methods have largely been abandoned because of high failure rates and significant morbidity, such as bowel injuries and peritonitis. Mechanical approaches involving various plugs have also been studied, the most notable being the technique that involves the formation of a silicone plug in-situ with success rates similar to traditional laparoscopic techniques. Complications, including uterine perforation, pelvic pain, plug fracture, and extravasation of silicone into the peritoneal cavity, have decreased the popularity and advisability of this technique. It is currently available only in parts of Europe.

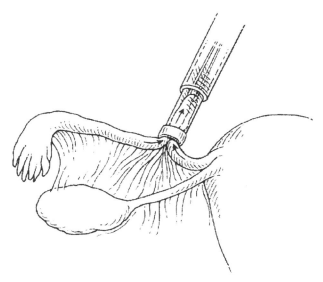

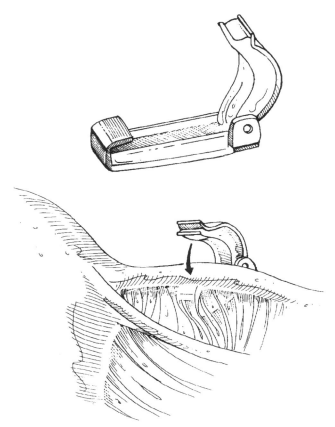

Figure 51. Falope ring application. (Rock JA, Jones HW. Te Linde's operative gynecology 10th edition. Philadelphia [PA]: Wolters Kluwer/Lippincott Williams & Wilkins; 2008.)

Sclerosing techniques involve a blind introduction of chemicals into the uterine cavity resulting in tubal occlusion. Disadvantages include the potential need for repeat applications to obtain tubal occlusion, use of caustic agents with possible spillage into the peritoneal cavity, and higher rates of failure. Multiple agents have been investigated over time, including phenol, tetracycline, methyl cyanoacrylate, and quinacrine.

Quinacrine, an intercalating agent that inhibits DNA repair, was used in the first reported method of chemical occlusion in the early 1970s and is the only chemical still being investigated today with more than 100,000 reported cases to date. The approach involves instillation of 252 mg of quinacrine hydrochloride into the uterine cavity using a modified intrauterine device inserter. The procedure has to be repeated in 1 month. Reported 10-year failure rates of sterilization with quinacrine are approximately 9–12% with significantly lower failure rates for women older than 35 years (7). In addition to this high failure rate, the safety of quinacrine is controversial because it is mutagenic with conflicting data about its potential carcinogenicity. Furthermore, confirmation of tubal occlusion with quinacrine is challenging. Confirmatory hysterosalpingography (HSG) cannot be performed because the imaging study itself may disrupt the occlusion. As a result of its high failure rate and unresolved safety issues, quinacrine currently is not available in the United States.

In 2002, the United States Food and Drug Administration (FDA) approved a contraceptive tubal occlusion device and delivery system (Essure). This was followed by the approval in July 2009 of another permanent contraception system (Adiana). These transcervical methods offer the advantage of no incision and no

Figure 52. Filshie clip application. (Rock JA, Jones HW. Te Linde's operative gynecology 10th edition. Philadelphia [PA]: Wolters Kluwer/Lippincott Williams & Wilkins; 2008.)

intraabdominal surgery and also can be performed in an office setting, often with minimal anesthesia required. They offer a permanent option for women with contraindications to surgery, such as medical comorbidities or pelvic adhesions that would interfere with transabdominal tubal ligation techniques. The failure rates of transcervical approaches are similar to traditional methods at 0.1–0.23% (8).

The major disadvantage to these transcervical sterilization methods is the 12-week delay required for the endotubal reaction to occur that accounts for the effectiveness of the procedure, necessitating the need for additional contraception during this time. These techniques also require a follow-up imaging study, such as HSG, to confirm complete tubal occlusion. For both procedures, proficiency at operative hysteroscopy is necessary to ensure expeditious and satisfactory placement of the devices into the internal tubal meatus.

Contraindications to transcervical sterilization include sensitivity to nickel, inability or unwillingness to undergo HSG, inability to access the tubal ostia bilaterally due to uterine or tubal pathology, such as submucosal fibroids or anomalies, recent or current pelvic infections, and recent pregnancy or abortion within the past 6 weeks (9).

Since the introduction of the first device in 2002 and its successful integration in practice, trends in sterilization techniques have indicated a relative decrease in laparoscopic methods and a resultant increase in hysteroscopic procedures (10). The use of this device involves a placement of a contraceptive insert into the interstitial portion of the fallopian tube under hysteroscopic guidance. The insert consists of an inner coil of stainless steel that is layered with polyethylene terephthalate fibers and an outer coil of nickel–titanium. The insert is loaded into a single-use device and inserted into the proximal fallopian tube in a coiled state. Once in the proper position, with a 5–10 mm tail left within the uterine cavity, the device is deployed and the coils expand, anchoring the insert into position. The polyethylene terephthalate fibers invoke a tissue response and fibrotic in-growth occludes the tube in 12 weeks. This device is easy to use with 94–99% of inserts successfully placed bilaterally (9, 11). The microinsert is cost-effective with reported savings over traditional laparoscopic tubal ligation methods (12, 13) (Fig. 53).

Patients need to be counseled that future surgery using unipolar coagulation is contraindicated after the placement of the insert and although magnetic resonance imaging studies are safe, artifact from the inserts may occur. Pregnancy is contraindicated after an endometrial ablation and it is possible to perform concomitant transcervical sterilization at the time of the ablation procedure. The uterine balloon therapy system, impedance controlled endometrial ablation system, and hydrothermal ablation are the most commonly reported methods of ablation combined with hysteroscopic sterilization (14). In theory, the energy used to perform the ablative procedure could be conducted through the nickel–titanium inserts and cause intraperitoneal thermal injury. This can be avoided by performing the ablation before the insertion of the implants. There have also been reported cases of inability to achieve a satisfactory HSG image due to intrauterine synechiae formed after the ablation procedure; however, most studies do not report any difficulties with the follow-up HSG studies.

The other transcervical permanent female contraception system currently available on the US market is a polymer matrix transcervical sterilization system that uses a combination of thermal injury caused by radiofrequency and the insertion of a silicone matrix to occlude the fallopian tubes. After the delivery system catheter is inserted into the tubal ostia under hysteroscopic guidance, proper placement is confirmed by the position detection array. Radiofrequency energy is then delivered through the tip of the catheter for 1 minute, causing a 5-mm thermal injury to the fallopian tube. A silicon matrix is then deployed within the thermal lesion and the catheter and hysteroscope are removed with no visible implant within the uterine cavity. The matrix stimulates a tissue reaction that leads to occlusion in 12 weeks. A follow-up HSG is conducted to confirm adequate sterilization. Early studies have shown a 95% bilateral placement success rate (15) (Fig. 54).

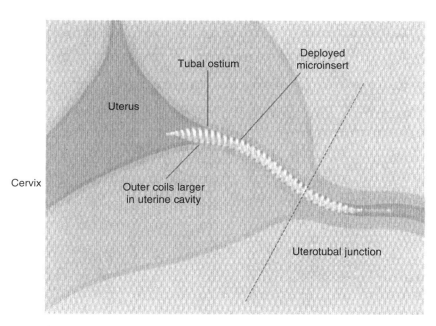

Figure 53. Microinsert placement. (Rock JA, Jones HW. Te Linde's operative gynecology 10th edition. Philadelphia [PA]: Wolters Kluwer/Lippincott Williams & Wilkins; 2008.)

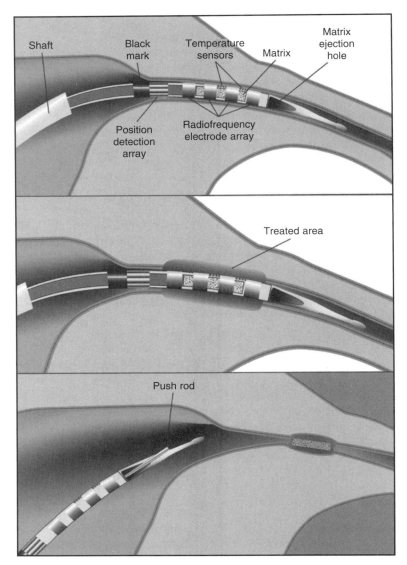

Figure 54. Illustration of the polymer matrix transcervical sterilization system procedure. This sequence of three sketches illustrates the stages of the intervention. The upper image shows the catheter in place, with the visual marker within the uterine cavity and thus visible by hysteroscopy. The middle image gives an idea of the lesion created, reaching approximately 0.5 mm into the tissue. The lower image shows the end result. (Vancaillie TG, Anderson TL, Johns DA. A 12-month prospective evaluation of transcervical sterilization using implantable polymer matrices. Obstet Gynecol 2008;112:1270–7.)

Transvaginal Techniques

Although no longer commonly performed for a variety of reasons (eg, inability to locate or ligate tubes and the risk of infection), interval tubal ligation procedures also can be performed transvaginally through a posterior colpotomy incision. This procedure has the advantage of avoiding an abdominal incision as well as reducing the reliance on technology and high maintenance, expensive equipment. Usually partial salpingectomies are performed with this approach but any of the described laparoscopic methods also could be used. According to one study, rates of failures and complications, including infections, may be similar to those of traditional approaches (16).

Anesthesia Selection

Tubal occlusion can be performed under general, regional, or local anesthesia. In the United States, postpartum sterilizations are generally provided using regional anesthesia, especially if the patient had an epidural anesthesia during labor. Minilaparotomy procedures, both postpartum and interval, also can be performed under local anesthesia with or without (in some developing countries) sedation. Laparoscopic techniques traditionally use general anesthesia but regional and local anesthesia with sedation also are cost-effective options. Transcervical approaches generally use a combination of local anesthesia with intravenous sedation. Procedures performed under local anesthesia, with or without intravenous sedation, offer the advantage of a decreased risk of complications from anesthesia, faster recovery times, and reduced cost.

Complications

Tubal sterilization procedures have a risk of death of 1–2 per 100,000 procedures (2). Most deaths in the United States are secondary to complications from general anesthesia. Risks of major morbidity after sterilization procedures performed postpartum are generally related to complications of the pregnancy or delivery itself, the only exception being the relative likelihood of a complication of general anesthesia in the postpartum setting.

The U.S. Collaborative Review of Sterilization (CREST) reported a range of major complications for interval procedures of 1.6–3.5% with the highest risks associated with interval minilaparotomy (3.5%) as compared with laparoscopic procedures (1.6%) (17). A more recent 2004 Cochrane database review did not reveal any difference in major morbidity rates in laparoscopic versus minilaparotomy procedures. However, there was a higher risk of minor morbidity associated with the minilaparotomy incisions (18). Overall complication rates were 0.9–1.6 per 100 procedures. The risk of complications was higher for women with diabetes, general anesthesia, previous abdominal or pelvic surgery, and obesity.

The major risks associated with transcervical sterilization include tubal perforation and hypovolemia during the procedure. Few long-term studies are available but reported risks of tubal perforation range from 1% to 3% (19). There have been no major adverse events reported to date with either FDA-approved transcervical method.

Tubal sterilizations are highly effective, but failures and resultant unintended pregnancies can occur. The U.S. Collaborative Review of Sterilization is the largest study to date on outcomes of sterilization techniques with an average of 8–14 years of follow-up for each subject (3). Of note, Filshie clips and transcervical sterilization techniques were not included in this study because they were introduced after the CREST study was published.

The overall failure rate of the CREST study was 13 per 1,000 procedures after 5 years of follow-up. This failure rate varies depending on the method of occlusion used and the patient's age at time of sterilization. Postpartum partial salpingectomies and unipolar interval methods have the lowest failure rates (1.1% and 0.37%, respectively), whereas the spring-loaded clip and bipolar coagulation have the highest failure rates (5%) for women aged 18–27 years at the time of sterilization. These failure rates decrease dramatically as women age, especially for patients older than 34 years. After 10 years, the probability of pregnancy for postpartum partial salpingectomy is 3.8 per 1,000 procedures for women in that age group. Bipolar coagulation failure rates also decreased in procedures performed in later years with the use of a current meter with 25W of power and the destruction of a continuous 3 cm segment of fallopian tube. The use of Filshie clip has largely replaced the spring-loaded clip in the United States and many other countries, and is also a highly effective method of sterilization with a 0.23% failure rate (Fig. 55, Table 19) (20).

Patients with successful bilateral transcervical micro-insert device placements have occlusion 96% of the time at the 3-month HSG follow-up. Repeat HSG studies in the phase III trials at 6 months confirmed 100% bilateral occlusion but other studies have reported a small rate of persistent tubal patency (21). The micro-insert currently has a reported mean failure rate of 1.28

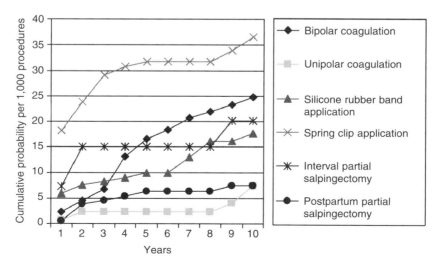

Figure 55. Life-table cumulative probability of pregnancy among women who had undergone tubal sterilization by method (cumulative probability per 1,000 procedures). (Modified from Peterson HB. Sterilization. Obstet Gynecol 2008;111:198–203.)

pregnancies per 1,000 procedures (8). Most failures are related to noncompliant patient or physician follow-up with the required HSG. Other causes of failures include pregnancy at the time of placement and misinterpretation of the HSG studies. There have been two isolated case reports of pregnancy after HSG verified tubal occlusion with perforation of the device later confirmed at the uterine cornua. The polymer matrix system is reported to carry a 1.82% failure rate at 2 years (22). Long-term follow-up studies are currently underway but initial reports indicate these procedures have at least comparable efficacy to more traditional methods.

Patients should be counseled regarding the risk of an unintended pregnancy after sterilization as previously detailed. They also should be counseled if they do become pregnant because there is a 33%-risk of an ectopic pregnancy. The crude overall 10-year probability of an ectopic pregnancy with all methods of tubal sterilization as described by the CREST study is 7.3 per 1,000 procedures. This risk is highest with bipolar coagulation and the spring-loaded clip at 17.1 and 8.5 per 1,000 procedures, respectively. The risk is lowest for postpartum partial salpingectomy and unipolar coagulation at less than 2 per 1,000 procedures for each method (2). Patients with a history of a tubal ligation and a subsequent positive pregnancy test result should be evaluated for a potential ectopic pregnancy at their initial presentation.

Long-Term Effects

Tubal sterilization is considered permanent contraception and most women who choose this method do not regret their decision. The CREST data revealed a 12.7% overall cumulative probability of regret with 14 years of follow-up. However, women older than 30 years had a 5.9% reported risk of regret whereas women aged 30 years and younger had a 20.3% rate of regret. Although age is a reliable predictor of regret, other risk factors include making the decision under pressure from a spouse or medical indication, marital discord at time of procedure, and subsequent change in marital status (23, 24). There also is no reported difference in rates of regret after tubal ligation or vasectomy (2).

There have been numerous reports of menstrual disturbances, including menorrhagia and dysmenorrhea, after sterilization. The term *posttubal ligation syndrome* has been coined for this phenomenon. Follow-up larger studies have contradicted these earlier reports. The largest analysis by the CREST data evaluated women 5 years after interval sterilization and compared them with those women whose partners underwent a vasectomy. Women with tubal occlusion were found to have a decrease in the amount and length of bleeding and decreased pain associated with menstruation. There was no difference in intermenstrual bleeding or cycle length. These women were more likely, however, to report cycle irregularities. Therefore, recent data argue strongly against the presence of the posttubal ligation syndrome and patients who ask about it should be counseled appropriately (2).

Women with a history of tubal ligation have an increased risk of a hysterectomy in the future (relative risk, 1.6–4.4) reported by several investigators (25). The CREST study reported that this increase risk persisted regardless of method of occlusion and age at time of sterilization. A comparison with women whose partners had a vasectomy confirmed this increased risk. The basis of this association is unclear, but women with a history of menstrual irregularities or benign pathology, such as leiomyomas or endometriosis predating the sterilization procedure, had a higher risk of hysterectomy in the future. These data are consistent with previously published studies. There is no known biologic causal etiology. It is possible that women with a history of sterilization are more likely to consider or be amenable to surgical options or, in light of their already-sterilized state, are more likely to be considered candidates for definitive surgical management of their gynecologic conditions (2).

Tubal sterilization has a long-term protective effect on ovarian cancer incidence (relative risk, 0.29–0.69) as reported in several observational studies. There also is a decreased risk of hospitalization for pelvic inflammatory disease; however, the procedure does not protect against sexually transmitted infections (2).

Most women (80%) report no change in sexual desire or interest after tubal sterilization. However, 17–18% of women do report an increase in interest or desire. There does not appear to be a negative impact on sexual function after a tubal occlusion procedure (2).

Women with a previous history of tubal ligation who undergo a subsequent endometrial ablation may have an increased risk of developing severe, cyclic pelvic pain. This phenomenon was first described after the introduction of rollerball endometrial ablation and rates of 6% have been reported with this ablative technique (26). This is likely related to residual endometrium in one or both cornua. Patients with a tubal ligation should be counseled regarding this potential complication.

Vasectomy

Vasectomy is the most effective method of male contraception and is widely used throughout the world. Approximately 500,000 vasectomies are performed yearly in the United States and it is the fourth most common form of contraception (1, 27). When combined with tubal sterilization, this is the most common method of birth control used in the United States.

Compared with female sterilization, vasectomy is safer because it is less invasive and commonly performed under local anesthesia alone. In addition, due to the feasibility of performing these procedures in an office setting, the minimal anesthesia needed and lack of required expensive equipment, vasectomy is more cost-effective than tubal sterilization. It is one of the most cost-effective contraceptive options available, comparable to the intrauterine device and system (28).

Methods

Vasectomy is a minor surgical procedure usually lasting 15 minutes and typically is performed by a urologist, family physician, or general surgeon. A vasectomy traditionally involves the surgical transection of the vas deferens with a combination of ligation; partial excision; and coagulation, fascial interposition, or both.

CONVENTIONAL VASECTOMY

Vasectomy traditionally employs bilateral scrotal incision and conventional scrotal dissection to isolate and transect the vas deferens. This procedure has been largely replaced in the United States and many other countries by the "no-scalpel" technique.

NO-SCALPEL TECHNIQUE

The no-scalpel technique was first described in China in 1973. After first isolating and grasping the vas deferens through the previously anesthetized scrotal skin (a specially designed no-scalpel vasectomy forceps is used for this), a single puncture is made with a sharp mosquito hemostat in lieu of bilateral incisions. The vas deferens is then easily retrieved from the grasp of the vasectomy forceps, brought through the puncture site, and transected. This technique has a decreased risk of side effects compared with conventional vasectomy (29).

Efficacy and Failure Rates

A semen analysis to confirm successful occlusion is required after a 3-month waiting period and 20 ejaculations because 80% of men will be azoospermic at that time. Patients need to be counseled to continue an alternative method of contraception during this timeframe until the confirmation of complete occlusion.

Reported failure rates of vasectomy are between 1% and 2%, with variation depending on the type of transection technique used. In the CREST study, the 5-year cumulative failure rate was 11.3 per 1,000 procedures (2).

Surgical Risks

Major complications and death are exceedingly rare after a vasectomy. Minor complications occur in less than 5% of procedures and include infection, sperm granu-

loma, hematoma, and persistent postoperative pain (2). Hematoma is the most common complication to occur. The risk of minor complications is lower with the no-scalpel technique, especially with regard to hematoma formation and infections. Surgeon experience appears to be the most important prognostic determinant of complications with those performing greater than 50 procedures a year having one third the rate of complications compared with those performing less than 10 procedures per year (30).

Long-Term Effects

There have been occasional reports of increased risk of atherosclerosis, prostate cancer, and testicular cancer after a vasectomy. However, more recent, rigorously conducted, larger studies have failed to prove any association of vasectomy with these long-term effects (2).

There has also been controversy regarding the existence of a postvasectomy pain syndrome, which has been reported in 0.1–15% of men after a vasectomy. This entity is poorly understood, but is thought to be due to chronic congestive epididymitis. If not relieved with supportive measures, surgical options, including a vasectomy reversal, may provide pain relief for some patients (2, 30).

References

1. Mosher WD, Martinez GM, Chandra A, Abma JC, Willson SJ. Use of contraception and use of family planning services in the United States: 1982-2002. Adv Data 2004;350:1–36.

2. Peterson HB. Sterilization. Obstet Gynecol 2008;111:189–203.

3. Peterson HB, Xia Z, Hughes JM, Wilcox LS, Tylor LR, Trussell J. The risk of pregnancy after tubal sterilization: findings from the U.S. Collaborative Review of Sterilization. Am J Obstet Gynecol 1996;174:1161–8; discussion 1168–70.

4. Zite N, Wuellner S, Gilliam M. Barriers to obtaining a desired postpartum tubal ligation. Contraception 2006;73:404–7.

5. Zite N, Wuellner S, Gilliam M. Failure to obtain desired postpartum sterilization: risk and predictors. Obstet Gynecol 2005;105:795–9.

6. Seibel-Seamon J, Visintine JF, Leiby BE, Weinstein L. Factors predictive for failure to perform postpartum tubal ligations following vaginal delivery. J Reprod Med 2009;54:160–4.

7. Sokal DC, Hieu T, Loan ND, Hubacher D, Nanda K, Weiner DH, et al. Contraceptive effectiveness of two insertions of quinacrine: results from 10-year follow-up in Vietnam. Contraception 2008;78:61–5.

8. Levy B, Levie MD, Childres ME. A summary of reported pregnancies after hysteroscopic sterilization. J Minim Invasive Gynecol 2007;14:271–4.

9. Essure: permanent birth control system. San Carlos (CA): Conceptus Inc.; 2002. Available at: http://www.accessdata.fda.gov/cdrh_docs/pdf2/P020014c.pdf. Retrieved December 7, 2010.

10. Shavell VI, Abdallah ME, Shade GH Jr, Diamond MP, Berman JM. Trends in sterilization since the introduction of Essure hysteroscopic sterilization. J Minim Invasive Gynecol 2009;16:22–7.

11. Arjona JE, Mino M, Cordon J, Povedano B, Pelegrin B, Castelo-Branco C. Satisfaction and tolerance with office hysteroscopic tubal sterilization. Fertil Steril 2008;90:1182–6.

12. Kraemer DF, Yen PY, Nichols M. An economic comparison of female sterilization of hysteroscopic tubal occlusion with laparoscopic bilateral tubal ligation. Contraception 2009;80:254–60.

13. Levie MD, Chudhoff SG. Office hysteroscopic sterilization compared with laparoscopic sterilization: a critical cost analysis. J Minim Invasive Gynecol 2005;12:318–22.

14. Donnadieu AC, Deffieux X, Gervaise A, Faivre E, Frydman R, Fernandez H. Essure sterilization associated with endometrial ablation. Int J Gynaecol Obstet 2007;97:139–42.

15. Vancaillie TG, Anderson TL, Johns DA. A 12-month prospective evaluation of transcervical sterilization using implantable polymer matrices. Obstet Gynecol 2008;112:1270–7.

16. Ayhan A, Boynukalin K, Salman MC. Tubal ligation via posterior colpotomy. Int J Gynaecol Obstet 2006;93:254–5.

17. Jamieson DJ, Hillis SD, Duerr A, Marchbanks PA, Costello C, Peterson HB. Complications of interval laparoscopic tubal sterilization: findings from the United States Collaborative Review of Sterilization. Obstet Gynecol 2000;96:997–1002.

18. Kulier R, Boulvain M, Walker DM, De Candolle G, Campana A. Minilaparotomy and endoscopic techniques for tubal sterilization. Cochrane Database of Systematic Review 2004, Issue 3. Art. No.: CD001328. DOI: 10.1002/14651858.CD001328.pub2.

19. Hurskainen R, Hovi SL, Gissler M, Grahn R, Kukkonen-Harjula K, Nord-Saari M, et al. Hysteroscopic tubal sterilization: a systematic review of the Essure system. Fertil Steril 2010;94:16–9.

20. Penfield J. The Filshie clip for female sterilization: a review of world experience. Am J Obstet Gynecol 2000;182:485–9.

21. Cooper JM, Carignan CS, Cher D, Kerin JF. Microinsert nonincisional hysteroscopic sterilization. Selective Tubal Occlusion Procedure 2000 Investigators Group. Obstet Gynecol 2003;102:59–67.

22. Adiana permanent contraception. Bedford (MA): Hologic; 2009. Available at: http://www.accessdata.fda.gov/cdrh_docs/pdf7/P070022c.pdf. Retrieved December 7, 2010.

23. Jamieson DJ, Kaufman SC, Costello C, Hillis SD, Marchbanks PA, Peterson HB. A comparison of women's regret after vasectomy versus tubal sterilization. US Collaborative Review of Sterilization Working Group. Obstet Gynecol 2002;99:1073–9.

24. Ludermir AB, Machado KM, Costa AM, Alves SV, Araujo TV. Tubal ligation regret and related risk factors: findings from a case-control study in Pernambuco State, Brazil. Cad Saude Publica 2009;25:1361–8.

25. Cohen MM. Long-term risk of hysterectomy after tubal sterilization. Am J Epidemiol 1987;125:410–9.

26. Mall A, Shirk G, Van Voorhis BJ. Previous tubal ligation is a risk factor for hysterectomy after rollerball endometrial ablation. Obstet Gynecol 2002;100:659–64.

27. Sheynkin YR. History of vasectomy. Urol Clin North Am 2009;36:285–94.

28. Trussell J, Lalla AM, Doan QV, Reyes E, Pinto L, Gricar J. Cost effectiveness of contraceptives in the United States [published erratum appears in Contraception 2009;80:229–30]. Contraception 2009;79:5–14.

29. Art KS, Nangia AK. Techniques of vasectomy. Urol Clin North Am 2009;36:307–16.

30. Adams CE, Wald M. Risks and complications of vasectomy. Urol Clin North Am 2009;36:331–6.

Pregnancy Termination

Anitra Beasley, Ana Cepin, and Carolyn Westhoff

Approximately one half of the pregnancies in the United States are unintended and more than 40% of these pregnancies are terminated (1). Overall, 22% of all pregnancies, excluding miscarriages, are terminated. At current rates, one third of women will have at least one induced pregnancy termination in their lifetimes (2). After peaking in the 1980's, the pregnancy termination rates persistently decreased, albeit more slowly after 2000, until 2005. Data collected for 2005 and 2006 reveal a 3.2% increase in these rates (3). Most terminations are performed for undesired pregnancies, but there are other maternal and fetal indications. Pregnancy is contraindicated in women with several medical conditions, including pulmonary hypertension, recent myocardial infarction, and other comparable major illnesses. Fetal anomalies and premature rupture of membranes in the early second trimester may be indications for terminations of pregnancy. Wide spread first-trimester screening results in the detection of fetal anomalies at an earlier stage and so pregnancy termination rates are affected.

Over time, some patterns of abortions have changed. From 1974 to 1989, women in their late teens had the highest abortion rates of all age groups, but now, more than one half of all abortions are performed for women in their twenties (Table 20). Almost 90% of all abortions are performed during the first 12 weeks of gestation, and the proportion performed before 9 weeks of gestation has increased to more than 60%. Most abortions are performed in non-hospital facilities, including freestanding clinics and office settings (4).

Patients and their health care providers can be reassured that abortion does not lead to problems in future pregnancies nor does it increase the risk of breast cancer, infertility, spontaneous abortion, ectopic pregnancy, early pregnancy failure, or birth defects in subsequent pregnancies (5). Even in the second trimester, gradual cervical dilation before dilation and evacuation (D&E) does not increase the future risk of preterm labor or delivery (6). Existing research does not support that abortion in itself increases the risk of poor psychologic outcomes (5).

Preprocedure Counseling and Evaluation

Counseling presents the patient with an opportunity to discuss her feelings and concerns regarding the pregnancy and available options and may include assistance with decision making, contraceptive choices, clarification of values, and referral for other health or social services. Once the health care provider is satisfied that the decision to terminate the pregnancy is not coerced, the evaluation may continue.

A pertinent history is obtained and physical examination performed as necessary. Before the procedure, gestational age must be accurately assessed, either by ultrasonography or bimanual examination in the first trimester and by ultrasonography in the second trimester. In the second trimester a patient with a suspected or actual placenta previa and prior uterine scarring should be evaluated for other placental abnormalities, such as placenta accreta. Rh-negative patients should receive Rh immune globulin regardless of gestational age (7).

Table 20. Characteristics of U.S. Women Obtaining Abortions, 2008

Characteristic	% of Abortions
Age	
Younger than 20 years	17.6
Aged 20–29 years	57.8
Aged 30 years or older	24.6
Parity	
0	39.1
1 or more	61
Marital status	
Unmarried	85.2
Married	14.8
Race or ethnicity	
Non-Hispanic white	36.1
Non-Hispanic black	29.6
Non-Hispanic other	9.4
Hispanic	24.9
Family income as percentage of federal poverty level	
Less than 100	42.4
100–199	26.5
200 or greater	31.1

Jones RK, Finer LB, Singh S. Characteristics of U.S. abortion patients, 2008, New York (NY): Guttmacher Institute, 2010. Available at: http://www.guttmacher.org/pubs/US-Abortion-Patients.pdf. Retrieved December 7, 2010.

Both medical and surgical approaches are available for terminating early gestations, whereas surgical methods and medical induction of labor are options for later gestations. The choices are affected by the availability of services. For example, 69% of metropolitan counties and 97% of nonmetropolitan counties have no trained abortion providers (2).

Medical Approach

Nonsurgical or medical pregnancy termination refers to the complete expulsion of the products of conception without surgical intervention and is widely available in the United States. Absolute contraindications for a medical approach are few and include suspicion of ectopic pregnancy, current anticoagulation or clotting disorder, concurrent long-term corticosteroid use, chronic adrenal failure, inherited porphyrias, and known hypersensitivity to misoprostol or mifepristone. First-trimester medical termination of pregnancy often includes heavy bleeding and passage of clots. Access to emergency care and follow-up care to ensure the abortion is complete also are indicated.

First-Trimester Gestations

The combination of mifepristone and misoprostol is the most commonly used regimen for termination of pregnancy. The regimen was approved for this indication by the U.S. Food and Drug Administration in 2000. The technique is highly effective, with published complete expulsion rates of up to 99%; however, effectiveness decreases slightly with advancing gestational age (8).

Mifepristone is a potent progesterone antagonist that acts on the pregnant uterus to cause decidual necrosis, detachment of the trophoblast, and cervical softening as well as uterine contractility and increased prostaglandin sensitivity. Misoprostol is a synthetic prostaglandin E_1 analogue that causes heightened uterine contractions and cervical softening, leading to expulsion of the products of contraception. The FDA-approved protocol is 200 mg of oral mifepristone followed 2 days later by 400 micrograms of oral misoprostol in gestations of up to 49 days. However, nearly all health care providers in the United States use an evidence-based regimen of 200 mg of mifepristone and 800 micrograms of buccal or oral misoprostol self-administered 6–72 hours after the administration of mifepristone. When oral misoprostol is used, this regimen is recommended up to 56 days of gestation and when misoprostol is given by the buccal route the regimen can be administered up to 63 days of gestation (7).

Bleeding heavier than menses and potentially severe cramping are to be expected and last for 4–6 hours; lighter bleeding and spotting may persist until the next spontaneous menses. Most health care providers encourage use of nonsteroidal antiinflammatory drugs (NSAIDs) for pain control and some also prescribe narcotic analgesics. Side effects, such as nausea, vomiting, diarrhea, warmth or chills, headache, dizziness, and fatigue, are common after misoprostol use.

Methotrexate, an antimetabolite that interferes with DNA synthesis and cell division, also may be combined with misoprostol to terminate a pregnancy, but it is less often used because of the greater availability of mifepristone. It is most commonly administered intramuscularly at the same dose used for the treatment of an early ectopic pregnancy, 50 mg/m^2, but other effective regimens include a standard intramuscular or oral dose (7). The use of combination of methotrexate and misoprostol results in complete termination rates of 92–96% in gestations up to 49 days, which decrease to 82% in gestations of between 50 days and 56 days (8). Therefore, this regimen is not recommended after 49 days of gestation (7). The use of 800 micrograms of misoprostol alone (moistened with water and placed vaginally) can result in complete pregnancy termination rates of 90% in women with pregnancies up to 56 days of gestation (8).

Patients return for follow-up with repeat ultrasonography or serial β-hCG testing 1–2 weeks later to evaluate the result of pregnancy termination. Presence of an intrauterine gestation with cardiac activity is considered a failed procedure. When medical protocol fails, surgical termination is strongly advised because of possible risk of fetal malformation from misoprostol use. If the gestational sac is present but without cardiac activity, the patient may elect to take additional misoprostol, have a suction curettage, or wait for spontaneous expulsion. However, no randomized studies have accessed the efficacy of additional doses of medication versus expectant management. After expulsion, the uterus often will contain substantial echogenic tissue consisting of blood, clots, and decidua. In the absence of excessive bleeding, these patients can be treated conservatively.

Second-Trimester Gestations

In the United States, greater than 97% of pregnancies in the second trimester are terminated using a surgical method (9). However, labor induction also may be used. In this method, medications are used to induce contractions, and the fetus and placenta are expelled in a manner similar to vaginal delivery. Routine curettage after medical induction is not necessary, but uterotonics or surgical intervention may be needed to complete the procedure in case of placental retention. Transient fetal survival can be a problem in second trimester medical terminations after 21 weeks of gestation. To prevent this complication, health care providers may use intracardiac potassium chloride or intrafetal or intraamniotic digoxin as feticidal agents before induction. Some practitioners believe that induced fetal demise facilitates second-trimester medical and surgical pregnancy termination; however, evidence supporting this claim is lacking.

Whether surgical or medical method is chosen will depend on patient preference and the medical services available. For an induction technique, personnel capable of surgical management, the necessary equipment, and a clinician for emergency care must be available throughout the process. If autopsy is desired, induction may provide the best chance for an intact specimen.

Intraamniotic solutions of hypertonic saline or urea were frequently used for induced termination of pregnancy until the 1980s, but misoprostol has largely succeeded instillation techniques due to safety concerns, the long induction to abortion time, and the frequent need for curettage after fetal expulsion (10). Still, the search for an optimal regimen for second trimester medical termination of pregnancy continues.

Mifepristone and Prostaglandin

Medical termination of pregnancy with mifepristone and a prostaglandin analogue is appropriate for second trimester abortions up to 24 weeks of gestation. The addition of mifepristone to a prostaglandin used alone increases the overall success rate, shortens the time to expulsion, and reduces the number of prostaglandin doses required for successful outcome. Current data support the use of 200 mg oral mifepristone followed by 600–800 micrograms of vaginal misoprostol 36–48 hours later; thereafter, 400 micrograms of oral or vaginal misoprostol may be used every 3 hours until complete termination of pregnancy or a maximum of five doses (7). Although the dose of mifepristone does not change with increasing gestational age, the dose of misoprostol may need to be increased. This regimen can be used in patients with previous cesarean deliveries. Available information suggests that the rate of uterine rupture in women with a scarred uterus is less than 0.3% (11).

Misoprostol

When given in combination, mifepristone and misoprostol act synergistically, and when both are available, both should be used. If mifepristone is not available, misoprostol alone may be used. Good evidence supports the use of 400 micrograms of vaginal misoprostol every 6 hours until complete termination of pregnancy (7).

High-Dose Oxytocin

The number of oxytocin receptors in the myometrium increases during gestation and, therefore, oxytocin is less effective at initiating uterine contractions in the midtrimester than in the third trimester. When com-

pared with misoprostol, oxytocin is associated with longer induction times and higher rates of serious side effects, including water intoxication. Therefore, the use of high-dose oxytocin as a means of second-trimester termination of pregnancy has substantially decreased.

Complications

The safety of medical agents used in pregnancy termination is well established, but risks include failure, incomplete expulsion of the products of conception, persistent bleeding, infection, and hemorrhage requiring transfusion or emergent uterine evacuation. As with any other method of pregnancy termination, complications increase with advancing gestational age. Because of the potential for heavy bleeding and other serious complications, it is advisable that second-trimester pregnancy terminations take place in facilities where emergent surgical uterine evacuation and blood transfusion are available.

Prolonged Bleeding and Hemorrhage

Heavy or prolonged bleeding is the principal side effect of terminations of early pregnancies. In a few cases, the bleeding may become excessive and clinically significant. Most of these women will have retained products of conception and will respond to vacuum aspiration. Surgical curettage must be available on a 24-hour basis for hemorrhage, but less than 1% of women will need emergency curettage (8). The need for transfusion is rare (in 0.05–0.25% of cases) (12).

Heavy bleeding requiring a transfusion increases with gestational age, but is reported to occur rarely—in less than 1% of second-trimester medical terminations. Hemorrhage is suggestive of lower genital tract lacerations, uterine atony, or retained placenta (13). In the rare case of hemorrhage before fetal expulsion, immediate surgical evacuation of the uterus and assessment for uterine rupture are indicated.

Infection

With rates of infection less than 1%, endometritis is a rare complication of medical termination of pregnancy (14). However, fatal cases of infection due to *Clostridium* species after mifepristone and misoprostol administration for medical termination of early pregnancies have occurred. The risk factors for the *Clostridium* infection are unclear, and such infections also may occur after miscarriage, birth, and nonpregnancy related events. In a recent retrospective analysis, routine use of prophylactic antibiotics and avoidance of the vaginal route for misoprostol administration decreased the risk of serious infection by up to 76% (15).

Infection in the setting of midtrimester medical termination of pregnancy also occurs rarely. Signs and symptoms of infection may include lower abdominal pain, bleeding, foul-smelling discharge, fever, and chills. In addition to antibiotic treatment, surgical evacuation of the uterus is warranted in the case of incomplete pregnancy termination. There are no data regarding use of prophylactic antibiotics in second-trimester medical pregnancy termination, but extrapolation from data regarding all other pregnancy termination-related care would suggest using such treatment.

Surgical Approach

Surgical methods for pregnancy termination are well established and currently are more widely available than the medical methods (2). By convention, suction procedures performed before 13 completed weeks of gestation are referred to as dilation and curettage (D&C) and later vaginal procedures are termed D&E. Suction curettage can safely be performed as early as 5 weeks from the last menstrual period, but failed procedures are slightly more likely if the gestational sac is small (eg, less than 1 cm).

A range of anesthesia options is available for early surgical pregnancy termination. A paracervical block using a local anesthetic in combination with an oral medication to reduce uterine cramping, such as a NSAID, often is acceptable. This regimen may be supplemented with oral or intravenous anxiolytics or narcotics. With intravenous medications, adequate respiratory support is essential to prevent hypoventilation and hypoxia that are rare but important causes of abortion related mortality.

Patients who have uneventful first-trimester vacuum aspiration pregnancy terminations with local anesthesia require only short recovery periods; administration of moderate or deep sedation may necessitate longer observation. Key elements of postprocedure care include monitoring of bleeding, pain management, provision of desired contraception, and discharge instructions. A routine follow-up visit is unnecessary after a suction termination of a first-trimester pregnancy.

Dilation and Evacuation

For a D&E, adequate cervical dilation for evacuation of fetal tissue requires gradually opening the cervix to a diameter greater than in the first trimester. This is usually accomplished using osmotic dilators over a period of 1–2 days, but prostaglandins may be used as an alternative or adjunct to osmotic dilators, especially early in the second trimester. Oral antibiotic prophylaxis is initiated after laminaria or a cervical dilator insertion and continued until after uterine evacuation. Nonsteroidal antiinflammatory drugs or narcotic analgesics are prescribed for associated uterine cramping. After dilation, narrow forceps and suction are used to remove the products of conception, and some clinicians use ultrasound guidance to facilitate evacuation of the uterus.

After the procedure, the operator should carefully examine the fetal parts to ensure they have been evacuated completely. If any fetal parts are retained in the uterus and general attempts at extraction fail, the procedure should be completed under ultrasound guidance. If ultrasonography is not available, it is best to stop, administer either an oxytocin infusion or misoprostol, and try again. Normally, by 2 hours, the remaining fetal parts will have been expelled or pushed into the internal cervical os, where they can be easily extracted.

Dilation and evacuation becomes progressively more challenging as gestational age advances, and after 20 weeks of gestation, the technique may vary. The intact D&E involves 2 days of successive cervical pretreatment with laminaria or a cervical dilator. During the procedure, a breech delivery is accomplished and the calvaria decompressed and delivered with the fetus otherwise intact. The choice of procedure should be dictated by provider comfort and intraoperative factors, such as amount of cervical dilation and fetal presentation. Some providers routinely use feticidal agents and confirm fetal demise before planned intact D&E procedures as a way to comply with the federal Partial-Birth Abortion Ban Act of 2003 (a nonmedical term that refers to the intact D&E), relevant state laws, or both.

The procedures cause discomfort despite a paracervical block, and most patients will benefit from moderate or deep sedation. Standard care and monitoring of the anesthetized patient must be provided, and the patient must be closely supervised until recovery from the anesthesia is complete.

Complications

The complications of first- and second-trimester surgical pregnancy terminations are similar but, as with medical terminations, occur with greater frequency at later gestations. Overall, complications rates are low, at 5% for second-trimester and 3–4% for first-trimester procedures (16, 17). Morbidity related to surgical pregnancy termination includes immediate or delayed hemorrhage, uterine perforation, incomplete procedure or hematometra requiring repeat aspiration, infection, and failed procedure with ongoing pregnancy. Abortion related causes of mortality include hemorrhage, infection, embolism, and complications of anesthesia.

Hemorrhage

Excessive bleeding may indicate uterine atony, trauma, abnormal placentation, retained products of conception, coagulopathy, or uterine vascular malformation. Initial management requires rapid reassessment of gestational age by examination of fetal parts already extracted and gentle exploration of the uterine cavity with a curette and possibly forceps. If necessary, the pregnancy termination is completed under ultrasound guidance. Uterine massage, misoprostol administered rectally, methylergonovine, and carboprost are important adjuncts to reduce bleeding due to atony. If available, intravenous oxytocin may be administered. The cervix also should be evaluated for lacerations. If bleeding does not improve, a Foley catheter with a 30-cc balloon inflated to 50–60 cc or a balloon catheter may tamponade bleeding, and radiographic uterine artery embolization may be helpful. Rarely, coagulopathy can be seen after D&E and in the setting of hemorrhage. Measures, such as adequate cervical dilation and the addition of vasopressin to the paracervical block may significantly reduce bleeding complications, especially in the second trimester and, thus, decrease the need for reaspiration (18).

UTERINE PERFORATION

Persistent postabortal bleeding, severe pain, and provider suspicion when an instrument passes further than anticipated are strongly suggestive of uterine perforation. The incidence of uterine perforation is less than 3 in 1,000 first-trimester pregnancy terminations (16). Perforations are more likely to occur with a marked uterine flexion, cervical stenosis, uterine anomalies, and difficult or prolonged uterine evacuation. Small perforations may be managed conservatively, but laparoscopy may be needed to determine the extent of the injury, including evaluation of injury to the abdominal viscera. With fundal injuries, the procedure can be completed under laparoscopic guidance if there is no active bleeding.

The clinical syndrome produced by uterine perforation depends on the anatomic location of the injury. Perforations at the junction of the cervix and lower uterine segment can lacerate the ascending branch of the uterine artery within the broad ligament, causing severe pain, broad ligament hematoma, and intraabdominal bleeding. Management requires ligation of the severed vessels and a repair of the uterine injury. Low cervical perforations, in contrast, may injure the descending branch of the uterine artery within the cardinal ligaments. In this case, the bleeding is usually external, through the cervical canal, and may subside temporarily as the artery goes into spasm. This complication usually is managed with hysterectomy, but consideration should be given to selective embolization. It also is important to consider the possibility of bowel injuries with perforations.

POSTABORTAL SYNDROME AND HEMATOMETRA

Postabortal syndrome refers to the accumulation of blood in the uterus and lower abdominal pain of increasing intensity after the procedure, which suggests

hematometra. Symptoms associated with postabortal syndrome are dizziness and nausea, in addition to the severe cramping. On examination, the uterus is large, globular, and firm. This condition may be confused with a broad ligament hematoma. However, with hematometra, the mass is midline, arises from the cervix, and is relieved with repeat aspiration. Milder versions of this problem can occur several days after the initial procedure.

INFECTION

A 1996 meta-analysis demonstrated that prophylactic antibiotics significantly reduce the risk of infection after termination of pregnancy (19). Antibiotic prophylaxis is now a standard approach for abortion, regardless of gestational age. Although the optimal regimen and dose are undefined, doxycycline is commonly used both for its effectiveness and the low cost (20).

When fever is present, intravenous antibiotic therapy is initiated, and uterine evacuation is performed shortly thereafter. Septic pregnancy termination, once common when pregnancy termination was illegal, is now rare. This condition requires prompt, intravenous antibiotics, uterine evacuation, and intensive cardiovascular support. If the patient develops hemolysis or fails to improve within 12–24 hours of uterine evacuation, hysterectomy may be necessary.

VASOVAGAL SYNCOPE

Vasovagal syncope produced by stimulation of the cervical canal can be seen with manipulation of the cervix or after paracervical block. Brief tonic–clonic activity may be noted and should not be confused with seizure activity. The procedure usually can be completed safely after administration of intravenous atropine.

Multifetal Pregnancy Reduction and Selective Termination

Multifetal pregnancy reduction and selective termination are two procedures developed to address problems unique to multifetal gestations. The goal of multifetal pregnancy reduction is to decrease the risk of adverse pregnancy outcomes associated with higher order multiple gestations whereas selective termination is used to terminate an anomalous fetus.

The most common approach for both procedures is transabdominal injection of potassium chloride into the fetal thorax. Pregnancy reduction with feticidal agents should be attempted only with multichorionic placentation because of the possibility of embolic phenomena and infarction in the surviving twin in monochorionic pregnancies. Maternal serum alpha-fetoprotein level may remain elevated for several weeks after reduction procedures.

Postprocedure Care

Contraceptive counseling is similar for women having first- or second-trimester procedures. A woman may ovulate and become pregnant again as soon as 2 weeks after a pregnancy termination. With the exception of cervical barriers, all contraceptive methods may be safely initiated immediately after a first- or second-trimester procedure, including hormonal contraception and the intrauterine device. Diaphragms and cervical caps may be fitted once bleeding has subsided and uterine involution is complete after later gestations. Postprocedure counseling is individualized, and those patients who have terminated desired pregnancies may have a greater need for counseling or counseling referrals.

Legal Issues

Pregnancy termination has been legal in the United States since 1973 when the U.S. Supreme Court decided in *Roe v Wade* (21). Since then, many states have enacted laws requiring that certain information be given to patients before the procedure or that a certain time period elapse after obtaining consent before performing the abortion. In some jurisdictions, minors must notify or obtain the consent of one or both parents or obtain judicial review (22). Furthermore, the Hyde Amendment currently forbids the use of federal funds for abortions except in cases of life endangerment, rape, or incest. Some states have chosen to use their own funds to cover pregnancy termination. Presidential Executive Order was signed making the Hyde Amendment applicable to the health insurance exchanges, which are expected to be operational in 2014. This order reiterates the provisions of the enacted health care reform legislation, which prohibits the use of tax credits and cost-sharing reduction payments to pay for abortion services (except in cases of rape and incest or when the life of the woman would be endangered). The legislation imposes strict payment and accounting requirements to ensure that federal funds are not used for abortion services in exchange plans (except in cases of rape or incest or when the life of the woman would be endangered).

The U.S. Congress passed the Partial-Birth Abortion Ban Act of 2003. This was upheld in 2007 in *Gonzales v Carhart* (23). The measure criminalizes the so-called *partial-birth abortion*, aimed at intact D&E. Providers of second-trimester pregnancy terminations must be familiar with the law and ensure that their surgical techniques are in adherence.

References

1. Finer LB, Henshaw SK. Disparities in rates of unintended pregnancy in the United States, 1994 and 2001. Perspect Sex Reprod Health 2006;38:90–6.

2. Jones RK, Zolna MR, Henshaw SK, Finer LB. Abortion in the United States: incidence and access to services, 2005. Perspect Sex Reprod Health 2008;40:6–16.

3. Pazol K, Gamble SB, Parker WY, Cook DA, Zane SB, Hamdan S. Abortion surveillance - United States, 2006. Centers for Disease Control and Prevention [published erratum appears in MMWR Morbid Mortal Wkly Rep 2010;59:561]. MMWR Surveill Summ 2009;58(SS-8):1–35.

4. Jones RK, Kost K, Singh S, Henshaw SK, Finer LB. Trends in abortion in the United States. Clin Obstet Gynecol 2009;52:119–29.

5. Paul M, Lichtenbert ES, Borgatta L, Grimes DA, Stubblefield PG, Creinin MD, editors. Management of unintended and abnormal pregnancy; comprehensive abortion care. West Sussex: Wiley-Blackwell; 2009. p. 252–63.

6. Chasen ST, Kalish RB, Gupta M, Kaufman J, Chervenak FA. Obstetric outcomes after surgical abortion at > =20 weeks' gestation. Am J Obstet Gynecol 2005;193:1161–4.

7. National Abortion Federation. 2010 clinical policy guidelines. Washington, DC; NAF; 2010. Available at: http://prochoice.org/pubs_research/publications/downloads/professional_education/CPG2010.pdf. Retrieved December 7, 2010.

8. Medical management of abortion. ACOG Practice Bulletin No. 67. American College of Obstetricians and Gynecologists. Obstet Gynecol 2005;106:871–82.

9. Gamble SB, Strauss LT, Parker WY, Cook DA, Zane SB, Hamdan S. Abortion surveillance--United States, 2005. Centers for Disease Control and Prevention. MMWR Surveill Summ 2008;57(SS-13):1–32.

10. Vargas J, Diedrich J. Second-trimester induction of labor. Clin Obstet Gynecol 2009;52:188–97.

11. Goyal V. Uterine rupture in second-trimester misoprostol-induced abortion after cesarean delivery: a systematic review. Obstet Gynecol 2009;113:1117–23.

12. Sitruk-Ware R. Mifepristone and misoprostol sequential regimen side effects, complications and safety. Contraception 2006;74:48–55.

13. Paul M, Lichtenbert ES, Borgatta L, Grimes DA, Stubblefield PG, Creinin MD, editors. Management of unintended and abnormal pregnancy; comprehensive abortion care. West Sussex: Wiley-Blackwell; 2009. p. 178–92

14. Paul M, Lichtenbert ES, Borgatta L, Grimes DA, Stubblefield PG, Creinin MD, editors. Management of unintended and abnormal pregnancy; comprehensive abortion care. West Sussex: Wiley-Blackwell; 2009. p. 111–34.

15. Fjerstad M, Trussell J, Sivin I, Lichtenberg ES, Cullins V. Rates of serious infection after changes in regimens for medical abortion. N Engl J Med 2009;361:145–51.

16. Zhou W, Nielsen GL, Moller M, Olsen J. Short-term complications after surgically induced abortions: a register-based study of 56 117 abortions. Acta Obstet Gynecol Scand 2002;81:331–6.

17. Paul M, Lichtenbert ES, Borgatta L, Grimes DA, Stubblefield PG, Creinin MD, editors. Management of unintended and abnormal pregnancy; comprehensive abortion care. West Sussex: Wiley-Blackwell; 2009. p. 157–77.

18. Schulz K, Grimes DA, Christensen DD. Vasopressin reduces blood loss from second-trimester dilatation and evacuation abortion. The Lancet 1985;326:353–6.

19. Sawaya GF, Grady D, Kerlikowske K, Grimes DA. Antibiotics at the time of induced abortion: the case for universal prophylaxis based on a meta-analysis. Obstet Gynecol 1996;87:884–90.

20. Antibiotic prophylaxis for gynecologic procedures. ACOG Practice Bulletin No. 104. American College of Obstetricians and Gynecologists. Obstet Gynecol 2009;113:1180–9.

21. Roe vs. Wade. 410 U.S. 113 (1973).

22. Guttmacher Institute. An overview of abortion laws. State policies in brief. New York (NY): Guttmacher; 2010. Available at http://www.guttmacher.org/statecenter/spibs/spib_OAL.pdf. Retrieved December 7, 2010.

23. Gonzales v. Carhart, 550 U.S. 124 (2007).

Chronic Pelvic Pain

Roger P. Smith

Chronic pelvic pain is common in women of reproductive age. It causes disability and distress and poses significant costs to health services and a challenge for the clinical gynecologist. The pathogenesis of chronic pelvic pain is poorly understood and efforts to establish a cause by diagnostic modalities, including laparoscopy, frequently reveal no obvious cause for pain. There are a number of possible pathologies that can cause chronic pelvic pain, including altered spinal cord and brain processing of peripheral and other stimuli. Treatment often is unsatisfactory and limited to the suppression of symptoms because the underlying pathophysiology of chronic pelvic pain is not well understood and a cause frequently is elusive. Despite this, strategies can be developed and a thoughtfully devised plan of treatment implemented that often will help relieve, if not eliminate, a good deal of the patient's distress.

Acute pelvic pain most often emanates from a single organ system, produces symptoms through known neural pathways, and follows in a recognizable sequence. When pain has become chronic, it may seem to emanate from all of the organs in the pelvis, in terms of both the symptoms and findings elicited during examination. Indeed, 25–50% of such women seen in primary care settings receive more than one diagnosis (1). Palpation of pelvic organs may produce pain in areas generally not considered to share a nerve supply with the organ being examined, and myofascial, neuropathic, affective, and psychosocial factors may add to the complexity of the problem. When evaluating pain that does not follow easily understood neural pathways, the clinician is tempted to label depression, stress, or a history of physical or sexual abuse as the major etiology. Although many times these components are important to understand when devising a treatment plan (2), it is more important to see the pain itself as the disease (Fig. 56) and one that requires multicomponent evaluation and therapy (3).

Etiologic Possibilities

Pain is defined as an unpleasant sensory and emotional experience associated with actual or potential tissue damage or is described in terms of such damage (4). Pain always is subjective and may not be tied to any specific stimulus. Patients may report pain in the absence of tissue damage or any likely pathophysiologic cause; in such cases, pain may have a psychologic basis or component, although one must avoid a premature assignment of cause to the exclusion of the diagnosis and treatment of other components of the problem.

One proposed definition of chronic pelvic pain is noncyclic pain lasting 6 months or longer that localizes to the anatomic pelvis, anterior abdominal wall at

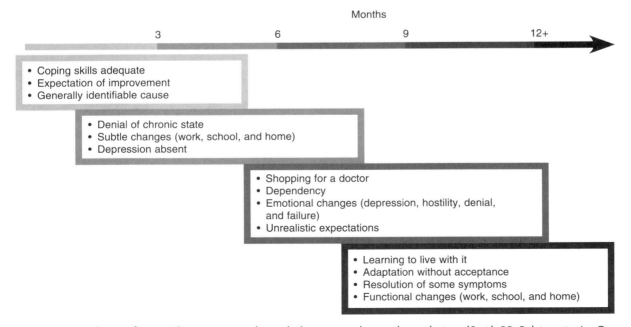

Figure 56. Evolution of pain. Chronic pain and pain behaviors tend to evolve with time. (Smith RP. Pelvic pain. In: Gynecology in primary care. Baltimore (MD): Williams and Wilkins; 1997. p. 471–99.)

or below the umbilicus, the lumbosacral back, or the buttocks and is of sufficient severity to cause functional disability or lead to medical care (5). A lack of physical findings does not negate the significance of a patient's pain, and normal examination results do not preclude the possibility of finding pelvic pathology.

The list of gynecologic and nongynecologic processes that can lead to chronic pelvic pain is long and often debated. Gynecologic causes (Box 30) may arise from processes intrinsic or extrinsic to the uterus. A number of processes affecting other organ systems also can provide the nexus of chronic pelvic pain syndromes (Table 21). A detailed discussion of these causes is beyond the scope of *Precis* and their diagnosis and treatment are well established. The difficulty comes when there is no apparent cause of the patient's symptoms.

There is growing evidence that chronic low-level neural stimulation can result in upregulation of the nervous system, hyperesthesia, and misinterpretation as painful, neural signals that might otherwise not be associated with painful sensations. In some settings, this has been referred to as a complex regional pain syndrome (previously referred to as reflex sympathetic dystrophy) (6, 7). Similar processes have been postulated to affect visceral neurologic pain reflexes and act as a component of chronic pelvic pain in some patients, explaining the observation that patients with one visceral pain disorder are more likely than the general population to have another visceral pain disorder. In some ways, this heightened pain perception and sensitivity parallel those seen in myofascial pain syndromes. Additionally, the self-propagating process suggests a need for early consideration of this component of pain perception and possible interventions to interrupt this cycle (see following discussion).

Diagnostic Strategies

Up to two thirds of women with chronic pelvic pain do not undergo diagnostic testing, never receive a diagnosis, and are never referred to a specialist for evaluation or treatment (8). A detailed history and physical examination are the basis for differential diagnosis and the planning of specific diagnostic studies. The general evaluation of the patient with chronic pelvic pain has been well documented elsewhere (5), but it is critical that this evaluation be wide ranging and include other organ systems, such as the urinary, gastrointestinal, and musculoskeletal. For this examination, a specialized single-hand pelvic examination has been advocated in which transvaginal palpation with only one finger, not using an abdominal hand at all, is used to detect areas of tenderness.

Diagnostic imaging, including ultrasonography, computed tomography, and magnetic resonance imaging, will be of assistance only when a physical exam-

ination is compromised, specific physical findings occur, or special pathologies are being considered where imaging is well documented to be of diagnostic significance. Based on the clinical suspicions provided by the patient's history and physical examination, a number

---

Box 30

Gynecologic Conditions That May Cause or Exacerbate Chronic Pelvic Pain, by Level of Evidence*

Level A[†]

- Endometriosis[‡]
- Gynecologic malignancies (especially late stage)
- Ovarian retention syndrome (residual ovary syndrome)
- Ovarian remnant syndrome
- Pelvic congestion syndrome
- Pelvic inflammatory disease[‡]
- Tuberculous salpingitis

Level B[§]

- Adhesions[‡]
- Benign cystic mesothelioma
- Leiomyomas[‡]
- Postoperative peritoneal cysts

Level C[||]

- Adenomyosis
- Atypical dysmenorrhea or ovulatory pain
- Adnexal cysts (nonendometriotic)
- Cervical stenosis
- Chronic ectopic pregnancy
- Chronic endometritis
- Endometrial or cervical polyps
- Endosalpingiosis
- Intrauterine contraceptive device
- Ovarian ovulatory pain
- Residual accessory ovary
- Symptomatic pelvic relaxation (genital prolapse)

*Level of evidence graded according to method outlined by the U.S. Preventive Services Task Force

[†]Level A: There is good and consistent scientific evidence of causal relationship to chronic pelvic pain.

[‡]Diagnosis is frequently reported in published series of women with chronic pelvic pain.

[§]Level B: There is limited or inconsistent scientific evidence of causal relationship to chronic pelvic pain.

[||]Level C: There is causal relationship to chronic pelvic pain based on expert opinions.

Data from Howard FM. Chronic pelvic pain. Obstet Gynecol 2003;101:594–611.

Table 21. Nongynecologic Conditions That May Cause or Exacerbate Chronic Pelvic Pain, by Level of Evidence*

Level of Evidence	Urologic	Gastrointestinal	Musculoskeletal	Other
Level A[†]	Bladder malignancy Interstitial cystitis Radiation cystitis Urethral syndrome	Carcinoma of the colon Constipation Inflammatory bowel disease Irritable bowel syndrome[‡]	Abdominal wall myofascial pain (trigger points) Chronic coccygeal or back pain[‡] Faulty or poor posture; Fibromyalgia Neuralgia of iliohypogastric, ilioinguinal, or genitofemoral nerves Pelvic floor myalgia (levator ani or piriformis syndrome) Peripartum pelvic pain syndrome	Abdominal cutaneous nerve entrapment in surgical scar Depression[‡] Somatization disorder
Level B[§]	Uninhibited bladder contractions (detrusor dyssynergia) Urethral diverticulum	N/A	Herniated nucleus pulposus Low back pain[‡] Neoplasia of spinal cord or sacral nerve	Celiac disease Neurologic dysfunction Porphyria Shingles Sleep disturbances
Level C[‖]	Chronic urinary tract infection Recurrent, acute cystitis Recurrent, acute urethritis Stone or urolithiasis Urethral caruncle	Colitis Chronic intermittent bowel obstruction Diverticular disease	Compression of lumbar vertebrae Degenerative joint disease Hernias—ventral, inguinal, femoral, and spigelian Muscular strains and sprains Rectus tendon strain Spondylosis	Abdominal epilepsy Abdominal migraine Bipolar personality disorders Familial Mediterranean fever

*Level of evidence graded according to method outlined by the U.S. Preventive Services Task Force
[†]Level A: There is good and consistent scientific evidence of causal relationship to chronic pelvic pain.
[‡]Diagnosis frequently is reported in published series of women with chronic pelvic pain.
[§]Level B: There is limited or inconsistent scientific evidence of causal relationship to chronic pelvic pain.
[‖]Level C: There is causal relationship to chronic pelvic pain based on expert opinions.
Data from Howard FM. Chronic pelvic pain. Obstet Gynecol 2003;101:594–611.

of diagnostic investigative paths may be appropriate (Table 22).

Specialized questionnaires that explore possible contributing or causal factors, such as depression or painful bladder syndrome, should be generously used in evaluating these patients. For example, the O'Leary–Sant IC Symptoms and Problem Index is a validated questionnaire that reliably predicts the diagnosis of painful bladder syndrome and may be used to help determine whether cystoscopy is indicated (9).

Chronic pelvic pain is the indication for at least 40% of all gynecologic laparoscopies. A new approach to diagnostic laparoscopy, "conscious laparoscopic pain mapping," has been suggested as a way to improve the diagnostic capability of laparoscopy. Conscious laparoscopic pain mapping is a diagnostic laparoscopy performed under local anesthesia, with or without conscious sedation, directed at the identification of sources of pain (10). Gentle probing or traction on tissues, lesions, and organs with a blunt probe or forceps

Table 22. Some of the Diagnostic Tests That May Be Useful in the Diagnostic Evaluation of Women With Chronic Pelvic Pain

Symptom, Finding, or Suspected Diagnosis	Potentially Useful Tests
Adenomyosis	Ultrasonography Hysterosalpingography Magnetic resonance imaging
Chronic urethral syndrome	Urodynamic testing
Compression or entrapment neuropathy	Nerve conducting velocities Needle electromyographic studies
Constipation	Anorectal balloon manometry and colonic transit time
Depression	Thyroid-stimulating hormone, thyroxine, and triiodothyronine levels Antithyroid antibody levels Complete blood count Renal function tests Hepatic function tests Electrolyte levels Rapid plasma reagin test
Diarrhea	Stool specimens for ova and parasites, polymorphonuclear leukocytes and red blood cells, cultures, *Clostridium difficile* toxin, and stool guaiac testing Barium enema radiography Colonoscopy Upper gastrointestinal series with follow-up Computerized tomography
Diverticular disease	Barium enema radiography
Dyspareunia	Urethral and cervical gonorrhea and chlamydia cultures Chlamydial polymerase chain reaction testing Vaginal cultures Urine cultures Vaginal wet preparations Vaginal pH
Endometriosis	Determination of CA 125 level Ultrasonography Barium enema radiography Hysterosalpingography Computed tomography Magnetic resonance imaging
Hernias	Abdominal wall ultrasonography Computed tomography Herniography
Painful blader syndrome	Cystourethroscopy Potassium chloride bladder challenge test Urine culture Urine cytologies Urodynamic testing Bladder biopsy

(continued)

Table 22. Some of the Diagnostic Tests That May Be Useful in the Diagnostic Evaluation of Women With Chronic Pelvic Pain (continued)

Symptom, Finding, or Suspected Diagnosis	Potentially Useful Tests
Ovarian remnant syndrome	Follicle-stimulating hormone and estradiol levels Gonadotropin-releasing hormone agonist stimulation Barium enema radiography Computed tomography
Pelvic congestion syndrome	Pelvic venography and ultrasonography with or without Doppler studies
Pelvic tuberculosis	Chest X-ray and tuberculin skin test
Porphyria	Urine porphobilinogen test
Urethral diverticulum	Vaginal ultrasonography Voiding cystourethrography Double-balloon cystourethrography Magnetic resonance imaging

Howard FM. Chronic pelvic pain. Obstet Gynecol 2003:101;595–611.

passed through a secondary trocar site is used to map possible pain sites. The diagnosis of an etiologic lesion or organ is based on the severity of pain elicited and on replication of the pain that is the patient's presenting symptom. No substantial data confirm improved diagnostic accuracy or improved clinical outcomes with conscious laparoscopic pain mapping (11).

Some authors have suggested the use of gonadotropin-releasing hormone (GnRH) agonists as both a diagnostic trial and therapeutic tool for patients with chronic pelvic pain. Authors of one clinical trial designed to evaluate empiric treatment of chronic pelvic pain with suspected endometriosis suggested that GnRH agonists have the same efficacy in women with symptoms consistent with endometriosis, whether or not they actually have endometriosis (12). Although the study was small, the results strongly suggest that empiric GnRH agonist therapy might be reasonable when there is sufficient suspicion of endometriosis as a cause of the patient's symptoms. It would also suggest that when there is a failure of the therapy to alter the symptoms reported, a gynecologic source is less likely. Some care must be exercised in drawing such conclusions, because symptoms of irritable bowel and painful bladder syndromes also vary with the menstrual cycle and may respond to GnRH agonist treatment. Often, a detailed 2–3 month pain diary can be just as revealing.

Therapeutic Options

The basic tenets of pain management are early intervention and treatment of the underlying process when possible. Because of the complex nature of chronic pelvic pain, such intervention may include nontraditional therapies and collaboration with a multitude of providers.

One Cochrane database review surveyed the literature regarding the treatment of chronic pelvic pain (13). Nineteen studies were identified of which fourteen were of satisfactory methodological quality. The review found that treatment with medroxyprogesterone acetate was associated with a reduction of pain during treatment, whereas goserelin gave a longer duration of benefit. A multidisciplinary approach to therapy was beneficial for some outcome measures, and adhesiolysis was not associated with an improved outcome apart from where adhesions were severe. The reviewers found that sertraline treatment was not beneficial. Intervention through counseling, supported by ultrasound scanning, was associated with reduced pain and improvement in mood. Because of the few studies performed and the incomplete reporting of others, the authors felt that strong recommendations based on this review were not possible and more research was needed.

When specific interventions are not possible, the short-term goal of therapy is achieving maximum function and the long-term goal should be gradual weaning of medications and other therapies over time while maintaining the ability to function more or less normally. For this plan to succeed, the patient needs to accept her responsibility for active participation in the rehabilitative process. The role of psychotropic and pain medications is critical to this process. Antidepressants are useful because depression very often complicates chronic pain. However, depression is rarely an important part of the origin of the problem and antidepressants are ineffective in isolation.

Analgesic therapy starts with nonsteroidal antiinflammatory agents. Inhibition of prostaglandin synthesis ameliorates the pain of dysmenorrhea as well as pain associated with endometriosis and fibroids, and can be very effective when these pathologies are present. No clinical trials have addressed chronic pelvic pain specifically, but moderate analgesic efficacy, as shown for other types of pain, would be anticipated.

If stronger medication is needed, narcotics can be helpful when prescribed and monitored carefully. Opioids are increasingly used in the treatment of chronic pain (14). Randomized clinical trials suggest significant analgesic effects, but not necessarily improvement in functional or psychologic status (15). The risk of addiction has been low in patients with chronic pain. If this represents a significant concern, methadone may be an option by virtue of its lack of mood effects, longer duration of action, and low cost. However, methadone as an option in opiate treatment for pain management is controversial. Recent analyses of the FDA data have demonstrated that the increased use of methadone as an analgesic has promoted increased methadone distribution with a subsequent increase in methadone-associated mortality. Methadone provides pain relief for 4–8 hours, but remains pharmacologically active for much longer periods, potentially leading to toxicity. Females are at an especially high risk for QT prolongation and *torsades de pointes*, which reinforces the need for a high degree of caution (16). A narcotic contract between the physician and patient should be used when controlled drugs are used for an indefinite period of time. Such a contract obligates the patient to obtain controlled medications from a single provider, at a specified pharmacy, and at set intervals. When opiates are used, they should be given on a scheduled basis. There are no published studies of opiate treatment for chronic pelvic pain. Adjuncts, such as amitriptyline and gabapentin or pregabalin, that have traditionally been used for neuropathic pain, may be worthwhile for some patients.

Surgical therapy for chronic pain should be limited to those processes that have been documented and are amenable to surgical therapy. Empiric hysterectomy for pelvic pain has not been associated with universal long-term success and may be associated with persistent pain in up to one third of patients after hysterectomy (17). Older proposed surgical therapies, such as uterine suspension, are associated with an even higher failure rates (50%) (18).

Newer and Experimental Therapeutic Options

In humans, prospective, placebo-controlled, double-blind studies have provided evidence for effectiveness of botulinum toxin therapy in a number of painful disorders (19). These disorders include neck and pelvic pain, low back pain, plantar fasciitis, postsurgical painful spasms, myofascial pain syndromes, migraine, and chronic daily headaches. Long-term studies on neck and low back pain have demonstrated safety and sustained efficacy after repeated injections. Recently, an Australian randomized controlled trial of botulinum toxin type A reported good success in patients with evidence of pelvic floor muscle spasm (20). The treatment was associated with a significant change from baseline for the parameters measured. Similar improvements in symptoms have been reported for patients with vulvodynia, although these results have come from case reports and small series (21). However, in the United States, the use of the botulinum toxin for chronic pain has not been approved by the U.S. Food and Drug Administration.

Another approach to muscle relaxation has been via the use of biofeedback. Biofeedback has been evaluated for the treatment of voiding and sexual dysfunction (22) but its efficacy for the treatment of chronic pain syndromes has been limited (23).

Transcutaneous nerve stimulation and physiotherapy have been shown to be effective in a number of pain settings, including chronic pelvic pain. Transcutaneous nerve stimulation has shown effectiveness in altering pain perception in primary dysmenorrhea (24) and certain models of chronic pain (25), although results often have been disappointing (26). Alternatively, the use of physiotherapy either alone or in combination with other interventions has demonstrated success in improving symptoms of chronic pelvic pain (27).

The idea of interrupting the neural pathways involved in transmitting nociceptive signals to the brain is an attractive one, but this strategy has produced disappointing results. Use of this treatment modality has been advocated for dysmenorrhea, but the evidence for efficacy is insufficient to recommend its use at this time (28, 29). In a parallel of this concept, the use of specialized spinal nerve stimulators for chronic pain has expanded (30). In the gynecologic setting, this approach has been applied with some success in a limited number of patients with vulvodynia (31) and visceral pain (32).

References

1. Zondervan KT, Yudkin PL, Vessey MP, Jenkinson CP, Dawes MG, Barlow DH, et al. Chronic pelvic pain in the community--symptoms, investigations, and diagnoses. Am J Obstet Gynecol 2001;184:1149–55.

2. Lampe A, Solder E, Ennemoser A, Shubert C, Rumpold G, Sollner W. Chronic pelvic pain and previous sexual abuse. Obstet Gynecol 2000:96;929–33.

3. Gunter J. Chronic pelvic pain: an integrated approach to diagnosis and treatment. Obstet Gynecol Surv 2003;58:615–23.

4. Pain terms: a current list with definitions and notes on usage. Revisions prepared by an Ad Hoc Subcommittee of the IASP Task Force on Taxonomy. In: Merskey H, Bogduk N, editors. Classification of chronic pain: descriptions of chronic pain syndromes and definition of pain terms. IASP Task Force on Taxonomy. 2nd ed. Seattle (WA): IASP Press; 1994. p. 207–13.

5. Chronic pelvic pain. ACOG Practice Bulletin No. 51. American College of Obstetricians and Gynecologists. Obstet Gynecol 2004;103:589–605.

6. Albazaz R, Wong YT, Homer-Vanniasinkam S. Complex regional pain syndrome: a review. Ann Vasc Surg 2008;22: 297–306.

7. Turner-Stokes L. Reflex sympathetic dystrophy--a complex regional pain syndrome. Disabil Rehabil 2002;24:939–47.

8. Zondervan KT, Yudkin PL, Vessey MP, Dawes MG, Barlow DH, Kennedy SH. Prevalence and incidence in primary care of chronic pelvic pain in women: evidence from a national general practice database. Br J Obstet Gynaecol 1999;106:1149–55.

9. Forrest JB, Mishell DR Jr. Breaking the cycle of pain in interstitial cystitis/painful bladder syndrome: toward standardization of early diagnosis and treatment: consensus panel recommendations. J Reprod Med 2009;54:3–14.

10. Howard FM, El-Minawi A, Sanchez RA. Conscious pain mapping by laparoscopy in women with chronic pelvic pain. Obstet Gynecol 2000;96:934–9.

11. Swanton A, Iyer L, Reginald PW. Diagnosis, treatment and follow up of women undergoing conscious pain mapping for chronic pelvic pain: a prospective cohort study. BJOG 2006;113:792–6.

12. Ling FW. Randomized controlled trial of depot leuprolide in patients with chronic pelvic pain and clinically suspected endometriosis. Pelvic Pain Study Group. Obstet Gynecol 1999;93:51–8.

13. Stones W, Cheong YC, Howard FM, Singh S. Interventions for treating chronic pelvic pain women. Cochrane Database of Systematic Reviews 205, Issue 2. Art. No.: CD000387. DOI: 10.1002/14651858.CD000387.

14. Dworkin RH, O'Connor AB, Audette J, Baron R, Gourlay GK, Haanpaa ML, et al. Recommendations for the pharmacological management of neuropathic pain: an overview and literature update. Mayo Clin Proc 2010;85:S3–14.

15. Jamison RN, Raymond SA, Slawsby EA, Nedeljkovic SS, Katz NP. Opioid therapy for chronic noncancer back pain. A randomized prospective study. Spine (Phila Pa 1976) 1998;23:2591–600.

16. Modesto-Lowe V, Brooks D, Petry N. Methadone deaths: risk factors in pain and addicted populations. J Gen Intern Med 2010;25:305–9.

17. Brandsborg B, Dueholm M, Nikolajsen L, Kehlet H, Jensen TS. A prospective study of risk factors for pain persisting 4 months after hysterectomy. Clin J Pain 2009;25:263–8.

18. Halperin R, Padoa A, Schneider D, Bukovsky I, Pansky M. Long-term follow-up (5-20 years) after uterine ventrosuspension for chronic pelvic pain and deep dyspareunia. Gynecol Obstet Invest 2003;55:216–9.

19. Jabbari B. Botulinum neurotoxins in the treatment of refractory pain. Nat Clin Pract Neurol 2008;4:676–85.

20. Abbott JA, Jarvis SK, Lyons SD, Thomson A, Vancaille TG. Botulinum toxin type A for chronic pain and pelvic floor spasm in women: a randomized controlled trial. Obstet Gynecol 2006;108:915–23.

21. Brown CS, Glazer HI, Vogt V, Menkes D, Bachmann G. Subjective and objective outcomes of botulinum toxin type A treatment in vestibulodynia: pilot data. J Reprod Med 2006;51:635–41.

22. Rivalta M, Sighinolfi MC, De Stefani S, Micali S, Mofferdin A, Grande M, et al. Biofeedback, electrical stimulation, pelvic floor muscle exercises, and vaginal cones: a combined rehabilitative approach for sexual dysfunction associated with urinary incontinence. J Sex Med 2009;6:1674–7.

23. Jensen MP, Barber J, Romano JM, Hanley MA, Raichle KA, Molton IR, et al. Effects of self-hypnosis training and EMG biofeedback relaxation training on chronic pain in persons with spinal-cord injury. Int J Clin Exp Hypn 2009;57:239–68.

24. Proctor M, Farquhar C, Stones W, He L, Zhu X, Brown J. Transcutaneous electrical nerve stimulation for primary dysmenorrhoea. Cochrane Database of Systematic Reviews 2002, Issue 1. Art. No.: CD002123. DOI: 10.1002/14651858. CD002123.

25. Koke AJ, Schouten JS, Lamerichs-Geelen MJ, Lipsch JS, Waltje EM, van Kleef M, et al. Pain reducing effect of three types of transcutaneous electrical nerve stimulation in patients with chronic pain: a randomized crossover trial. Pain 2004;108:36–42.

26. Warke K, Al-Smadi J, Baxter D, Walsh DM, Lowe-Strong AS. Efficacy of transcutaneous electrical nerve stimulation (tens) for chronic low-back pain in a multiple sclerosis population: a randomized, placebo-controlled clinical trial. Clin J Pain 2006;22:812–9.

27. Montenegro ML, Vasconcelos EC, Candido Dos Reis FJ, Nogueira AA, Poli-Neto OB. Physical therapy in the management of women with chronic pelvic pain. Int J Clin Pract 2008;62:263–9.

28. Latthe PM, Proctor ML, Farquhar CM, Johnson N, Khan KS. Surgical interruption of pelvic nerve pathways in dysmenorrhea: a systematic review of effectiveness. Acta Obstet Gynecol Scand 2007;86:4–15.

29. Proctor M, Latthe P, Farquhar C, Khan K, Johnson N. Surgical interruption of pelvic nerve pathways for primary and secondary dysmenorrhoea. Cochrane Database of Systematic Reviews 2005, Issue 4. Art. No.: CD001896. DOI: 10.1002/14651858.CD001896.pub2.

30. Simpson EL, Duenas A, Holmes MW, Papaioannou D, Chilcott J. Spinal cord stimulation for chronic pain of neuropathic or ischaemic origin: systematic review and economic evaluation. Health Technol Assess 2009;13:iii, ix–x, 1–154.

31. Nair AR, Klapper A, Kushnerik V, Margulis I, Del Priore G. Spinal cord stimulator for the treatment of a woman with vulvovaginal burning and deep pelvic pain. Obstet Gynecol 2008;111:545–7.

32. Kapural L, Narouze SN, Janicki TI, Mekhail N. Spinal cord stimulation is an effective treatment for the chronic intractable visceral pelvic pain. Pain Med 2006;7:440–3.

Benign Breast Disease

Catherine Takacs Witkop

Conditions of the breast are common and cause a great deal of concern for many women. Evaluation involves a thorough history and physical examination and often includes assessment by ultrasonography or mammography. Women's health care providers need to be well versed in these disorders, including an understanding of when and how to refer the patient to other specialists.

Mastalgia

Mastalgia can be divided into three categories: 1) cyclic mastalgia, 2) noncyclic mastalgia, and 3) extramammary (nonbreast) pain (1). Cyclic mastalgia begins with the luteal phase of the menstrual cycle and resolves after the onset of menses. The pain usually is bilateral and often involves the upper outer quadrants, radiating to the upper arm and axillary region (1). Women commonly seek care once the pain interferes with activities of daily living, such as work, sleep, or physical or sexual activity. The precise etiology often is unknown.

By definition, noncyclic mastalgia is not associated with the menstrual cycle and includes such etiologies as tumors, trauma, mastitis, cysts, or history of breast surgery. A number of women present with idiopathic noncyclic mastalgia. Furthermore, noncyclic mastalgia has been associated with certain medications (Box 31). Nonmammary pain includes a variety of conditions, such as Tietze syndrome, chest wall trauma, rib fracture, fibromyalgia, cervical radiculopathy, shoulder pain, herpes zoster, coronary artery disease, and pericarditis (1). Treatment for the musculoskeletal disorders often includes antiinflammatory medications, but more serious causes of chest pain (eg, angina) need to be ruled out first.

The workup for breast pain includes a thorough history and physical examination. Performing an examination of the spine, chest wall, shoulders, arms, heart, and lungs, as well as the breasts, will help narrow the differential diagnosis and allow for appropriate referrals if necessary. Mammography, breast ultrasonography, or both, are necessary to evaluate any masses (see later discussion on the workup of masses). Mammography also should be considered in a woman with focal breast pain who is older than 30 years or who has significant risk factors for breast cancer. Ultrasonography may be considered in a woman with focal breast pain, even if a mass is not palpable. Because a negative radiologic result does not rule out malignancy, a patient should be reevaluated if the focal breast pain is persistent.

Some nonpharmacologic measures to help relieve breast pain include a properly fitted brassiere or sports

---

Box 31

Medications Associated With Breast Pain in Women

Hormonal Medications
- Estrogens
- Progestogens
- Oral contraceptives
- Menopausal hormonal therapy
- Diethylstilbestrol
- Clomiphene
- Cyproterone

Antidepressant, Antipsychotic, and Anxiolytic Medications
- Sertraline (and other serotonin reuptake inhibitors)
- Venlafaxine
- Mirtazapine
- Chlordiazepoxide
- Amitriptyline*
- Doxepin*
- Haloperidol (and other antipsychotic agents)

Antihypertensive and Cardiac Medications
- Spironolactone*
- Methyldopa
- Minoxidil
- Digoxin*
- Reserpine*

Antimicrobial Agents
- Ketoconazole*
- Metronidazole*

Miscellaneous Agents
- Cimetidine*
- Cyclosporine
- Domperidone
- Penicillamine
- Methadone*
- Carboprost, dinoprostone (and other prostaglandins)
- Estramustine

Information obtained from MEDLINE, MICROMEDEX, and discussion with breast specialists and pharmacists

*Medications causing galactorrhea and gynecomastia and believed to be associated with breast pain. Other medications (not listed) also may be associated with breast pain and should be considered according to clinical circumstances.

Smith RL, Pruthi S, Fitzpatrick LA. Evaluation and management of breast pain. Mayo Clin Proc 2004;79:353–72. Used with permission.

bra worn throughout the day or during exercise, weight reduction, a regimen of regular exercise, and smoking cessation. Although no randomized controlled trials have demonstrated the utility of these interventions, they are conservative measures worth recommending. Oral contraceptives also may be helpful in women with fibrocystic changes.

Results of studies examining the effect of reduced caffeine intake on mastalgia have been mixed, with the possibility of a placebo effect. However, a reduction in caffeine has no side effects and may be recommended. No evidence currently supports the efficacy of vitamin supplementation for the treatment of mastalgia (1). A study evaluating evening primrose oil versus fish oil in a randomized double-blinded study using wheat oil and corn oil as controls found that the number of days with pain decreased 10–16% in all four groups (2). Because all four groups received vitamin E, the authors concluded that either all the oils or vitamin E had an equal effect or "time and care" was responsible for the improvement (2).

The only medication approved by the U.S. Food and Drug Administration for treating mastalgia is danazol, but its use is limited by significant side effects. Other hormonal therapies with some efficacy include bromocriptine, lisuride maleate, and gonadotropin-releasing hormone agonists, but they too have side effects that prevent widespread clinical use.

Selective estrogen receptor modulators may have a role in treating severe mastalgia. A meta-analysis of trials for treatment of mastalgia demonstrated a beneficial effect of tamoxifen, with the best side effect profile (3). The most common side effects are hot flushes and vaginal discharge, although other known risks include increased endometrial hyperplasia and thromboembolic disease. Studies also are ongoing in newer medications from this class, such as toremifene, which may have fewer side effects. At this time, given the potential side effects, selective estrogen receptor modulators should be reserved for patients with severe, unremitting mastalgia and treatment should be limited to the lowest possible dose for 3–6 months.

Infections

Postpartum mastitis occurs in approximately 10% of women during lactation. The cause of infectious mastitis is typically milk stasis, leading to bacterial contamination, inflammation, edema, and the potential for abscess formation. The most common pathogens are *Staphylococcus aureus* and coagulase-negative staphylococci. Diagnosis usually is clinical and symptoms include fevers, chills, myalgia, malaise, and unilateral breast pain. Examination may be significant for a well-demarcated erythematous area on the breast, which is tender and warm to palpation. Management includes

supportive therapy (rest and pain control) and empiric treatment with dicloxacillin, cephalexin, clindamycin, or another antibiotic that covers gram-positive organisms. Breastfeeding, pumping, or both should continue to allow continual breast emptying. If a fluctuant mass is palpable under the skin or if the infection does not respond to initial antibiotics, an abscess is likely and breast ultrasonography can be used for diagnosis. Abscess may occur in approximately 5–11% of women with infectious mastitis and treatment is drainage and antibiotic therapy (4). There are no alternative therapies that have evidence to support use in prevention or treatment of mastitis. More details on management of postpartum mastitis can be found in *Precis: Obstetrics,* Fourth Edition.

Inflammation and infection also can occur in women who are not breastfeeding. The etiology in some cases is thought to be the dilation and rupture of subareolar ducts and subsequent acute and chronic inflammation in periductal tissues (5). Local skin infections or trauma also can result in nonlactational mastitis as in the case of nipple piercing. Diagnosis and treatment are similar to those in postpartum women. However, it is critical that if a woman does not respond to antibiotics and an abscess is not found, inflammatory carcinoma should be considered and referral to a breast surgeon expedited.

Intertriginous candidiasis may occur, appearing as pruritic and erythematous patches beneath the breasts. Keeping the skin dry and exposed to air may help prevent this condition, but this is difficult to achieve. Drying agents and powdered topical antifungal formulations are useful in treatment. Because of the difficulty in treating this condition, oral antifungals, such as fluconazole, may be indicated for a long time period in cases of severe or extensive intertriginous candidiasis.

Trauma

One etiology of breast trauma, nipple piercing, has become widespread in the past several years. Although not extensively studied, it has been shown to be associated with infection and abscess, pain, bleeding, hematoma, cyst formation, allergic reaction, and keloid formation, as well as increased risk of hepatitis B, hepatitis C, and human immunodeficiency virus (HIV) (6). Healing time for nipple piercing is approximately 3–6 months, which often results in delayed diagnosis of complications related to the procedure. Given that most individuals do not seek medical advice before or related to nipple piercing, health care providers need to be particularly attentive to the possibility that piercing may be the cause of a breast problem. Treatment of infection related to nipple piercing includes antibiotics and removal of the foreign body.

Other sources of breast trauma include breast biopsy or surgery, sports trauma, accidents (motor vehicle and other), and abuse. If a patient presents with pain, redness, or bruising, it is critical that a thorough history be taken to evaluate for possible trauma. Contusions, abrasions, lacerations, and hematomas can all be types of trauma to the breast. Treatment usually is similar to that elsewhere on the body, but adequate analgesia and firm support (including a supportive bra) often are helpful for such injuries in the breast (7). A complication of trauma can be fat necrosis. A patient who has fat necrosis may present with a tender mass or induration. Fat necrosis typically has a specific appearance on mammography (5).

Other causes of breast trauma include sports-related trauma, due to either cold temperatures or friction from clothing during repetitive activities, or blunt trauma during sporting activities (7). Symptoms often include raw, painful, and bloody nipple or nipples. Prevention can include a bandage or petroleum jelly during exercise and use of a fitted sports bras and wind breaking material over the chest.

Breast Implants

More than 1 million women have undergone breast augmentation in the United States. Complications that can lead to further surgery include capsular contraction, implant rupture, hematoma, and wound infection (8). Other potential risks of breast implants include postoperative asymmetries; changes due to pregnancy, breastfeeding, or weight fluctuations; permanent changes in sensation to the nipples or breasts; wrinkling of the implant; or deflation (8). The number of adolescent women who request breast augmentation surgery has increased in the past several years. There are unique considerations in this population. The American Society for Plastic Surgery has produced guidelines for this patient population, including the recommendations that candidates should be aged at least 18 years and undergo extensive counseling concerning risks, activity restrictions, and recovery time (6).

Breast implants also may complicate evaluation of a breast mass or cancer screening. Magnetic resonance imaging is a useful adjunct in the workup of a woman with breast implants in whom mammographic or ultrasound results are inconclusive. It also is useful in a patient in whom rupture of the implant is a concern.

Breast Masses

It is imperative to obtain a thorough history in any woman who presents with a breast mass. Associated symptoms, such as pain, nipple discharge, changes in appearance of the breast, and relationship with the menstrual cycle, should be noted. The health care provider should document onset of symptoms or date of detection of the mass and interval changes in size and consistency of the mass. The cancer risk profile of the patient includes historical factors and past tissue diagnoses (Box 32). Atypical ductal hyperplasia, the most common pathologic lesion associated with an increased risk of breast cancer, increases the risk of cancer fourfold.

The patient's breast cancer risk profile can be calculated using the Breast Cancer Risk Assessment Tool, developed by the National Cancer Institute and the National Surgical Adjuvant Breast and Bowel Project (see Appendix A). This tool allows the provider or the patient to project a woman's estimated breast cancer risk over a 5-year period and up to age 90 years. It also allows for comparison of an individual woman's risk with that of a woman of her age from general population. The National Comprehensive Cancer Network (see Appendix A) also provides a useful resource for screening, surveillance, and treatment guidelines. Regardless of risk assessment, all masses should be evaluated.

Physical examination can sometimes be challenging, especially in younger women. A dominant mass usually can be distinguished from the surrounding tissue and will not change throughout the menstrual cycle. Features suggesting possible malignancy include firmness, poorly defined margins, immobility, skin dimpling or color change, unilateral retraction or change in the nipple, nipple scaling, bloody nipple discharge, and associated lymphadenopathy (9).

For a patient with a report of a breast lump or finding of a new mass, the clinician is responsible for documenting the findings and providing appropri-

---

Box 32

Risk Factors for Breast Cancer

- Age
- Personal history of breast cancer
- History of atypical hyperplasia (ductal or lobular) on past biopsies
- Inherited genetic mutations
- First-degree relatives with breast cancer or ovarian cancer diagnosed at an early age
- Early menarche (younger than 12 years)
- Late cessation of menses (older than 55 years)
- No term pregnancies
- Late age at first live birth (older than 30 years)
- Never breastfed
- Alcohol consumption
- Recent oral contraceptive use
- Use of hormone therapy
- Personal history of endometrial, ovarian, or colon cancer
- Jewish heritage

ate follow-up care or referrals. Figure 57 provides an algorithm for the evaluation of a breast mass. If a mass is thought to be cystic, an office cyst aspiration can be performed. If clear fluid is aspirated and the mass disappears, the fluid can be discarded and the patient should return for repeat examination in 4–6 weeks. If the mass returns, the patient should be referred for further diagnostic workup.

Evaluation by ultrasonography or mammography is indicated if no fluid can be aspirated, no mass is palpable on initial clinical breast examination despite patient reporting a lump, a solid mass is palpable, or the clinician is not comfortable performing cyst aspiration. In a

woman younger than 40 years, if no dominant mass is visualized on ultrasonography and if the clinical breast examination reveals vague nodularity, the finding is most likely due to fibroglandular changes and repeat clinical breast examination in 2–4 months is sufficient. If a mass can be distinguished from normal breast tissue, the patient should be referred to a breast surgeon. Other situations requiring referral to a surgeon include patients with history of breast surgery, extremely fibrocystic breasts, persistent localized pain, or a request for a second opinion.

In women younger than 40 years, ultrasonography is the recommended modality to evaluate a palpable breast

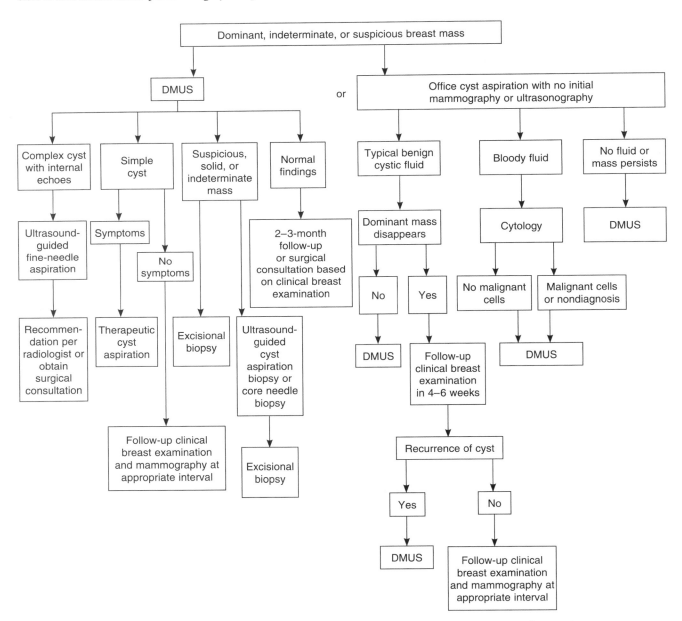

Figure 57. Workup of dominant, indeterminate, or suspicious breast mass. Abbreviation: DMUS indicates diagnostic mammography and ultrasonography. (Pruthi S. Detection and evaluation of a palpable breast mass. Mayo Clin Proc 2001;76:641–7. Used with permission.)

mass because mammography is not as sensitive in the denser breast tissue of young woman. Ultrasonography also can be used to differentiate between a cystic lesion and a solid lesion. A lesion that is anechoic on ultrasound examination is consistent with a simple cyst and can be drained for symptomatic relief or can be observed without intervention.

In women older than 40 years, mammography often is the first-line study in evaluating a patient presenting with a mass. Whereas screening mammography includes two standard views, craniocaudal and mediolateral, diagnostic mammography may include other views as recommended by the radiologist who is present during the examination. Additionally, ultrasonography, spot-compression views, and magnification views may be used to localize a mass that cannot be detected by standard mammography and are essential for the surgeon performing biopsy.

A patient with a solid mass should be referred for diagnostic procedure, such as fine-needle aspiration, core needle biopsy, stereotactic biopsy, incisional biopsy, or excisional biopsy. If a palpable area of nodularity is present, without a discrete mass, mammography or ultrasonography should be performed. If no abnormality is detected, close clinical follow-up or referral to a breast specialist is necessary. The American College of Obstetricians and Gynecologists (the College) provides guidelines for making referrals to other physicians or diagnostic testing and recommends that documentation of the referral be clear in the medical record (Box 33) (10).

Box 33

Guidelines for Referral for Diagnostic Testing

When a patient is referred to another physician for diagnostic testing or consultation, the obstetrician-gynecologist should ensure that the patient is provided with the following information:

- An explanation that she needs further care
- The names of qualified physicians from whom the patient can receive care
- An opportunity to have her questions answered
- A summary of the history, physical examination, and diagnostic tests performed
- Information for the consultant if diagnostic imaging is required for a reason of clinical concern rather than merely routine screening

Documentation of these steps and a description of the clinical findings should be included in the medical record.

American College of Obstetricians and Gynecologists. Guidelines for women's health care. 3rd ed. Washington, DC: ACOG; 2007. p. 164.

In adolescents, most masses are benign fibroadenomas, followed by a small proportion diagnosed as fibrocystic changes. Rarely are abscesses or mastitis diagnosed (6). Most studies demonstrate that most fibroadenomas decrease in size or even resolve, especially in young women. Nonsurgical management, with follow-up radiographic evaluation every 6 months for 1 year, and then annual follow-up, usually is reasonable in most young women (5). Excisional biopsy or surgery can be considered if the mass is enlarging or changing, there are overlying skin changes, infection or abscess develops, or the woman has a history of malignancy (6). Conservative management does require certainty that the diagnosis is fibroadenoma; phyllodes tumor often is similar in presentation and requires complete excision.

Nipple Discharge

Nipple discharge usually is a benign finding, but can indicate either endocrine dysfunction or cancer. Hyperprolactinemia is the most common endocrinologic cause of nipple discharge and can result in galactorrhea, even in a nulligravid or postmenopausal woman. Hypothyroidism also can cause galactorrhea; therefore, measurements of both serum prolactin and thyroid-stimulating hormone are useful initial tests.

Nonendocrine etiologies of nipple discharge include ductal ectasia and fibrocystic changes, which usually cause bilateral nipple discharge, as well as intraductal papilloma, intraductal carcinoma, and invasive ductal carcinoma, each of which usually present as unilateral and uniductal. When the discharge is nonbloody, greenish-black in appearance, and comes from multiple ducts, the cause is most likely ductal ectasia, and the patient can be reassured of the benign nature. If fibrocystic changes are present and no dominant mass is identified, the patient also may be reassured (11). If a bloody discharge is present or if a nonbloody discharge is unilateral or otherwise differs from ductal ectasia or fibrocystic disease, carcinoma cannot be ruled out and duct excision is necessary. An intraductal papilloma is the most common etiology for a bloody, uniductal nipple discharge and is treated with duct excision. The patient should be referred to a specialist who is credentialed in this procedure.

Breast Cancer Screening

The American College of Obstetricians and Gynecologists recommends that mammography be performed every 1–2 years in women aged 40–49 years and annually thereafter (12). The American Medical Association, American College of Radiology, and American Cancer Society (ACS) recommend annual screening beginning at age 40 years, based on concerns that examinations every 2 years will miss opportunities to detect early cancer (13). The adverse consequences of mammography include the need for additional studies or biopsies for false-positive findings and impact on psychologic and physical welfare. The most recent guidelines from the U.S. Preventive Services Task Force (USPSTF) recommend biennial as opposed to annual screening mammography between in women aged 50–74 years (14). The recommendations also state that "the decision to start regular, biennial screening mammography before 50 years should be an individual one and take patient context into account, including the patient's values regarding specific benefits and harms" (14). The American College of Obstetricians and Gynecologists and other organizations have not changed their recommendations based on these USPSTF guidelines (15).

Communication of mammographic results is regulated by the Mammography Quality Standards Act. One method of reporting the results is the Breast Imaging Reporting and Data System, which specifies assessment categories (16).

In examining newer technologies for screening, the USPSTF found the evidence is insufficient to assess the additional benefits or harms of digital mammography or MRI in breast cancer screening (14). Although digital mammography may be better than film mammography in detecting cancer in premenopausal women younger than 50 years or women with dense breasts (17), there are no formal guidelines from the College or ACS concerning digital mammography. The American Cancer Society does address the use of magnetic resonance imaging (MRI) in high-risk women.

The value of clinical breast examination also has come under scrutiny. Several analyses have supported the use of clinical breast examination. The American College of Obstetricians and Gynecologists continues to recommend annual clinical breast examination (10, 12). The American Cancer Society's recommendations include clinical breast examination every 3 years for women aged 20–39 years and annually thereafter (13). The United States Preventive Services Task Force concluded that evidence was insufficient to recommend for or against clinical breast examination alone (14).

Recommendations concerning breast self-examination have been similarly mixed. The American College of Obstetricians and Gynecologists continues to support breast self-examination because of the potential to detect palpable breast cancer (10, 12). The United States Preventive Services Task Force recommends against teaching women breast self-examination (14). Further details on screening, diagnosis, and treatment of breast cancer can be found in *Precis: Oncology*, Third Edition.

Special Considerations in Screening

Women with inherited mutations of *BRCA1* and *BRCA2* have the highest risk of breast cancer comprising 5–10% of all women with diagnosed breast cancer. The mean age of these women at diagnosis is 50 years, nearly a decade younger than of those with sporadic breast cancer. Current surveillance recommendations for *BRCA* carriers include monthly breast self-examination (beginning at age 18–20 years), clinical breast examination, and mammography beginning after age 25 years or 5–10 years before the diagnosis was made in an affected relative (18). Consultation with a genetic counselor is recommended whenever there is a possibility of an inherited predisposition to breast and ovarian cancer.

Magnetic resonance imaging has been found to be superior to mammography in delineating masses in young women with dense breasts and may be helpful in surveillance of postsurgical breasts and in women with implants. In studies comparing MRI with other screening modalities in women with genetic or familial predisposition to breast cancer, MRI was found to have a higher sensitivity and perform better as a screening tool (19).

The use of MRI in women at low risk of breast cancer is still being evaluated. The American Cancer Society recommends screening with MRI in high-risk women, including women with a known genetic mutation, who have a first-degree relative with a high-risk mutation, who have a greater than 20–25% lifetime risk, or who received chest irradiation (therapeutic) between ages 10 years and 30 years (20). Where available, MRI also is being used in patients in whom the mammographic and ultrasound examination results are indeterminate to help determine the extent of disease and presence of multifocal disease, contralateral disease, or both, especially in high-risk women and women with dense breasts.

References

1. Smith RL, Pruthi S, Fitzpatrick LA. Evaluation and management of breast pain. Mayo Clin Proc 2004;79:353–72.

2. Blommers J, de Lange-De Klerk ES, Kuik DJ, Bezemer PD, Meijer S. Evening primrose oil and fish oil for severe chronic mastalgia: a randomized, double-blind, controlled trial. Am J Obstet Gynecol 2002;187:1389–94.

3. Srivastava A, Mansel RE, Arvind N, Prasad K, Dhar A, Chabra A. Evidence-based management of mastalgia: a meta-analysis of randomised trials. Breast 2007;16:503–12.

4. Barbosa-Cesnik C, Schwartz K, Foxman B. Lactation mastitis. JAMA 2003;298:1609–12.

5. Miltenburg DM, Speights VO. Benign breast disease. Obstet Gynecol Clin North Am 2008;35:285–300, ix.

6. Breast concerns in the adolescent. ACOG Committee Opinion No. 350. American College of Obstetricians and Gynecologists. Obstet Gynecol 2006;108:1329–36.

7. Greydanus DE, Matytsina L, Gains M. Breast disorders in children and adolescents. Prim Care 2006;33:455–502.

8. Antoniuk PM. Breast augmentation and breast reduction. Obstet Gynecol Clin North Am 2002;29:103–15.

9. Pruthi S. Detection and evaluation of a palpable breast mass. Mayo Clin Proc 2001;76:641–7.

10. American College of Obstetricians and Gynecologists. Guidelines for women's health care. 3rd ed. Washington, DC: ACOG; 2007. p. 164.

11. Falkenberry SS. Nipple discharge. Obstet Gynecol Clin North Am 2002;29:21–9.

12. Breast cancer screening. ACOG Practice Bulletin No. 42. American College of Obstetricians and Gynecologists. Obstet Gynecol 2003;101:821–31.

13. Smith RA, Saslow D, Sawyer KA, Burke W, Costanza ME, Evans WP 3rd, et al. American Cancer Society guidelines for breast cancer screening: update 2003. American Cancer Society High-Risk Work Group; American Cancer Society Screening Older Women Work Group; American Cancer Society Mammography Work Group; American Cancer Society Physical Examination Work Group; American Cancer Society New Technologies Work Group; American Cancer Society Breast Cancer Advisory Group. CA Cancer J Clin 2003;53:141–69.

14. Screening for breast cancer: U.S. Preventive Services Task Force recommendation statement. U.S. Preventive Services Task Force [published errata appear in Ann Int Med 2010;152:688; Ann Intern Med 2010;152:199–200]. Ann Int Med 2009;151:716–26, W-236.

15. American College of Obstetricians and Gynecologists statement on revised U.S. Preventive Services Task Force Recommendations on breast cancer screening. Washington, DC: ACOG; 2009. Available at: http://www.acog.org/from_home/publications/press_releases/nr11-16-09.cfm. Retrieved December 7, 2010.

16. American College of Radiology. ACR BI-RADS Mammography. ACR breast imaging reporting and data system, breast imaging atlas. 4th ed. Reston (VA): ACR; 2003.

17. Pisano ED, Gatsonis C, Hendrick E, Yaffe M, Baum JK, Acharyya S, et al. Diagnostic performance of digital versus film mammography for breast-cancer screening. Digital Mammographic Imaging Screening Trial (DMIST) Investigators Group [published erratum appears in N Engl J Med 2006;355:1840]. N Engl J Med 2005;353:1773–83.

18. National Comprehensive Cancer Network. Genetic/familial high-risk assessment: breast and ovarian. NCCN Clinical Practice Guidelines in Oncology. 1. Fort Washington (PA): NCCH; 2010. Available at: http://www.nccn.org/professionals/physician_gls/PDF/genetics_screening.pdf. Retrieved December 7, 2010.

19. Kriege M, Brekelmans CT, Boetes C, Besnard PE, Zonderland HM, Obdeijn IM, et al. Efficacy of MRI and mammography for breast–cancer screening in women with a familial or genetic predisposition. Magnetic Resonance Imaging Screening Study Group. N Engl J Med 2004;351:427–37.

20. Saslow D, Boetes C, Burke W, Harms S, Leach MO, Lehman CD, et al. American Cancer Society guidelines for breast screening with MRI as an adjunct to mammography. American Cancer Society Breast Cancer Advisory Group [published erratum appears in CA Cancer J Clin 2007;57:185]. CA Cancer J Clin 2007;57:75–89.

Pediatric Gynecology

Samantha Schon and Diane F. Merritt

Pediatric gynecology is a distinct specialty involving the unique gynecologic problems of the neonate and prepubertal child. A practicing obstetrician–gynecologist may be asked to recognize, treat, or triage some of the most common office-based problems that arise in this discipline. Knowledge of the normal appearance of the genitalia and basic pediatric pathophysiology can alert the practitioner to abnormal findings and well as prevent misinterpretation of normal variants as pathologic.

Physical Examination of the Neonate

Estrogen is transiently elevated in the neonate due to maternal and placental sources. Estrogenic effects noticeable in the newborn include breast buds, prominent labia majora, and a white vaginal discharge. The labia minora and hymen may protrude slightly from the vestibule. The clitoris may appear large in proportion to the other genital structures, especially in premature infants. Visualization of the vaginal orifice in a neonate may be difficult because of edema and redundancy of the hymen or to location of the vaginal orifice with a slit-like opening just beneath the urethra. Presence of a discharge confirms vaginal patency. Once newborn levels of estrogen decrease, the breast buds flatten and the vaginal discharge ceases until peripuberty when they are stimulated by endogenous estrogen production. In childhood, the hymenal membrane thins, becoming shiny or translucent, and is easily injured by trauma. Endogenous estrogen production with puberty initiates growth and elongation of the labia minora, maturation of the uterus and vagina, production of vaginal secretions (physiologic leukorrhea), and increased distensibility of the hymen and introitus. The impact of estrogen (or lack of) plays a direct role in the physical examination of the external and internal genital structures of newborns, infants, children, and adolescents, and in the response of the reproductive organs to disease and trauma. Because endogenous estrogen production is under neuroendocrine control, factors that impact the central nervous system (congenital anomalies, tumors, and trauma) may directly affect the child's reproductive health.

Examination of the Prepubertal Child

Physical Examination

The external genital examination in prepubertal girls requires a gentle, patient approach to minimize fear or embarrassment. Before beginning the external genital examination, the procedure should be explained to the child and parent and a permission to examine the child should be obtained. Forcible restraint is never indicated and sedation is rarely necessary. Different examination techniques may be used that include the following methods:

- A young child can be placed on the parent's lap with the child's legs straddling the parent's thighs.
- If the child permits, she may be positioned on the table in the supine position with the hips fully abducted and the feet together in the "frog-leg" position.
- An older child may prefer to use foot stirrups.
- The child may be placed in the knee-chest position with elevation of the buttocks and hips. This position provides exposure of the inferior portion of the hymen, the lower vagina, and possibly the upper vagina and cervix.
- If there is an acute problem (injury or bleeding) or if the child is unable to cooperate for evaluation, an examination under anesthesia may be more appropriate and less traumatic for the child.

The labia majora should be evaluated for symmetry, size, presence of rashes or traumatic changes, and presence or absence of pubic hair. The labia majora and minora may then be retracted laterally to expose the vaginal orifice and hymen. Careful attention should be paid to ensuring the patency of the hymen, as well as the presence or absence of vaginal discharge.

Vaginoscopy

If the circumstances require an evaluation of the vagina of a prepubertal girl, a useful technique is vaginoscopy. An endoscope (cystoscope or hysteroscope) is placed in the vagina and the labia are gently opposed, allowing the vagina to distend with water or saline. This technique permits visualization of the vagina and cervix allowing for full evaluation of an anatomical variant, tumor, injury, or presence of a foreign body. The prepubertal vagina is pink with faint rugae. The cervix is flat with a slit-like opening and nearly flush at the apex of the vagina. Adult-sized specula are not to be used to examine children.

Imaging Studies

Ultrasonography is a widely accepted initial screening tool for pelvic masses and a superior modality for ovarian visualization. It is, however, operator- and technique-dependent. Young children cannot be examined transvaginally, so the transabdominal view requires that the bladder be full. Poor images will result from attempts to view pelvic structures transabdominally without adequate bladder distention, and the obese patient also presents challenges. More recently, three-dimensional ultrasonography has been shown to have potential as a useful diagnostic tool.

Pelvic anomalies are best viewed by magnetic resonance imaging (MRI). This is the most sensitive and specific imaging technique used for evaluating müllerian anomalies because of its ability to image nearly all reproductive structures, blood flow, external contours, junctional zone resolution on T2 weighted images, as well as associated renal and other associated anomalies. Magnetic resonance imaging also has a high correlation with surgical findings because of its multiplanar capabilities and high spatial resolution. Sedation may be needed.

Gynecologic Concerns

Common pediatric disorders include vulvovaginitis (nonspecific and specific pathogens), labial adhesions, acute genital ulcers, lichen sclerosus, human papillomavirus (HPV) infection, psoriasis, and urethral prolapse. Less common are neoplasms, especially ovarian cancer. Of concern also is vaginal bleeding in a pediatric patient. It can be a result of an underlying gynecologic or endocrine condition or trauma, accidental or inflicted.

Vulvovaginitis

Poor or excessive hygiene and chemical irritants are the most common causes of vulvovaginitis. Children are especially prone to nonspecific vulvovaginitis due to their hypoestrogenic state, poor perianal hygiene, and the proximity of the vagina to the anus. If culture indicates a sexually transmitted infection (STI), a prompt evaluation for sexual abuse is indicated (1, 2).

Under the influence of estrogen, the normal adult vaginal epithelium cornifies and produces glycogen. This acts as a substrate for lactobacilli and results in an acidic pH, which protects reproductive-aged women against vaginal infections. The normal pH of the prepubertal vagina is more alkaline due to absence of lactobacilli and a relative lack of estrogen. As a result, in pediatric patients, the vagina is more susceptible to irritation and infection. Children with vulvovaginitis may present with perianal redness and inflammation of the introitus. If caused by a bacterial infection, a yellow–green or brown vaginal discharge may occur and improved hygiene or antibiotics should result in relief of symptoms. A foul-smelling serosanguineous discharge may be the presenting symptom of a foreign

body in the vagina. Girls may present with dysuria, vaginal spotting, or bleeding. The bleeding may be one time, intermittent, or continuous in nature. Other conditions (ie, pinworms or lichen sclerosus) can cause irritation and pruritus and examination of the external genitals is necessary to make a proper diagnosis. Infectious vulvovaginitis may be caused by fecal or respiratory bacteria. These organisms generally are transmitted to the genital area as a result of poor handwashing or improper toilet hygiene. Many parents and physicians assume that vulvar itching and vaginal discharge in children is due to a yeast infection and incorrectly diagnose and treat with antifungal preparations. Although *Candida albicans* is a fungus that normally lives on the skin and mucous membranes (mouth, nose, and bowels) it is less likely to be a cause of vulvovaginitis in children. Under certain clinical settings, *Candida* infection may cause a red, raised, patchy rash with sharp borders, mostly over the genitalia but with satellite spots sprinkled around the diaper area. Risk factors include antibiotics that alter the bacterial flora of the bowels, immunosuppression, and debilitating medical conditions. Although a trial of topical antifungals might improve a diaper rash caused by the *Candida* species, it would not benefit children with a purulent discharge caused by bacterial pathogens. Sexually transmitted infections also may cause vaginal discharge or vulvovaginal irritation. Occasionally, children may acquire these infections via vertical transmission from their mothers during childbirth. However, if these infections arise after the neonatal period, they are likely sexually acquired. Sexually transmitted infections in children and minors should be reported to authorities according to established protocol.

The diagnosis of vulvovaginitis is based on history, clinical findings, microscopic evaluation of vaginal secretions (wet mount examination), pH testing, and cultures. Screening questions should reference hygiene practices (type of soap used and direction of wiping motion employed). The clinical examination should include an external inspection of the perineal area, including the vaginal introitus using lateral traction of the labia majora. If a discharge is present, microscopic analysis may be performed by a wet preparation, with or without culture.

Cultures may be obtained with cotton swabs or urethral swabs moistened with nonbacteriostatic saline. A topical anesthetic can be applied before placing the swab into the vagina. If a discharge is present, an aerobic vaginal culture and gonorrhea and chlamydia testing may be done. Alternatively, a small tube attached to a syringe with a small amount of saline for vaginal wash and aspiration can be used.

Highly specific tests should be used when the diagnosis of an STI might lead to initiation of an investigation for child abuse. Testing for gonorrhea and chlamydia in children may be done by culture or by nucleic acid amplification testing, depending on institutional or state and Centers for Disease Control and Prevention guidelines.

Although nucleic acid amplification tests (NAATs) are recommended for detection of reproductive tract infections caused by *Chlamydia trachomatis* and *Neisseria gonorrhoeae* in women with and without symptoms, use in children is under investigation. Nucleic acid amplification tests have been used in cases of pediatric sexual abuse with superior sensitivity and specificity for the detection of *Chlamydia* species. Positive test results for gonorrhea from NAATs have significant cross-reaction with nongonococcal *Neisseria* species. As a result, NAAT results positive for gonorrhea should be retested for confirmation by culture. Clinical trials are needed to further evaluate use of NAATs in children.

Optimal specimens for NAATs include first catch urine. There is little need or evidence for urethral swab specimens. Vaginal swab specimens are preferred and self-obtained swabs are undergoing investigation (3, 4). Treating children with vulvovaginitis requires extensive parent and patient education. The condition usually is improved by educating the caregivers and the child about the importance of consistently wiping in a front to back direction (from urethra to anus). If the problem persists or recurs, it is beneficial to follow the use of toilet tissue with a pre-moistened cloth or paper wipe to decrease fecal contamination. Counseling also should include proper hygiene and avoidance of prolonged time in wet or soiled diapers. Chemicals, such as perfumed or deodorant soap products, bubble baths, harsh detergents, scented dryer sheets or fabric softeners, and chemically treated water in swimming pools and hot tubs, may cause irritation. Wearing tights, leotards, swimsuits, and other constrictive clothing should be limited to the related activity, and loose-fitting cotton undergarments and clothing are preferred to minimize the problem.

Labial Adhesions

Labial adhesions (agglutination) occur when the adjacent edges of the labia adhere to each other. The etiology is not well understood but believed to be associated with inflammation, and perpetuated by irritation of urine leakage from behind the obstructing adhesions. Labial agglutination may be asymptomatic; however, urinary dribbling, urinary tract infections, urethritis, and vulvitis can be presenting symptoms. Labial adhesions appear as attachments of the opposing labia with a fine avascular line visible in the midline. The urethral orifice and hymen may be difficult to see if they are posterior to the labial adhesions. Labial adhesions need to be treated only if they are symptomatic or adversely affect urination. Treatment involves applying a small amount of topical estrogen to the affected

semi-translucent line of adhesions. Steroid creams may function as second-line therapy. In both cases, the cream should be rubbed along the line of the adhesions using a cotton swab while applying gentle labial traction. The adhesions will often resolve within 2–3 months; however, they frequently recur. Application of small amount of lubricating ointment daily can help to prevent the reformation of the adhesions in the initial months after separation. Surgical treatment rarely is indicated and should not be done in the office setting. If mechanical separation is done under anesthesia, the adhesions may reform within 24 hours unless topical estrogen, ointments, or barriers are applied.

Acute Genital Ulcers

Acute genital ulcers, also known as aphthous or virginal ulcers, are thought to be associated with cytomegalovirus, Epstein–Barr virus, and influenza A viral infections. These lesions usually present in conjunction with systemic viral symptoms, and initially appear on the inner vulvar surface as very painful red areas, which then ulcerate with sharply demarcated edges and develop a purulent or escharotic base. Patients with acute genital ulcers often report severe dysuria. If patients are treated for a urinary tract infection without a visual examination of the introitus, the proper diagnosis may be delayed. A purulent vaginal discharge usually accompanies the lesions. These young patients may receive a wrong diagnosis of herpes simplex virus (HSV), but the clinical appearance is not typical of HSV and HSV test results (if obtained) will be negative. Acute genital ulcers can be treated with topical anesthetics, oral or parenteral pain management, and antibiotics if a bacterial superinfection is present. At this time, it is unclear if prophylactic influenza vaccinations or antiviral medications could prevent or ameliorate the symptoms of acute viral ulcers. The usual time course until the lesions resolve is 7–14 days. If the patient cannot urinate due to pain or swelling, admission to the hospital and placement of a Foley catheter are necessary to avoid urinary retention. If the lesions recur, an immunologic workup is indicated to exclude Behçet disease. Other causes of ulcerative lesions in children include HSV, Epstein–Barr virus, Crohn disease, and fixed drug eruptions (5).

Lichen Sclerosus

Lichen sclerosus generally manifests itself with intense vulvar pruritus and occasionally with spotting or bleeding. The skin is hypopigmented, surrounding the vulva, rectum, or both in a keyhole fashion. Scratching can lead to petechiae or blood blisters. In long-term untreated cases, the vulvar anatomy can be lost due to scarring. Unlike in elderly adults whose white pruritic lesions may be a sign of vulvar malignancies, biopsies of lichen sclerosus lesions are rarely necessary in children.

Lichen sclerosus should be treated with administration of a high-potency steroid ointment, such as clobetasol 0.05%, to the affected area up to twice daily until the symptoms and signs regress and then the steroids need to be tapered. Once the diagnosis of lichen sclerosus is established, the child needs to be monitored for signs of recurrence and repeat treatment if necessary.

Human Papillomavirus

Low-risk types, such as HPV 6 and HPV 11 are responsible for almost all cases of genital warts and additional abnormal Pap test results (6). High-risk oncogenic types are associated with cervical intraepithelial neoplasia. Human papillomavirus types 16 and 18 are responsible for 99.7% of all cases of cervical cancer. In 2006, the quadrivalent vaccine was approved by the U.S. Food and Drug Administration for vaccination against HPV types 6, 11, 16, and 18 and in 2009, a bivalent vaccine was approved by the U.S. Food and Drug Adinistration for vaccination against HPV types 16 and 18. Both the Centers for Disease Control and Prevention's Advisory Committee on Immunization Practices and the American College of Obstetricians and Gynecologists currently recommend routine vaccination of girls aged between 11 years and 12 years, although vaccination may be administered as early as age 9 years (7). Although the vaccine is now widely marketed and administered, data evaluating the natural history and long-term outcomes in the pediatric population are lacking. The assessment of HPV infection in children has been limited to highly selective small population studies, which also include sexually abused groups in which the transmitters of HPV may be different from typical adolescent-acquired populations.

For the population as a whole, the acquisition of HPV is predominately related to sexual activity; however, children also may acquire the virus through vertical transmission. Other suggested modes of transmission include autoinoculation, heteroinoculation, and indirect transmission via fomites (8). Sequelae of vertically transmitted HPV in children include recurrent laryngeal papillomatosis and anogenital condylomata. Screening for sexual abuse should be considered in children first presenting with anogenital warts after age 3 years, or children presenting with laryngeal papillomas after age 5 years (8). In 2007, a study evaluated the prevalence of HPV DNA in the oral cavity or oropharynx in a cross-section of children aged from 2 weeks to 20 years. The authors found a bimodal distribution with the highest HPV prevalence in the youngest and oldest groups (ages younger than 1 year and 16–20 years). Results from this study suggest that acquisition of HPV before age 1 year most likely occurs by a vertical transmission with clearance of the infection or reduction to undetectable viral loads with the increasing age. Prevalence increases again with sexual debut in the 16–20-year age group (9). This study is one of only a few that examines the prevalence of HPV in the pediatric population. More research is needed because the long-term effects of HPV infection in infancy and children are not known.

Vaginal Bleeding

As maternal estrogen levels decrease in the neonate, any endometrial proliferation that occurred in utero due to placental transfer of maternal estrogen may slough, leading to vaginal spotting or bleeding in newborn females. The most common causes of vaginal bleeding in children are vulvovaginitis (see "Vulvovaginitis" earlier in this section), foreign bodies in the vagina, urethral prolapse, and dermatologic conditions; less common are tumors. Each structure in the genital tract is a possible source of vaginal bleeding. A thorough external genital examination will help to determine the cause or source of bleeding. If a cause cannot be identified in the office setting, an examination under anesthesia may be needed.

URETHRAL PROLAPSE

Urethral prolapse (when the distal end of the urethra everts) may cause bleeding and generally appears with a red or dusky mass at the vaginal introitus. Predisposing factors include low-estrogen states, trauma, chronic cough, and constipation. Urethral prolapse typically resolves with application of topical estrogen cream to the affected area for 2–6 weeks.

FOREIGN BODIES

Foreign bodies in the vagina can cause vaginal bleeding that generally is accompanied by a foul smelling serosanguineous discharge. The objects, most commonly pieces of toilet paper, can stay in the vagina for weeks to months and can be difficult to see on examination. Foreign bodies should be removed for resolution of the bleeding and any associated symptoms. This may be accomplished by vaginal irrigation with warm water or by vaginoscopy.

PRECOCIOUS PUBERTY AND HORMONAL DISORDERS

When vaginal bleeding in a young girl is accompanied by other signs of reproductive maturity, such as breast development and terminal hair growth, precocious puberty should be considered. In children, early maturation of the hypothalamic–pituitary–gonadal axis and related release of follicle-stimulating hormone and luteinizing hormone to stimulate the production of estrogen can result in endometrial proliferation and bleeding. Also known as central precocious puberty or gonadotropin-dependent precocious puberty, approximately 10–20% of cases are due to a central nervous system lesion but most cases are idiopathic. Gonadotropin independent estrogen sources include exogenous intake and steroid producing tumors of the ovaries and adrenal glands. When precocious puberty is suspected as the cause of the vaginal bleeding, a thorough physical examination determining Tanner staging and diagnostic studies, including growth charts and bone age, are helpful in establishing this diagnosis. An elevated serum estradiol level or an adnexal mass diagnosed by pelvic ultrasonography can suggest an ovarian tumor. The gonadotropin-releasing hormone stimulation study typically is used to diagnose precocious puberty. Magnetic resonance imaging can rule out a hypothalamic tumor as a cause of the precocious puberty.

Neoplasms

Hemangiomas are benign growths of blood vessels that generally regress with time. They blanche with compression. Large perineal hemangiomas may be associated with spinal cord anomalies. Polyps can be found on the hymen and in the vagina and, like hemangiomas, are generally benign. Neoplasms are uncommon causes of vaginal bleeding in prepubertal girls. Maturation of an isolated follicle can produce enough estradiol to cause breast budding and endometrial proliferation. As the follicle resolves and the estradiol levels decrease, the breast buds dissipate and the endometrium sloughs resulting in a limited episode of vaginal bleeding. *Rhabdomyosarcomas* and endodermal sinus tumors (germ cell tumors) are malignant lesions that can be found in the genital tract. They are very rare and require tissue diagnosis and collaboration with pediatric oncologists for appropriate treatment. Ovarian granulosa cell tumors can produce estrogen and stimulate precocious secondary sexual development and vaginal bleeding in children. Neoplasms are rare and should be suspected based on the findings of physical examination, imaging studies, and other diagnostic markers.

Genital Trauma

Genital trauma may be the result of an accidental injury or sexual abuse. Straddle-type injuries, which often result in only minor lacerations or abrasions of the labia, account for most accidental genital injuries in children. Straddle injuries occur as the soft tissues of the vulva are compressed between the bones of the pelvis and an object. Common sources of injury include playground equipment, bicycles frames, and edges of swimming pools or bathtubs. These injuries usually affect the mons pubis, clitoris, and labia, whereas the hymen and the vagina rarely are involved. Ecchymoses, lacerations, and abrasions are common. If there is active bleeding, these injuries may require suturing. If a straddle injury or trauma causes a vulvar hematoma, conservative management (bed rest and ice packs) is recommended for small, nonexpanding hematomas.

Expanding hematomas, especially if there is mottling of the skin, require incision and drainage to prevent a prolonged recovery or necrosis of the overlying vulva. The child must be able to void or a Foley catheter should be placed (10). Accidental penetrating injuries may occur when the girl falls onto a sharp or pointed object.

Pediatric sexual abuse includes verbal, physical, and sexual mistreatment of children. Although in most cases of sexual abuse there are no clinical findings, suspicion of abuse is raised when the hymen is transected. Because it is difficult to determine if trauma is accidental or inflicted, an eyewitness to the event or a history that fits with the clinical findings and injury may be helpful in determining the etiology. Multiple or conflicting versions of the etiology of the injury should raise suspicions of child maltreatment. Vulvar lesions also may be confused with child abuse, so the examiner must be familiar with the appearance of typical lesions, such as lichen sclerosus or labial adhesions.

References

1. Dei M, Di Maggio F, Di Paolo G, Bruni V. Vulvovaginitis in childhood. Best Pract Res Clin Obstet Gynaecol 2010; 24:129–37.

2. Workowski KA, Berman S. Sexually transmitted diseases treatment guidelines, 2010. Centers for Disease Control and Prevention. Division of STD Prevention National Center for HIV/AIDS, Viral Hepatitis, STD, and TB Prevention. Rep 2010;59(RR-12):1–110.

3. Black CM, Driebe EM, Howard LA, Fajman NN, Sawyer MK, Girardet RG, et al Multicenter study of nucleic acid amplification tests for detection of Chlamydia trachomatis and Neisseria gonorrhoeae in children being evaluated for sexual abuse. Pediatr Infect Dis J 2009;28:608–13.

4. Girardet RG, Lahoti S, Howard LA, Fajman NN, Sawyer MK, Driebe EM, et al. Epidemiology of sexually transmitted infections in suspected child victims of sexual assault. Pediatrics 2009;124:79–86.

5. Van Eyk N, Allen L, Giesbrecht E, Jamieson MA, Kives S, Morris M, et al. Pediatric vulvovaginal disorders: a diagnostic approach and review of the literature. J Obstet Gynaecol Can 2009;31:850–62.

6. Ault K. Epidemiology and natural history of human papillomavirus infections in the female genital tract. Infect Dis Obstet Gynecol 2006;2006 Suppl:40470.

7. Ault K. Human papillomavirus vaccines: an update for gynecologists. Clin Obstet Gynecol 2008;51:527–32.

8. Sinal SH, Woods CR. Human papillomavirus infections of the genital and respiratory tracts in young children. Semin Pediatr Infect Dis 2005;16:306–16.

9. Smith E, Swarnavel S, Ritchie JM, Wang D, Haugen TH, Turek LP. Prevalence of human papillomavirus in the oral cavity/oropharynx in a large population of children and adolescents. Pediatr Infect Dis J 2007;26:836–40.

10. Merritt DF. Genital trauma in the pediatric and adolescent female. Obstet Gynecol Clin North Am 2009;36:85–98.

Appendix
Information Resources

Hysteroscopy and Other Transcervical Procedures

American College of Obstetricians and Gynecologists
http://www.acog.org

American College of Surgeons
http://www.facs.org

American Society for Reproductive Medicine
http://www.asrm.org

Society of Obstetricians and Gynaecologists of Canada
http://www.sogc.org/index_e.asp

Society of Reproductive Surgeons
http://www.reprodsurgery.org

Laparoscopy

American Association of Gynecologic Laparoscopists
http://www.aagl.org/index.php

American College of Obstetricians and Gynecologists
http://www.acog.org

Society of Laparoendoscopic Surgeons
http://www.sls.org/i4a/pages/index.cfm?pageid = 1

Society of Obstetricians and Gynaecologists of Canada
http://www.sogc.org/index_e.asp

Society of Reproductive Surgeons
http://www.reprodsurgery.org

Gynecologic Imaging

American College of Obstetricians and Gynecologists
http://www.acog.org

American Institute of Ultrasound in Medicine
http://www.aium.org

American College of Radiology
http://www.acr.org

RadiologyInfo
http://www.radiologyinfo.org

Cervical Cytology and Cervical Intraepithelial Neoplasia

American Cancer Society
http://www.cancer.org/docroot/home/index.asp

American College of Obstetricians and Gynecologists
http://www.acog.org

American Social Health Association
http://www.ashastd.org

American Society for Colposcopy and Cervical Pathology
http://www.asccp.org

Centers for Disease Control and Prevention
http://www.cdc.gov

National Breast and Cervical Cancer Early Detection Program
http://www.cdc.gov/cancer/nbccedp

National Cervical Cancer Public Education Campaign
http://www.cervicalcancercampaign.org

National Cancer Institute
http://www.cancer.gov

Society of Gynecologic Oncologists
http://www.sgo.org

Perioperative Care

Agency for Healthcare Research and Quality
http://www.ahrq.gov

American College of Obstetricians and Gynecologists
http://www.acog.org

American College of Surgeons
http://www.facs.org

American Society of Anesthesiologists
http://www.asahq.org

American Society for Reproductive Medicine
http://www.asrm.org

Association of periOperative Registered Nurses
http://www.aorn.org

Benign Disorders of the Vulva

American College of Obstetricians and Gynecologists
http://www.acog.org

Centers for Disease Control and Prevention
http://www.cdc.gov

International Society for the Study of Vulvovaginal Disease
http://www.issvd.org

National Vulvodynia Association
http://www.nva.org

Vulvar Pain Foundation
http://www.vulvarpainfoundation.org

Vulvovaginitis

American College of Obstetricians and Gynecologists
http://www.acog.org

American Social Health Association
http://www.ashastd.org

Centers for Disease Control and Prevention
http://www.cdc.gov

International Society for the Study of
Vulvovaginal Disease
http://www.issvd.org

National Institute of Allergy and Infectious Diseases
http://www.niaid.nih.gov/Pages/default.aspx

Pelvic Support Defects

American College of Obstetricians and Gynecologists
http://www.acog.org

American Society of Colon and Rectal Surgeons
http://www.fascrs.org

American Urogynecologic Society
http://www.augs.org/Default.aspx

American Urogynecologic Society Foundation:
Patient Resources
http://www.mypelvichealth.org

American Urological Association
http://www.auanet.org/content/homepage/
homepage.cfm

American Urological Association Foundation
http://www.urologyhealth.org/auafhome.asp

The Pelvic Floor Disorders Network
www.pfdnetwork.org

The Urinary Incontinence Treatment Network
www.uitn.net

Society of Pelvic Reconstructive Surgeons (SPRS)
http://www.sprs.org

Surgical Management of Incontinence

American College of Gastroenterology
http://www.gi.org

American College of Obstetricians and Gynecologists
http://www.acog.org

American Society of Colon and Rectal Surgeons
http://www.fascrs.org

American Urogynecologic Society
http://www.augs.org/Default.aspx

American Urological Association
http://www.auanet.org/content/homepage/
homepage.cfm

National Association for Continence
http://www.nafc.org

National Institute of Diabetes and Digestive and
Kidney Disease
http://www2.niddk.nih.gov

Society of Pelvic Reconstructive Surgeons
http://www.sprs.org

Management of Uterine Leiomyomas

American College of Obstetricians and Gynecologists
http://www.acog.org

American College of Radiology
http://www.acr.org

American Society for Reproductive Medicine
http://www.asrm.org

Brigham and Women's Hospital, Center for Uterine
Fibroids
http://www.fibroids.net

National Uterine Fibroids Foundation
http://www.nuff.org

Radiology Society of North America
http://www.rsna.org

Society of Pelvic Reconstructive Surgeons
http://www.sprs.org

First-Trimester Management of Nonviable Pregnancy

American College of Obstetricians and Gynecologists
http://www.acog.org

American Society for Reproductive Medicine
http://www.asrm.org

The Compassionate Friends
http://www.compassionatefriends.org/home.aspx

March of Dimes
http://www.marchofdimes.com

National Institute of Child Health and Human
Development
http://www.nichd.nih.gov

Management of Ovarian Cysts and Adnexal Masses

American College of Obstetricians and Gynecologists
http://www.acog.org

Agency for Healthcare Research and Quality
http://www.ahrq.gov

American Society for Reproductive Medicine
http://www.asrm.org

National Cancer Institute
http://www.cancer.gov

Society of Gynecologic Oncologists
http://www.sgo.org

Society of Obstetricians and Gynaecologists of Canada
http://www.sogc.org/index_e.asp

Women's Cancer Network
http://www.wcn.org

Recognition and Management of Surgical Injuries

Agency for Healthcare Research and Quality
http://www.ahrq.gov

American College of Obstetricians and Gynecologists
http://www.acog.org

American College of Surgeons
http://www.facs.org

Centers for Disease Control and Prevention
http://www.cdc.gov

The Joint Commission
http://www.jointcommission.org

National Institute for Occupational Safety and Health
http://www.cdc.gov/niosh

National Patient Safety Foundation
http://www.npsf.org

Postoperative Complications

Agency for Healthcare Research and Quality
http://www.ahrq.gov

American College of Obstetricians and Gynecologists
http://www.acog.org

American College of Surgeons
http://www.facs.org

American Society of Anesthesiologists
http://www.asahq.org

Association of periOperative Registered Nurses
http://www.aorn.org

Institute for Healthcare Improvement: Patient Safety
http://www.ihi.org/IHI/Topics/PatientSafety

The Joint Commission
http://www.jointcommission.org

National Heart, Lung and Blood Institute
http://www.nhlbi.nih.gov

Surgical Site Infections

American College of Obstetricians and Gynecologists
http://www.acog.org

American College of Surgeons
http://www.facs.org

Centers for Disease Control and Prevention
http://www.cdc.gov

Centers for Disease Control and Prevention: Infection Control in Healthcare Settings
http://www.cdc.gov/ncidod/dhqp/index.html

Institute for Healthcare Improvement: Patient Safety
http://www.ihi.org/IHI/Topics/PatientSafety

The Joint Commission: Patient Safety
http://www.jointcommission.org/PatientSafety

Surgical Infection Society
http://www.sisna.org

Sterilization

American College of Obstetricians and Gynecologists
http://www.acog.org

American College of Surgeons
http://www.facs.org

Association of Reproductive Health Professionals
http://www.arhp.org

Family Health International
http://www.fhi.org/en/index.htm

National Family Planning & Reproductive Health Association
http://www.nfprha.org/main/index.cfm

Planned Parenthood
http://www.plannedparenthood.org

Pregnancy Termination

American College of Obstetricians and Gynecologists
http://www.acog.org

Association of Reproductive Health Professionals
http://www.arhp.org

National Abortion Federation
http://www.prochoice.org

National Family Planning & Reproductive Health Association
http://www.nfprha.org/main/index.cfm

Planned Parenthood
http://www.plannedparenthood.org

Chronic Pelvic Pain

American College of Obstetricians and Gynecologists
http://www.acog.org

American Society for Reproductive Medicine
http://www.asrm.org

International Pelvic Pain Society
http://www.pelvicpain.org

Interstitial Cystitis Association
http://www.ichelp.org/Page.aspx?pid = 329

National Institutes of Health Pain Consortium
http://painconsortium.nih.gov

National Vulvodynia Association
http://www.nva.org

Vulvar Pain Foundation
http://www.vulvarpainfoundation.org

Benign Breast Disease

American Academy of Family Physicians
http://www.aafp.org/online/en/home.html

American Cancer Society
http://www.cancer.org/docroot/home/index.asp

American College of Obstetricians and Gynecologists
http://www.acog.org

National Breast and Cervical Cancer Early
  Detection Program
http://www.cdc.gov/cancer/nbccedp

National Cancer Institute
http://www.cancer.gov

National Cancer Institute: Breast Cancer Risk
  Assessment Tool
http://www.cancer.gov/bcrisktool

U.S. Preventive Services Task Force
http://www.ahrq.gov/clinic/USpstfix.htm

National Comprehensive Cancer Network
http://www.nccn.org/index.asp

Pediatric Gynecology

American College of Obstetricians and Gynecologists
http://www.acog.org

American Academy of Pediatrics
http://www.aap.org

North American Society for Pediatric and
  Adolescent Gynecology
http://www.naspag.org

Society for Adolescent Health and Medicine
http://www.adolescenthealth.org//AM/Template.cfm?
  Section = Home

Index

Note: Page numbers followed by *b, f,* and *t* indicate boxes, figures, and tables, respectively.

A

Abdominal wall, cross-sectional anatomy of, 10*f*
Abortion
  complete, 110
    evaluation (diagnostic testing in), 108*t*
    management of, 108*t*
    physical findings in, 108*t*
    signs and symptoms, 108*t*
  incomplete, 111
    evaluation (diagnostic testing in), 108*t*
    management of, 108*t*
    physical findings in, 108*t*
    signs and symptoms, 108*t*
  induced. *See also* Pregnancy termination
    antibiotic prophylaxis for, 141, 142*t*
    outcomes with, 157
    patient characteristics, 157, 157*t*
  inevitable
    evaluation (diagnostic testing in), 108*t*, 111
    management of, 108*t*, 111
    physical findings in, 108*t*, 111
    signs and symptoms, 108*t*, 111
  missed
    evaluation (diagnostic testing in), 108*t*, 109
    management of, 108*t*, 109–110
    physical findings in, 108*t*, 109
    signs and symptoms, 108*t*, 109
  partial-birth, criminalization of, 162
  sepsis associated with, 115
  spontaneous, 108, 108*t*, 109–110
  threatened
    adverse prognostic factors in, 112
    evaluation (diagnostic testing in), 108*t*, 112
    management of, 108*t*, 112
    physical findings in, 108*t*, 112
    signs and symptoms, 108*t*, 111–112
Abscess
  Bartholin gland, 62
  pelvic, postoperative, 144
  wound, postoperative, 144
Acne inversa. *See* Hidradenitis suppurativa
Activated partial thromboplastin time, in surgical patient, 42
Acute kidney injury
  definition of, 48
  mortality rate for, 48
  risk factors for, 48

Acyclovir, for herpes simplex virus infection, 74, 75, 75*t*
  in fetus, 76
  in infant, 76
  in pregnancy, 76
Adenocarcinoma in situ (AIS), 30
  epidemiology, 35
  management of patient with, 33, 35
Adenomyosis
  diagnosis of, sonohysterography for, 20
  diagnostic strategies for, 167*t*
  magnetic resonance imaging of, 23
Adhesiolysis, small bowel injury in, 128
Adhesion(s)
  labial, pediatric, 180
  laparoscopic removal of, 13
  prevention of, in laparoscopy, 9
Adiana system, for sterilization, 4, 150
Adnexal masses
  in adolescents, 117–118, 121*t*
  benign *versus* malignant, discrimination between, 18–19, 22
  cystic, 18
    complex, 18
    simple, 18
  imaging of, 18, 18*t*
  information resources, 184–185
  magnetic resonance imaging of, 22
  malignant, in young females, 117
  papillary projections, magnetic resonance imaging of, 22
  in postmenopausal women, 119–122
    differential diagnosis, 119–120, 121*t*
    expectant management of, 121
    preoperative risk assessment with, 120–121
    prevalence of, 119
    surgical intervention for, 121–122
  in premenarchal females, 117–118, 121*t*
  in premenopausal women, 118–119
    differential diagnosis, 121*t*
    expectant management of, 119
    management of, 118, 118*b*
    preoperative risk assessment with, 118–119
    signs and symptoms, 118
  prevalence of, 117
  risk of malignancy for, 120, 122*b*
  solid, 18
  ultrasonography of, 18–19, 18*t*, 22
Adolescent(s)
  breast masses in, 175
  with cervical cytologic and histologic abnormalities, management of, 31, 31*f*
  sexually active, counseling and testing of, 26–27

Adrenal insufficiency, perioperative management of, 50
Age. *See also* Older patients
  and cervical cancer screening, 26–27, 28
  and morbidity and mortality after gynecologic surgery, 52
  and perioperative care, 52
  and prevalence of human papillomavirus (HPV) infection, 28
  and surgical site infection, 141
Air embolism, in hysteroscopy, 7
Airway management, postoperative, 138
AIS. *See* Adenocarcinoma in situ
Albumin, serum levels, as surgical risk predictor, 42
Alendronate, perioperative management of, 40*t*
Allodynia, 63
American Cancer Society
  recommendations on breast cancer screening, 175–176
  recommendations on cervical cancer screening, 26–27, 28
American College of Obstetricians and Gynecologists
  cervical cancer screening guidelines, 26–27, 28
  guidelines for fluid monitoring, 6
  guidelines for referral to gynecologic oncologist, 118–119, 119*b*
  recommendations on breast cancer screening, 175
American College of Radiology
  accreditation standards for ultrasound, 21–22
  recommendations on breast cancer screening, 175–176
American Institute of Ultrasound in Medicine (AIUM)
  accreditation standards for ultrasonography, 21–22
  certification of ultrasound technicians, 22
American Medical Association, recommendations on breast cancer screening, 175–176
American Registry for Diagnostic Medical Sonography, credentialing of ultrasound technicians, 22
American Society for Colposcopy and Cervical Pathology
  guidelines for management of cervical cytologic abnormalities, 26, 30
  guidelines for Pap test specimen adequacy and patient management, 29
Amitriptyline
  and breast pain, 171*b*
  for chronic pelvic pain, 169
  for vulvar pain, 64

Ampicillin, for postoperative infection, 143
Anaerobes, of vaginal flora, 67
Analgesia
    for chronic pelvic pain, 168–169
    renal dysfunction and, 49
Anemia. *See also* Iron-deficiency anemia
    and perioperative risk, 46
    in surgical patient, 41
    treatment of, 46–47
Anesthesia
    neuraxial, and prophylactic anticoagulation, 47
    pulmonary complications of, in older patients, 52
    for surgical pregnancy termination, 160
    for tubal sterilization, 152–153
Anesthetic(s), topical, and vulvar allergic contact dermatitis, 56, 56b
Angiotensin-converting enzyme inhibitors, perioperative management of, 39t, 48
Angiotensin II receptor blockers, perioperative management of, 40t, 48
Antiarrhythmics, perioperative management of, 39t
Antibiotic(s)
    prophylactic, 44
        with laparoscopy, 8
        in nonviable pregnancy management, 115
        in operative management of nonviable first-trimester pregnancy, 111
        regimens for, by procedure, 141, 142t
        for surgical site infection, 141, 142t
    and pseudomembranous enterocolitis, 138
    for surgical site infection, 142–144
    topical, and vulvar allergic contact dermatitis, 56, 56b
Anticholesterol drugs, perioperative management of, 40t
Anticoagulation
    bridging therapy, 47, 48b
    for deep vein thrombosis (DVT), 134–135, 134t
    perioperative, 47, 48b
    for pulmonary embolism, 134t, 135
    reversal, for emergent surgery, 47
Antidepressants
    associated with breast pain, 171b
    for chronic pelvic pain, 168
Antifungals, topical, and vulvar allergic contact dermatitis, 56, 56b
Antihistamines, for vulvar pruritus, 56, 57
Antihypertensive agents, associated with breast pain, 171b
Antimicrobial agents, associated with breast pain, 171b

Antiphospholipid syndrome
    and arterial thrombosis, 44
    and venous thrombosis, 45
Antipsychotics, associated with breast pain, 171b
Antithrombotic therapy, perioperative, 47, 48b
Antithyroid medication, perioperative management of, 51–52
Antiviral therapy, for human papillomavirus (HPV) infection, 60
Anxiety, and vulvar pain syndromes, 63
Anxiolytics, associated with breast pain, 171b
Aorta, injury, in laparoscopy, 13–14
Aphthous ulcers, in pediatric patient, 180
Aspiration, 138
Aspirin, perioperative management of, 40t
Atrophic vaginitis
    clinical features of, 76
    diagnosis of, 76
    pathogenesis of, 76
    prevalence of, 76
    treatment of, 76
Atypical glandular cells
    favor neoplasia, 30
    management of patient with, 33
    not otherwise specified, 30, 33
Atypical squamous cells, 29–30
    cannot exclude high-grade SIL, 29–30
    favor high grade, management of patient with, 32
    undetermined significance, 29–30
        adolescent patient with, management of, 31, 31f
        age distribution of, 26
        management of patient with, 31–32
        triage of patients with, 31–32
        undetermined significance human papillomavirus (HPV)-positive, management of patients with, 32–33
Autoimmune disorders
    and lichen planus, 59
    and lichen sclerosus, 57–58
Azathioprine, for vulvovaginal lichen planus, 59
Azole(s)
    for candidal vulvovaginitis, 71–72, 72t
    resistance to, candidal, 71–72
    topical, reaction to, 72

B

Bacteria, of vaginal flora, 67
Bacterial infection(s), vulvovaginitis caused by, 67, 69b
Bacterial vaginosis
    associated infections, 69
    clinical features, 68–69, 70t
    complications of, 68, 69
    diagnosis of, 69

Bacterial vaginosis *(continued)*
    epidemiology, 68
    microbiology, 67, 68, 69
    pathogenesis of, 68–69
    in pregnancy, 68–69
    prevalence of, 68
    recurrence, 69
    risk factors for, 69
    and surgical site infection, 140–141
    treatment of, 69, 70t
Balloon thermal endometrial ablation, 5
Bartholin gland(s)
    abscess of, 62
    cancer of, 62
    cysts of, 62, 62f
Beta-blockers
    perioperative management of, 39, 39t, 44
    withdrawal, 39
Bethesda System, 2001 revision, 29–30
Biofeedback therapy
    for chronic pain, 169
    for vulvar pain, 64, 65
Bladder. *See also* Painful bladder syndrome
    assessment of, after laparoscopic surgery, 13, 14
    injury
        in laparoscopy, 14
        surgical, 124–127, 127b
Bleeding
    abnormal uterine
        postmenopausal, 20, 21f, 30
        premenopausal, workup for, 20, 21f
        workup for, sonohysterography in, 20, 21f
    after medical pregnancy termination, 159
    after surgical pregnancy termination, 160–161
    after termination of nonviable first-trimester pregnancy, 110
    hysteroscopy-related, 6
    leiomyomas and, 105, 106
    ovarian vessel, postoperative, 132
    postmenopausal, evaluation by transvaginal ultrasonography, 18
    postoperative, 132–133
    retroperitoneal, postoperative, 133
    uterine vessel, postoperative, 132
    vaginal
        in pediatric patients, 178, 179, 180, 181, 182
        postoperative, 132
Blood glucose, perioperative management of, in diabetes mellitus, 50
Blood transfusion
    guidelines for, in perioperative care, 47
    for postoperative hemorrhage, 132
Blood vessel(s), injury, in laparoscopy, 13–14
BMI. *See* Body mass index
Boari–Ockerblad bladder flap, 125, 126f

Body mass index (BMI), and surgical site infection, 140. *See also* Obesity

Body weight, and medication dosages, 46. *See also* Obesity

Boric acid, for candidal vulvovaginitis, 72

Botulinum toxin therapy, for chronic pain, 169

Bowel injury, surgical, 127–131

Bowel obstruction, postoperative, 137

Bowel preparation
  perioperative, 52
  and prevention of surgical complications, 128

BRCA1 and *BRCA2* gene mutations, and breast cancer screening, 176

Breast(s)
  clinical examination of, 176
  infections in, 172
  self-examination, 176
  trauma to, 172–173

Breast cancer
  risk factors for, 173, 173*b*
  screening for, 175–176

Breast disease(s), benign, 171–177, 186

Breast implants, complications of, 173

Breast masses
  in adolescents, 175
  and referral of patient for diagnostic testing, guidelines for, 175, 175*b*
  workup for, 173–175, 174*f*

Breast pain. *See also* Mastalgia
  medications associated with, 171, 171*b*
  treatment of, 171–172
  workup for, 171

Bubble test, 130, 130*f*

Burch colposuspension, 97–98, 97*f*, 103

Butoconazole, for candidal vulvovaginitis, 72*t*

C

Caffeine, and mastalgia, 172

Calcineurin inhibitors, for vulvar lichen sclerosus, 58. *See also* Cyclosporine; Tacrolimus

Calcipotriene, for vulvar psoriasis, 58–59

Calcium-channel blockers, perioperative management of, 39*t*

CAM. *See* Complementary and alternative medicine

Cancer
  breast. *See* Breast cancer
  cervical. *See* Cervical cancer
  endometrial. *See* Endometrial cancer
  lymph node metastases, imaging of, 23–24
  magnetic resonance imaging of, 23–24, 23*f*
  ovarian. *See* Ovarian cancer
  positron emission tomography of, 24
  response to treatment, magnetic resonance imaging evaluation of, 24

Candida albicans, in vaginal flora, 67. *See also* Candidiasis

Candida glabrata. See also Candidiasis
  azole resistance, 72
  vaginitis caused by, 71
  treatment of, 72

Candidiasis
  intertriginous, 172
  vulvovaginitis caused by, 67, 69–72, 69*b*

Carbon dioxide (CO$_2$)
  embolism, in hysteroscopy, 6–7
  insufflation, for hysteroscopy, 3–4
  and shoulder pain after laparoscopy, 14–15

Carboprost, and breast pain, 171*b*

Carcinoma in situ, cervical, 30

Cardiac care, for noncardiac surgery, 42–44, 43*f*

Cardiac disease. *See* Heart disease

Cardiac evaluation, for noncardiac surgery, 42–44, 43*f*

Cardiac index, 48

Cardiac medications, associated with breast pain, 171*b*

Cardiac status, perioperative evaluation and management of, 42–44, 43*f*, 52

Cardiovascular evaluation, perioperative, 42–44, 43*f*, 52

Cefazolin, prophylactic, 142*t*

Cephalosporins
  for postoperative infection, 143
  prophylactic, with laparoscopy, 8

Cervical cancer
  lymph node metastases, imaging of, 23–24
  magnetic resonance imaging of, 23, 23*f*
  in older women, 27
  precursors, management of, 26, 30
  response to treatment, magnetic resonance imaging evaluation of, 24
  screening for, 26
    cost-effective strategy for, 27–28
    discontinuation of, age for, 27
    initiation of, age for, 26–27
    and interval between tests, 27–28
    in older women, indications for, 27
  staging, positron emission tomography for, 17, 17*f*

Cervical cytology. *See also* Pap test
  abnormalities
    after hysterectomy for benign disease, 27
    management of, 26, 30–36
  conventional methods
    sensitivity and specificity, 26, 28
    test interval for, 28
  information resources, 183
  with liquid-based methods
    advantages of, 26
    and human papillomavirus cotesting, 26
    sensitivity and specificity, 26, 28
    test interval for, 28

Cervical cytology *(continued)*
  plus human papillomavirus testing, 26, 28–29
  in posttreatment follow-up, 35–36
  results, reproducibility of, 33–34
  screening, American College of Obstetricians and Gynecologists guidelines for, 26
  sensitivity and specificity
    in cervical cancer screening, 26
    with conventional methods, 26, 28
    with liquid-based methods, 26, 28
  specimen adequacy, 29

Cervical intraepithelial neoplasia
  age distribution of, 27
  follow-up for, 34
  grade 1, 30
    in adolescent, management of, 31
    epidemiology, 34
    management of, 26, 34
  grade 2, 30
    in adolescent, management of, 31
    with atypical squamous cell, undetermined significance, 31
    and cervical cancer screening, 27–28
    epidemiology, 34
    with high-grade squamous intraepithelial lesions, 33
    with human papillomavirus-positive atypical squamous cell—undetermined significance, 32
    with low-grade squamous intraepithelial lesions, 32
    management of, 26, 35
    presenting cytologic result for, 30
  grade 3, 30
    with atypical squamous cell—undetermined significance, 31
    and cervical cancer screening, 27–28
    epidemiology, 34
    with high-grade squamous intraepithelial lesions, 33
    with human papillomavirus-positive atypical squamous cell—undetermined significance, 32
    with low-grade squamous intraepithelial lesions, 32
    management of, 35
    presenting cytologic result for, 30
  information resources, 183
  in low-risk women, and cervical cancer screening, 27–28
  persistence after treatment, 35–36
  with positive margins postprocedure, 35–36
  recurrence, tests for, 35–36
  treatment of, and adverse pregnancy outcomes, 34

Cesarean delivery
  for herpes simplex virus-infected patient, 76
  leiomyomas and, 105
  and surgical site infection, 140

Chest radiography
  postoperative, 138
  for surgical patient, 42
Child(ren)
  genital trauma in, 182
  prepubertal, physical examination
    of, 178
  sexual abuse of, 178, 180, 181, 182
Child abuse
  and vulvar pain syndromes, 63
  workup for, 179–180
Chlamydia trachomatis
  and Bartholin gland cysts, 62
  infection, diagnosis of, 73
Chlordiazepoxide, and breast pain,
  171*b*
Cholestyramine, perioperative management of, 40*t*
Chromotubation, antibiotic prophylaxis
  for, 141, 142*t*
Chronic urethral syndrome, diagnostic
  strategies for, 167*t*
Cimetidine, and breast pain, 171*b*
Ciprofloxacin, prophylactic, 141
Clindamycin
  adverse effects and side effects of,
    69
  for bacterial vaginosis, 69, 70*t*
  plus aztreonam, prophylactic, 142*t*
  plus gentamicin, prophylactic, 142*t*
  plus quinolone, prophylactic, 142*t*
  for postoperative infection, 143
  for trichomoniasis, 73, 73*t*
Clobetasol propionate, for vulvar lichen
  sclerosus, 58
Clomiphene, and breast pain, 171*b*
Clonidine
  perioperative management of, 39, 39*t*
  withdrawal, 39
Clopidogrel, perioperative management
  of, 40*t*
Clostridium difficile, pseudomembranous enterocolitis, 138
Clotrimazole, for candidal vulvovaginitis,
  71, 72*t*
Clotting factors, postoperative replacement, 132
CMV. *See* Cytomegalovirus (CMV)
  infection
CO₂. *See* Carbon dioxide
Coagulation studies, in surgical patient,
  42
Colonic obstruction, postoperative,
  137–138
Colpopexy, sacrospinous, 89–90
Colposcopy, 30–31
  with endocervical sampling, indica-
    tions for, 33
  with endometrial sampling, indica-
    tions for, 33
  indications for, 35–36, 60
  in patients with atypical squamous
    cell, cannot exclude high-grade
    SIL, 32

Colposcopy *(continued)*
  in patients with atypical squamous
    cell—undetermined significance,
    31–32
  in patients with atypical glandular
    cells, 33
  in patients with human papillomavi-
    rus-positive atypical squamous
    cell—undetermined significance,
    32–33
Complementary and alternative medicine, perioperative
  management of, 39, 40
Complex regional pain syndrome, 165
Compression neuropathy, diagnostic
  strategies for, 167*t*
Computed tomography (CT)
  of adnexal masses, 18*t*
  clinical applications of, 18
  of incisional hernia, 15
  of lymph node metastases, 23–24
  postoperative, 18
  principles of, 18
Conscious laparoscopic pain mapping,
  166–168
Constipation, diagnostic strategies for,
  167*t*
Contrast agent(s), renal dysfunction
  and, 49
Corticosteroid(s). *See also* Steroid(s)
  vaginal side effects of, 60
  for vulvar dermatitis, 56
  for vulvar lichen simplex chronicus,
    57
  for vulvar psoriasis, 58–59
  for vulvovaginal lichen planus,
    59–60
  withdrawal, 39
Cotton swab test, for vulvar pain, 64
CT. *See* Computed tomography
COX-2 inhibitors. *See*
  Cyclooxygenase-2 inhibitors
Cyclooxygenase-2 (COX-2) inhibitors,
  perioperative management of,
  40*t*
Cryoablation, endometrial, 5
Culdoplasty, McCall, 89–90, 90*f*
Cyclophosphamide, for vulvovaginal
  lichen planus, 59
Cyclosporine
  and breast pain, 171*b*
  for vulvar psoriasis, 59
  for vulvovaginal lichen planus, 59
Cyproterone, and breast pain, 171*b*
Cystadenoma(s), ovarian, 119
Cystocele, 82*f*, 87*f*, 88–89, 88*f*
Cytomegalovirus (CMV) infection, and
  acute genital ulcers in pediatric
  patient, 180

D
Dalteparin, therapeutic dosages of,
  134–135, 135*b*
Danazol, for mastalgia, 172

Deep vein thrombosis (DVT)
  diagnosis of, 134
  erythropoietin therapy and, 47
  obesity and, 46
  prevention of, 44, 45*t*
  risk factors of, 44, 44*b*
  treatment of, 134–135, 134*t*
Defecation, obstructed, pelvic support
  defects and, 80
Depression
  diagnostic strategies for, 167*t*
  and vulvar pain syndromes, 63
Dermatitis
  definition of, 55
  endogenous, 55
  exogenous, 55
  subtypes of, 55
  vulvar
    allergic contact, 55–56, 56*b*
    atopic, 55
    contact, 55–56, 55*f*, 56*b*, 71
    irritant contact, 55–56, 55*f*, 56*b*
    prevalence of, 55
    seborrheic, 55
Dermatoses, vulvar, 57–60, 64
Dermoid cyst(s), ovarian, ultrasonography of, 19, 19*f*
Diabetes mellitus
  and perioperative care, 50, 50*b*
  and surgical site infection, 141
Diabetic ketoacidosis, in surgical
  patient, 50
Diarrhea
  diagnostic strategies for, 167*t*
  postoperative, 138
Diethylstilbestrol, and breast pain, 171*b*
Digoxin
  and breast pain, 171*b*
  perioperative management of, 39, 39*t*
Dilation and curettage
  for nonviable first-trimester preg-
    nancy, 109–111
  for pregnancy termination, 160
Dilation and evacuation
  antibiotic prophylaxis for, 141, 142*t*
  legal considerations in, 162
  for pregnancy termination, 160
Dinoprostone, and breast pain, 171*b*
Diuretics, perioperative management
  of, 39*t*
Diverticular disease, diagnostic strategies
  for, 167*t*
Domperidone, and breast pain, 171*b*
Double decidual sac sign, 112
Doxepin
  and breast pain, 171*b*
  for vulvar pruritus, 56
Doxycycline, prophylactic, 142*t*
Drug(s). *See* Medication(s)
DVT. *See* Deep vein thrombosis
Dysmenorrhea, and leiomyomas, 105.
  See also Pelvic pain
Dyspareunia, diagnostic strategies for,
  167*t*. *See also* Pelvic pain

E

Echinacea, potential perioperative effects of, 41*t*

Education and training, about first-trimester management of non-viable pregnancy, 115–116

Electrocardiography, for surgical patient, 42

Electrolyte testing, in surgical patient, 42

Endocarditis, prophylaxis, 44

Endocrinopathy(ies)
and hidradenitis suppurativa, 61
in pediatric patients, 181–182
and perioperative care, 50–52

Endodermal sinus tumor, in pediatric patient, 182

Endometrial ablation, 4
balloon thermal ablation technique for, 5
cryoablation technique for, 5
global, nonresectoscopic methods of, 4–5
for leiomyomas, 106
microwave ablation technique for, 5
radiofrequency ablation technique for, 5
thermal fluid ablation technique for, 5

Endometrial biopsy
guidance, sonohysterography for, 20
insufficient tissue for, 18

Endometrial cancer
lymph node metastases, imaging of, 23–24
magnetic resonance imaging of, 23, 23*f*
recurrence, positron emission tomography of, 17–18
transtubal spillage of malignant cells in, sonohysterography and, 20–21

Endometrial stripe
assessment, by transvaginal ultrasonography, 18
thickness, 18

Endometrioma(s), ovarian, 119
magnetic resonance imaging of, 22
ultrasonography of, 19

Endometriosis
diagnostic strategies for, 167*t*
laparoscopic treatment of, 13

Endometrium, perioperative thinning of, 4

Endopelvic fascia, anatomy of, 78, 79*f*

Enoxaparin, therapeutic dosages of, 134–135, 135*b*

Enterocele, 82*f*, 92–93

Enterotomy, repair of, 128, 129*f*

Entrapment neuropathy, diagnostic strategies for, 167*t*

Ephedra, potential perioperative effects of, 41*t*

Epigastric vessels, inferior, 100*f*
anatomy of, 12–13, 13*f*
injury, in laparoscopy, 13–14

Epoetin alfa, preoperative therapy with, 47

Epstein–Barr virus, and acute genital ulcers in pediatric patient, 180

Erythropoietin therapy, preoperative, 47

Essure system, for sterilization, 4, 150–151

Estramustine, and breast pain, 171*b*

Estrogen
and breast pain, 171*b*
for vaginal atrophy, 76

European Society of Hysteroscopy, classification of leiomyomas, 104, 105*b*

F

Factor V Leiden, and venous thromboembolism, 44

Famciclovir, for herpes simplex virus infection, 75*t*

Fecal incontinence
evaluation of patient for, 81, 82
surgery for, 102–103, 184

Feticide, selective, in multifetal pregnancy, 161

Fever, postoperative, 142–143

Fibroma(s), ovarian, magnetic resonance imaging of, 22

Fimbriectomy, for tubal sterilization, 149*t*

Fluconazole, for candidal vulvovaginitis, 71

Flucytosine, for candidal vulvovaginitis, 72

Fluorine-18 deoxyglucose, in positron emission tomography, 17

Fluoroquinolones, for postoperative infection, 143

Folate, deficiency of, treatment of, 47

Folate deficiency, and venous thromboembolism, 45

Foreign body(ies), vaginal, in pediatric patients, 181

Fresh frozen plasma, postoperative therapy with, 132

Functional capacity, and perioperative care, 42–43, 43*f*

Fungal infection(s), vulvovaginitis caused by, 67, 69*b*

G

Gabapentin
for chronic pelvic pain, 169
for vulvar pain, 64

Garlic, potential perioperative effects of, 41*t*

Gas embolism, in hysteroscopy, 6–7

Gastrointestinal complications, postoperative, 136–138

Gastrointestinal disease, pain caused by, 166*t*

Gastrointestinal injury(ies), surgical, 127–131

Genital trauma, in pediatric patient, 182

Genital ulcer(s), acute, in pediatric patient, 180

Genital warts. *See* Human papillomavirus

Gentamicin, for postoperative infection, 143

Gentian violet, for candidal vulvovaginitis, 72

Germ cell tumor
malignant, ovarian, 119
in pediatric patient, 182

Ginkgo biloba, potential perioperative effects of, 41*t*

Ginseng, potential perioperative effects of, 41*t*

Gonadotropin-releasing hormone agonists
in chronic pelvic pain, 168
for leiomyomas, 106

Gonorrhea
and Bartholin gland cysts, 62
diagnosis of, 73

Goserelin, for chronic pelvic pain, 168

Graded compression stockings
combined with low-dose unfractionated heparin, for prevention of venous thromboembolism, 46
for prevention of venous thromboembolism, 45

Graft(s), in pelvic reconstructive surgery, 86–87, 86*b*, 90, 91*f*

Graves disease, perioperative management of, 51–52

Gynecologic disorders, pain caused by, 165*b*

Gynecologic oncologist, referral to
American College of Obstetricians and Gynecologists guidelines for, 118–119, 119*b*
Society of Gynecologic Oncologists guidelines for, 118–119, 120*b*

H

Haloperidol, and breast pain, 171*b*

hCG. *See* Human chorionic gonadotropin

Heart disease
and perioperative monitoring, 133
and surgical risk, 42–44, 52

Hemangioma(s), vaginal bleeding caused by, in pediatric patient, 182

Hematometra, after surgical pregnancy termination, 161

Hemoglobin, testing, in surgical patient, 41

Hemorrhage
after medical pregnancy termination, 159
after surgical pregnancy termination, 160–161
postoperative, 132–133

Heparin
  bridging therapy with, 47, 48*b*, 49*f*
  for deep vein thrombosis, 134–135, 134*t*
  low molecular weight
    bridging therapy with, protocol for, 49*f*
    for prevention of venous thrombo-embolism, 46
    therapeutic dosages of, 134–135, 134*t*, 135*b*
  for pulmonary embolism, 134*t*, 135
  unfractionated
    for bridging therapy, 47
    low-dose, 45, 46
Herbal remedies, perioperative manage-ment of, 39, 40–41, 41*t*
Hernia(s), diagnostic strategies for, 167*t*
Herpes simplex virus (HSV)
  genital infection
    clinical features of, 74
    complications of, 74
    diagnosis of, 73
    pathogenesis of, 73–74
    prevalence of, 73
    primary (first clinical episode), treatment of, 74, 75*t*
    recurrent, treatment of, 74–76, 75*t*
    treatment of, 74–76
  neonatal infection, 74, 76
  in pediatric patient, misdiagnosis of, 180
  in pregnant patient, 76
  transmission to sexual partners, pre-vention of, 75–76
  vulvovaginitis caused by, 67, 69*b*
Hidradenitis suppurativa, vulvar, 61–62, 61*f*
High-grade squamous intraepithelial lesions, 30
  age distribution of, 26, 27
  management of patients with, 33–34
Homocysteine, elevated levels, and venous thrombosis, 44
Hormonal disorders, in pediatric patients, 181–182
Hormonal medications, associated with breast pain, 171*b*
Hormone therapy, perioperative man-agement of, 40*t*
Hospitalization, preoperative, and surgi-cal site infection, 141
HPV. *See* Human papillomavirus
HSV. *See* Herpes simplex virus
Human chorionic gonadotropin (hCG), beta subunit
  levels of
    in ectopic pregnancy, 113
    in medical management of ectopic pregnancy, 113–115, 113*b*, 114*b*
    in missed abortion, 109
  therapy with, in threatened abortion, 112

Human leukocyte antigen(s), and vulvo-vaginal lichen planus, 59
Human papillomavirus (HPV)
  anogenital subtypes, 60
  DNA testing
    with cervical cytology, 28–29
    guidelines for, 28–29
  genotyping assay, 26, 28–29
  high-risk genotypes, 28–29, 30, 32, 60
  infection
    cervical, 30
    cytopathic effects of, 30
    in pediatric patient, 181
    prevalence of, age-related changes in, 28
    recurrence, 60
    spontaneous regression of, 60
    vulvar, 60–61
  negative test for, management of patient with, 29
  oncogenic subtypes, 60
  positive test for
    with atypical squamous cell—undetermined significance, man-agement of patient with, 32–33
    management of patient with, 29, 30–31
  testing for
    indications for, 32
    in patients with atypical squamous cell—undetermined significance, 32
    in patients with atypical glandular cells, 33
    in patients with atypical glandular cells—not otherwise specified, 33
  vaccine against, 26, 181
Hydroxychloroquine, for vulvovaginal lichen planus, 59
Hydroxyzine, for vulvar pruritus, 56
Hyperalgesia, 63
Hyperosmolar hyperglycemic nonketo-sis, in diabetic surgical patient, 50
Hypertension
  perioperative management of, in older patients, 52
  in renal dysfunction, perioperative management of, 48
Hyperthyroidism, perioperative man-agement of, 51–52
Hypotension, intraoperative, in older patients, 52
Hypothyroidism, perioperative manage-ment of, 50–51
Hysterectomy
  antibiotic prophylaxis for, 141, 142*t*
  for benign disease, cytologic screen-ing abnormalities after, 27
  benign glandular cytology after, man-agement of, 33
  bladder injury in, 125–126

Hysterectomy *(continued)*
  bowel injury in, 127–128
  for leiomyomas, 106
  risk of, after tubal sterilization, 154
  and risk of pelvic organ prolapse, 79
  and surgical site infection, 140
  ureteral injury in, 124–125
Hysterosalpingography, 3–4, 141, 142*t*
Hysteroscope(s), 3
  continuous-flow, 3, 4
  diagnostic, 3
  flexible, 3
  operative, 3
  rigid, 3
Hysteroscopy
  antibiotic prophylaxis for, 141, 142*t*
  bleeding caused by, 6
  complications of, 5–7
  contraindications to, 4
  diagnostic, clinical applications of, 3
  equipment for, 3
  fluid distending media for, 3–4, 6
  gas embolism in, 6–7
  in gynecologic practice, 3
  information resources, 183
  of leiomyomas
    diagnostic, 105
    therapeutic, 104, 105*b*, 106
  office, 3–4
  for sterilization, 150–151, 151*f*
  surgical procedures, 4
  uterine perforation in, 5–6

I

Icodextrin solution, for adhesion pre-vention, 9
Ileus, postoperative, 136–137
Iliac vessels, injury, in laparoscopy, 13–14
Iliococcygeus muscle, 78
Imaging
  of adnexal masses, in premenopausal women, 118
  gynecologic, 17–25. *See also specific imaging modality*
  information resources, 183
  of leiomyomas, 105
  of ovarian cyst, in premenopausal women, 118
  in prepubertal girl, 178–179
Imiquimod
  for human papillomavirus (HPV) infection, 60–61
  for vulvar intraepithelial neoplasia, 61
Incisional hernia, after laparoscopy, 15, 15*f*
Incontinence. *See* Fecal incontinence; Urinary incontinence
Indigo carmine
  for assessment of abdominal organs, after laparoscopic surgery, 13, 14
  in diagnosis of ureterovaginal fistula, 136

Infection(s)
  after medical pregnancy termination, 159–160
  after surgical pregnancy termination, 161
  breast, 172
  gynecologic, life-threatening, 144–145
  life-threatening
    microbiology of, 144–145
    treatment of, 144–145
  obstetric, life-threatening, 144–145
  pelvic, postoperative, 143
  postoperative, life-threatening, 144–145
  surgical site, 140–146
Infertility, leiomyomas and, 105, 106
Influenza A, and acute genital ulcers in pediatric patient, 180
Infracoccygeal sacropexy, 90, 91*f*
INR. *See* International normalized ratio
Interferon, intralesional, for human papillomavirus infection, 61
International normalized ratio, monitoring
  in perioperative care, 47
  in warfarin therapy, 135
Interstitial cystitis, and vulvodynia, 63
Intradecidual sign, 112
Intrauterine device, progestin-bearing, for leiomyomas, 106
Intrauterine synechiae, hysteroscopic lysis of, 4
Iron, supplementation, for anemic patient, 47
Iron-deficiency anemia, 47
Irritable bowel syndrome, and vulvodynia, 63
Irving procedure, for tubal sterilization, 149*t*
Itraconazole, for candidal vulvovaginitis, 71

K

Kava, potential perioperative effects of, 41*t*
Ketoconazole
  and breast pain, 171*b*
  for candidal vulvovaginitis, 71

L

Labial adhesions, pediatric, 180
Beta-lactamase inhibitors, for postoperative infection, 143
Beta-lactam inhibitors, for postoperative infection, 143
Lactobacilli, vaginal, 67
Laparoscopy
  for abscess drainage, 144
  access (entry) for
    anatomic considerations in, 9, 10*f*, 11*f*
    approaches for, 9
    complications of, 13–14, 13*b*

Laparoscopy, access (entry) for (*continued*)
    direct trocar insertion in, 11
    intraumbilical incision for, 9, 11*f*
    radially expanding system for, 12
    trocar method for, 10–11
    Veress needle placement for, 9–10
    visual system for, 12
  advantages of, 8
  anatomic considerations in, 9, 10*f*, 11*f*, 12–13, 13*f*
  antibiotic prophylaxis for, 141, 142*t*
  antibiotic use with, 8
  bladder injury in, 14
  for chronic pelvic pain, 166–168
  complications of, 9, 10, 12, 13–15, 13*b*
  for cryomyolysis, 107
  diagnostic evaluation in, 13
  incisional hernia after, 15, 15*f*
  information resources, 183
  insufflating pressure for, 10
  large bowel injury in, 14
  for myolysis, 107
  open, 11–12
  patient positioning for, 8–9, 8*f*, 10, 13
  patient preparation for, 8
  for pelvic reconstruction, 86, 88, 88*f*, 90–92, 91*f*, 92*f*
  pneumoperitoneum for, 10, 11
  renal dysfunction and, 49
  robot-assisted, 15–16
  for sacrocervicopexy, 91–92, 92*f*
  for sacrocolpopexy, 90, 91*f*
  shoulder pain after, 14–15
  single port access technique for, 12
  small bowel injury in, 14
  trocars for, 12–13
  for tubal sterilization, 148–154, 149*t*
  ureteral injury in, 14
  ureter management in, 14
  uterine artery ligation, for leiomyomas, 107
  vascular injury in, 13–14
Laparotomy
  for abscess drainage, 144
  antibiotic prophylaxis for, 141, 142*t*
Large bowel, injury
  in laparoscopy, 14
  surgical, 130–131
Laser therapy
  for human papillomavirus infection, 60
  for vulvar intraepithelial neoplasia, 61
LeFort procedure, for pelvic floor defects, 93, 94*f*
Leiomyoma(s)
  asymptomatic, 104, 105
  and bleeding, 105, 106
  and cesarean delivery, 105

Leiomyoma(s) (*continued*)
  classification of
    anatomic, 104, 105*b*
    European Society of Hysteroscopy, 104, 105*b*
    traditional, 104, 104*b*
  diagnosis of, 105
  diagnostic hysteroscopy for, 3–4
  epidemiology, 104
  etiology of, 104
  genetics of, 104
  imaging of, 105
  information resources, 184
  intracavitary, 104, 104*b*, 105*b*
  intramural, 104, 104*b*
  magnetic resonance imaging of, 23
  operative hysteroscopy for, 4
  and pain, 105, 106
  pedunculated, 104, 104*b*, 105*b*
  and pregnancy, 105
  signs and symptoms, 105
  sonohysterography of, 20*f*
  submucosal, 104*b*
  subserosal, 104, 104*b*
  treatment of, 105–106
  ultrasonography of, 105
  urinary tract symptoms caused by, 105–106
Leiomyosarcoma(s), imaging of, 23
Levator ani muscle, anatomy of, 78, 79*f*
Lichen planus
  erosive, 59, 59*f*
  human leukocyte antigen association, 59
  oral, 59
  vulvar, 59–60, 59*f*
Lichen sclerosus
  in pediatric patient, 180–181
  vulvar, 55*f*, 57–58, 57*f*, 64
Lichen simplex chronicus, vulvar, 55, 57, 64
Liver function test(s), for surgical patient, 42
Loop electrosurgical excision procedure, 26
Low-grade squamous intraepithelial lesions, 30
  adolescent patient with, management of, 31, 31*f*
  age distribution of, 26
  management of patients with, 32–33

M

Magnetic resonance imaging
  of adnexal masses, 18*t*, 22
  advantages of, 22
  in breast cancer screening, 176
  of cancer, 23–24, 23*f*
  dynamic contrast agent enhanced, in cancer, 24
  gadolinium contrast for, 22
  high-field strength, 24
  image acquisition speed, 22
  image resolution, 22

Magnetic resonance imaging *(continued)*
  of leiomyomas, 23
  of lymph node metastases, 23–24
  of müllerian anomalies, 22
  in prepubertal girl, 179
  technical considerations in, 22
  T1 weighted, 22
  T2 weighted, 22
Magnetic resonance venography, in
    diagnosis of deep vein thrombo-
    sis, 134
Malignancy. *See* Cancer; *specific malig-
    nancy*
Mammography
  of breast mass, 174–175
  screening, 175–176
Marshall–Marchetti–Krantz procedure,
    97
Mastalgia, 171–172
  cyclic, 171–172
  noncyclic, 171–172
Mastitis
  nonlactational, 172
  postpartum, 172
McCall culdoplasty, 89–90, 90*f*
Medication(s)
  breast pain caused by, 171, 171*b*
  dosages, body weight and, 46
  perioperative management of, 39–41,
      39*t*–40*t*, 52
  topical, and vulvar allergic contact
      dermatitis, 56
  for vulvar dermatitis, 56
  vulvar dermatitis caused by, 56, 56*b*
Medroxyprogesterone acetate, for
    chronic pelvic pain, 168
Mesh, in pelvic reconstructive surgery,
    86–87, 86*b*, 88–89, 90, 91, 91*f*
Metabolic equivalent tasks, and func-
    tional capacity, 42–44
Metabolic syndrome, and surgical risk,
    46
Methadone
  adverse effects and side effects of,
      169
  and breast pain, 171*b*
  for chronic pelvic pain, 169
Methicillin-resistant *Staphylococcus
    aureus* (MRSA), 144
Methotrexate
  for ectopic pregnancy, 113–115
    contraindications to, 113*b*
    protocols for, 114–115, 114*b*
  for nonviable first-trimester preg-
      nancy, 110
  for vulvar psoriasis, 59
  for vulvovaginal lichen planus, 59
Methyldopa, and breast pain, 171*b*
Metronidazole
  for bacterial vaginosis, 69, 70*t*
  and breast pain, 171*b*
  plus gentamicin, prophylactic, 142*t*
  plus quinolone, prophylactic, 142*t*
  for postoperative infection, 143

Metronidazole *(continued)*
  prophylactic, 8, 142*t*
  for trichomoniasis, 73, 73*t*
Miconazole, for candidal vulvovaginitis,
    72*t*
Microwave endometrial ablation, 5
Mifepristone
  for nonviable first-trimester pregnancy,
      110
  plus prostaglandin, for pregnancy
      termination, 159
Minoxidil, and breast pain, 171*b*
Mirtazapine, and breast pain, 171*b*
Miscarriage. *See* Abortion
Misoprostol, for pregnancy termination,
    110, 110*b*, 111, 159
Monitoring, perioperative
  central, 133
  in older patients, 52
MRSA. *See* Methicillin-resistant
    Staphylococcus aureus
Müllerian anomalies
  magnetic resonance imaging of, 22
  ultrasonography of, 19
Multifetal pregnancy, reduction, 161
Musculoskeletal disorders, pain caused
    by, 166*t*
Myomectomy, 106–107

N

Narcotics, for chronic pelvic pain, 169
Necrotizing fasciitis, 145
Neonate(s), physical examination of,
    178
Neoplasia, 64
Nerve stimulation, for chronic pain, 169
Nipple discharge, 173, 175
Nipple piercing, complications of, 172
Nitrates, perioperative management of,
    39*t*
Nonsteroidal antiinflammatory drugs
    (NSAIDs)
  for chronic pelvic pain, 168–169
  perioperative management of, 39, 40*t*
  renal dysfunction and, 49
NSAIDs. *See* Nonsteroidal antiinflam-
    matory drugs
Nucleic acid amplification tests, 180
Nutrition, and surgical site infection, 141
Nystatin, for candidal vulvovaginitis,
    72, 72*t*

O

Obesity
  and deep vein thrombosis, 46
  and hidradenitis suppurativa, 61
  and medication dosages, 46
  and postoperative complications, 46
  and postoperative pulmonary compli-
      cations, 138
  and pulmonary embolism, 46
  and surgical risk, 46
  and surgical site infection, 140, 141
  and venous access, 46

Obstructive sleep apnea
  obesity and, 46
  perioperative management of, 46
Older patients, perioperative care for, 52
Opioids, for chronic pelvic pain, 169
Oral contraceptives
  and breast pain, 171*b*
  for leiomyomas, 106
  perioperative management of, 40*t*
Ovarian cancer
  age-related risk for, 117
  magnetic resonance imaging of, 24
  positron emission tomography of, 17
  in premenopausal women, 118
  risk of, algorithm for, 118, 119*b*
  signs and symptoms, 120
Ovarian cyst(s). *See also* Adnexal
    masses
  hemorrhagic, ultrasonography of, 19
  information resources, 184–185
  laparoscopic treatment of, 13
  postmenopausal, transvaginal ultra-
      sonography of, 19
  in postmenopausal women, 119–122
  in premenopausal women, 118–119
    expectant management of, 119
    signs and symptoms, 118
  prevalence of, 117
Ovarian granulosa cell tumor, in pediat-
    ric patient, 182
Ovarian remnant syndrome, diagnostic
    strategies for, 165*b*, 168*t*
Ovarian torsion, in young women, 117
Oxytocin, high-dose, for pregnancy
    termination, 159

P

Pain
  breast. *See* Breast pain; Mastalgia
  definition of, 164
  neuropathic, 63
  pelvic. *See* Pelvic pain
  vulvar. *See* Vulvar pain; Vulvodynia
Pain behaviors, evolution of, 164*f*
Painful bladder syndrome, diagnostic
    strategies for, 167*t*
Palmer's point, 9
Pap test. *See also* Cervical cytology
  atypical endocervical cells on, man-
      agement of patient with, 33
  endometrial cells on
    management of patient with, 33
    in older women, 30
  epithelial cell abnormalities on, 30
  glandular cell abnormalities on, 30
  negative for intraepithelial lesions or
      malignancy, 29
  repetition of, guidelines for, 29
  results reporting, 29
  and specimen adequacy, 29
  squamous intraepithelial lesions on,
      30
  unsatisfactory result, management
      of, 29

Parkland procedure, for tubal sterilization, 147, 148f, 149t
Partial thromboplastin time, in surgical
patient, 42
Pediatric gynecology, 178–182,
186. See also Adolescent(s);
Child(ren)
Pelvic congestion syndrome, diagnostic
strategies for, 168t
Pelvic floor, anatomy of, 78, 79f
Pelvic floor disorders. See also Pelvic
organ prolapse; Pelvic support
defects
  prevalence of, 78
  and vestibulodynia, 63
Pelvic infection, postoperative, 143
Pelvic organ prolapse. See also Pelvic
support defects
  asymptomatic, 79
  diagnosis of, 79–82
  epidemiology, 78
  imaging of, 81–82
  lifestyle changes and, 82–83
  nonsurgical management of, 82–84
  pessaries for, 83–84, 83f, 84t, 85t,
  93
  physical examination of patient with,
  Baden–Walker system for, 80,
  81b
  quantification of, 80–81, 81b, 81f
  recurrences, 84
  risk factors for, 78–79
  signs and symptoms, 80
  stages of, 81, 81b, 81f
  surgical management of, 84–94
    approach for, selection of, 85–86,
    85b
    candidates for, 84–85, 85b
    graft materials for, 86–87, 86b
    site-specific repairs, 87–89
    symptom-directed therapy for,
    82–83
  uterine, surgical repair, 90–92
  vaginal vault, surgical repair, 89–90
Pelvic pain
  acute, 164
  after tubal ligation and endometrial
  ablation, 154
  chronic, 164–170
    definition of, 164–165
    diagnostic strategies for, 165–168,
    167t–168t
    etiologic possibilities, 164–165,
    165b, 166t
    evaluation of, 164
    evolution of, 164f
    information resources, 185–186
    pathogenesis of, 164
    therapeutic options for, 168–169
  leiomyomas and, 105, 106
Pelvic support
  anatomy of, 78, 79f
  levels of, 78, 79f, 80b
  quantitation of, 80–81, 81b, 81f

Pelvic support defects, 78–96. See also
Pelvic floor disorders; Pelvic
organ prolapse
  anterior compartment, 80, 82f
  apical, 80, 82f
  asymptomatic, 79
  diagnosis of, 79–82
  examination of patient with, 80–81
  information resources, 184
  lifestyle changes and, 82–83
  nonsurgical management of, 82–84
  paravaginal, surgical repair, 87f,
  88–89, 88f, 89f
  pessaries for, 83–84, 83f, 84t, 85t, 93
  posterior compartment, 80, 82f, 93,
  93f
  recurrences, 84
  risk factors for, 78–79
  signs and symptoms, 80
  surgical management of, 84–94
  surgical repair
    LeFort procedure, 93, 94f
    obliterative procedures, 93, 94f
  symptom-directed therapy for, 82–83
Penicillamine, and breast pain, 171b
Penicillins, for postoperative infection,
143
Perineal body, 78, 79f
Perineal membrane, 78, 79f
Perineorrhaphy, 93
Perioperative care
  adrenal insufficiency and, 50
  anemia and, 46–47
  bowel preparation in, 52
  cardiovascular evaluation in, 42–44
  endocrine dysfunction and, 50–52
  information resources, 183
  medication management in, 39–41,
  39t–40t
  metabolic syndrome and, 46
  obesity and, 46
  for older patients, 52
  and prevention of venous thromboembolism, 45–46
  and pulmonary function testing, 44
  renal dysfunction and, 48–49
  testing in, 41–42
  transfusion guidelines for, 47
Pessaries, 83–84, 83f, 84t, 85t, 93
Physical therapy, for vulvar pain, 64–65
Physiotherapy, for chronic pain, 169
Platelet count, in surgical patient, 42
Platelet transfusion, postoperative, 132
Pneumatic compression, for prevention
of venous thromboembolism, 45
Pneumonia, hospital-acquired, 138
Podofilox, for human papillomavirus
infection, 60–61
Polyp(s)
  sonohysterography of, 20f
  vaginal bleeding caused by, in pediat-
  ric patient, 182
Pomeroy procedure, for tubal steriliza-
tion, 147, 147f, 149t

Porphyria, diagnostic strategies for,
168t
Positron emission tomography, 17–18
  of adnexal masses, 18t
  of cancer, 24
  clinical applications of, 17–18
  technical considerations in, 17
Postabortal syndrome, 161
Precocious puberty, 181–182
Prednisone, and perioperative care, 50,
51f
Pregabalin, for chronic pelvic pain, 169
Pregnancy
  anembryonic, 109
  ectopic
    assisted reproductive technology
    and, 113
    evaluation (diagnostic testing in),
    108t, 112–113
    incidence of, 113
    management of, 108t, 112–115
    medical management of, 113–114,
    113b
    mortality rate for, 113
    physical findings in, 108t, 112
    prevalence of, 108
    signs and symptoms, 108t, 112
    sites of, 112–113
  extrauterine, prevalence of, 108
  nonviable
    expectant management of, 110–
    111
    first-trimester management of,
    108–116, 184
    intrauterine, 108, 109–110
    resident education about, 115–116
Pregnancy loss, first-trimester. See also
Abortion, 108, 108t, 115–116
  causes of, 108, 108t
  resident education about, 116
Pregnancy termination, 157–163
  in first trimester
    medical, 110, 110b
    surgical approaches, 110–111
    by vacuum aspiration, 110–111
  indications for, 157
  information resources, 185
  legal considerations in, 162
  medical, 158–160
    agents for, 159
    complications of, 159–160
    in first trimester, 158
    in second trimester, 158–159
  patient characteristics, 157, 157t
  patient evaluation for, 157
  postprocedure patient care, 162
  preprocedure patient counseling
  about, 157
  rates, 157
  selective, in multifetal gestation, 161
  surgical, 160–161
    complications of, 160–161
    legal considerations in, 162
Pregnancy testing, for surgical patient, 42

Progestin(s), for leiomyomas, 106
Progestogens, and breast pain, 171b
Prothrombin *G20210A* mutation, and deep vein thrombosis (DVT), 44
Pruritus, vulvar, 55, 63–64
    acute, 55
    chronic, 55
Pseudomembranous enterocolitis, *Clostridium difficile*, 138
Psoriasis, vulvar, 58–59, 58f, 64
Pubococcygeus muscle, 78
Puborectalis muscle, 78
Pulmonary artery catheterization, with thrombolytic agent administration, for pulmonary embolism, 135
Pulmonary complications, postoperative, 138
Pulmonary disorders
    in older patients, and perioperative care, 52
    and perioperative monitoring, 133
Pulmonary embolectomy, 135
Pulmonary embolism
    diagnosis of, 135
    obesity and, 46
    prevention of, for obese patient, 138
    in surgical patients
        prevalence of, 44
        risk factors of, 44, 44b
    treatment of, 134t, 135
Pulmonary function testing, perioperative, 44, 52

Q
Quinacrine, sterilization using, 150
Quinolones, for postoperative infection, 143

R
Radiofrequency endometrial ablation, 5
Rectal injury, surgical, 130–131
Rectocele, 82f
Rectosigmoid repair, 130–131
Rectum, assessment of, after laparoscopic surgery, 13
Renal dysfunction, perioperative management of, 48–49
Renal function test(s), for surgical patient, 42
Renal insufficiency, as surgical risk predictor, 42
Reserpine, and breast pain, 171b
Respiratory complications, postoperative, 138
Respiratory papillomatosis, 61
Retinoids
    for vulvar psoriasis, 59
    for vulvovaginal lichen planus, 59
Retropubic colposuspension, 97–98, 97f, 103
Rhabdomyosarcoma, in pediatric patient, 182
Richter hernia, after laparoscopy, 15, 15f

Risk of malignancy index, 120, 122b
Robotics
    da Vinci surgical system, 15–16
    and laparoscopy, 15–16
    in pelvic reconstructive surgery, 86

S
Sacrocervicopexy, 91–92, 92f
Sacrocolpopexy
    abdominal, 89–90, 90f
    laparoscopic, 90, 91f
Sacropexy, infracoccygeal, 90, 91f
Sacrospinous colpopexy, 89–90
St John's wort, potential perioperative effects of, 41t
Sedatives, for vulvar pruritus, 56, 57
Selective estrogen receptor modulators
    adverse effects and side effects of, 172
    for mastalgia, 172
Selective reduction, in multifetal pregnancy, 161
Selective serotonin reuptake inhibitors (SSRIs)
    and breast pain, 171b
    for vulvar pruritus, 56, 57
    withdrawal, 39
Septic abortion, 115
Septic shock, 144–145
Sertraline, and breast pain, 171b
Sex cord stromal tumors, malignant, ovarian, 117, 119, 121t
Sexual abuse
    pediatric, 182
    and vulvodynia, 63
Shaving, preoperative, and surgical site infection, 141
Shock, perioperative, management of, 133
Shoulder pain, after laparoscopy, 14–15
Sinecatechins, for human papillomavirus (HPV) infection, 60–61
Sling procedure(s), for urinary incontinence, 97, 98–101, 100f, 101t, 102, 102t, 103
Small bowel
    injuries
        crush, 128
        in laparoscopy, 14, 128
        surgical, 128–130
        thermal, 128–130
    obstruction, postoperative, 137
Smoking
    and surgical site infection, 141
    and vulvar intraepithelial neoplasia, 61
Society of Gynecologic Oncologists, guidelines for referral to gynecologic oncologist, 118–119, 120b
Sonohysterography, 3, 4, 18, 20–21
    contraindications to, 20
    for guidance of endometrial biopsy, 20

Sonohysterography (*continued*)
    indications for, 20, 20b
    of leiomyoma(s), 20f, 105
    of polyps, 20f
    three-dimensional, 19
    and transtubal spillage of cancer cells, 20–21
Sphincteroplasty, for fecal incontinence, 102–103
Spironolactone, and breast pain, 171b
SSRIs. *See* Selective serotonin reuptake inhibitors
Statins, withdrawal, 39
Sterilization, 147–156. *See also* Vasectomy
    Essure for, 4, 150–151
    hysteroscopic, 4, 150–151, 151f
    implantable polymer matrix for, 151, 152f
    information resources, 185
    patient counseling about, 147
    patient selection for, 147
    quinacrine for, 150
    transvaginal techniques for, 152
    tubal. *See also* Tubal sterilization
        occlusion methods, 147–154
        rate of, 147
        worldwide rate of, 147
Steroid(s). *See also* Corticosteroid(s)
    perioperative administration of, guidelines for, 50, 51f
    and surgical site infection, 141
    for vulvar lichen sclerosus, 58
Strawberry cervix, 70t, 72
Stress response, to surgery, 50
Suburethral sling procedure(s), 97, 98–101, 103
    autologous tissues for, 98, 99f
    outcomes with, 101, 101t, 102t
    retropubic synthetic tension-free sling for, 98–99, 100f, 101, 101t, 102, 102t, 103
    synthetic transobturator sling for, 99–100, 100f, 102t
        complications of, management of, 101
        outcomes with, 101, 101t, 102t
    technique for, 98–100
    trocarless slings for, 100
Surgery. *See also specific procedure*
    for adnexal masses, in postmenopausal women, 121–122
    for chronic pelvic pain, 169
    duration of, and surgical site infection, 140
    for fecal incontinence, 102–103
    for human papillomavirus infection, 60
    pelvic, and risk of pelvic organ prolapse, 79
    postoperative complications of, 132–139
    stress response to, 50
    for stress urinary incontinence, 97–102

Surgery *(continued)*
  urogynecologic, antibiotic prophy-
      laxis for, 141, 142*t*
  for vulvar intraepithelial neoplasia,
      61
Surgical complications
  postoperative, 132–139, 185. *See also*
      Surgical site infection(s)
  recognition and management of,
      124–131
Surgical injury(ies), recognition and
      management of, 124–131, 185
Surgical site infection(s)
  antibiotics for, 142–143
  evaluation for, 142–143
  failure of initial treatment, 143–144
  information resources, 185
  life-threatening, 144–145
  microbiology of, 140–141, 143
  pathophysiology of, 140
  prevention of, 141, 142*t*
  rates, 140
  risk factors of, 140–141
  risk of, by procedure, 140
  workup of, 142–143
Swan–Ganz catheter, perioperative use,
      133
Systemic lupus erythematosus, and
      venous thromboembolism, 45

T

Tacrolimus, for vulvovaginal lichen
      planus, 59
Tamoxifen
  adverse effects and side effects of, 172
  for mastalgia, 172
Teratoma(s), ovarian, 22, 119
Terconazole, for candidal vulvovaginitis,
      72*t*
Theophylline, perioperative manage-
      ment of, 39
Thermal fluid endometrial ablation, 5
Thromboembolism. *See* Venous throm-
      boembolism
Thrombophilias, and venous thrombo-
      embolism, 44–45
Thyroid hormone therapy, perioperative
      management of, 50–51
Thyroid storm, perioperative, 52
Tinidazole
  for bacterial vaginosis, 70*t*
  for trichomoniasis, 73, 73*t*
Tioconazole, for candidal vulvovaginitis,
      72*t*
Toremifene, for mastalgia, 172
Toxic shock syndrome, 145
Transcutaneous electrical nerve stimula-
      tion, for chronic pain, 169
Trauma
  to breasts, 172–173
  genital, in pediatric patient, 182
Trichomoniasis
  associated infections, 72
  clinical features of, 70*t*, 72–73

Trichomoniasis *(continued)*
  diagnosis of, 72–73
  epidemiology, 72
  and human immunodeficiency virus
      infection, 72
  metronidazole-resistant, 73
  pathogenesis of, 72
  in pregnancy, complications of, 72
  treatment of, 73, 73*t*
  vulvovaginitis caused by, 67, 69*b*
Tricyclic antidepressants, for vulvar
      pain, 64
Trocar(s), laparoscopic, 12–13
  direct insertion of, 11
  disposable shielded, 12
  endoscopic threaded imaging port
      type, 12
  entry into peritoneal cavity, technique
      for, 10–11
  optical, with cutting knife, 12
  secondary (accessory), 12
Tubal sterilization
  anesthesia for, 152–153
  complications of, 153–154
  efficacy of, 149*t*, 153, 153*f*
  electrocoagulation for, 148, 149*t*
      bipolar, 149*t*
      unipolar, 149*t*
  failure of, 149*t*, 153, 153*f*
  Falope ring for, 148, 149*t*, 150*f*
  Filshie clip for, 148, 149*t*, 150*f*
  fimbriectomy for, 149*t*
  hysteroscopic, 4
  interval methods, 148–154, 149*t*
  Irving procedure, 149*t*
  long-term effects of, 154
  mechanical methods, 148, 149*t*
  occlusion methods, 147–154
  Parkland procedure, 147, 148*f*,
      149*t*
  Pomeroy procedure, 147, 147*f*,
      149*t*
  postpartum, 147–148, 149*t*
  pregnancy after, 149*t*, 153–154,
      153*f*
  rate of, 147
  spring-loaded (Hulka–Clemens) clip
      for, 148, 149*t*
  transcervical approaches for, 148–
      151
  Uchida procedure, 149*t*
Tuberculosis, pelvic, diagnostic strate-
      gies for, 168*t*
Tumor markers, in evaluation of adnexal
      masses
  in postmenopausal women, 120–121
  in premenopausal women, 118
  in young women, 117, 120*b*

U

Uchida procedure, for tubal steriliza-
      tion, 149*t*
Ulcer(s), acute genital, in pediatric
      patient, 180

Ultrasonography
  accreditation
      Internet resources for, 21, 21*b*
      standards for, 21–22
  of breast mass, 174–175
  certification, 22
  Doppler
      of adnexal masses, 18*t*
      in diagnosis of deep vein thrombo-
          sis, 134
  of ectopic pregnancy, 112–113
  of embryonic development, in first
      trimester, 109*t*
  endoanal, indications for, 82
  fetal, first-trimester findings, 109*t*
  four-dimensional, 19
  of leiomyomas, 105
  magnetic resonance imaging-guided
      focused surgery, for leiomyomas,
      107
  pelvic, 18
  in prepubertal girl, 178–179
  renal, indications for, 82
  three-dimensional, 19
      advantages of, 19
      data acquisition for, 19
  training
      Internet resources for, 21*b*
      requirements for, 21
  transvaginal
      of adnexal masses, 18–19, 18*t*, 118
      in antepartum patient with bleed-
          ing, 3
      for endometrial stripe assessment,
          18
      of intrauterine pregnancy, 112
      of ovarian cyst, in premenopausal
          women, 118
      of postmenopausal ovarian cysts,
          19
United States Preventive Services Task
      Force
  recommendations on breast cancer
      screening, 176
  recommendations on cervical cancer
      screening, 26–27
Ureter(s)
  assessment of, after laparoscopic
      surgery, 13, 14
  injury
      computed tomography of, 18
      in laparoscopy, 14
      surgical, 124–125, 125*b*, 126*f*,
          127*t*, 136
      intraoperative management of, in
          laparoscopy, 14
      obstruction, secondary to surgical
          injury, management of, 125
Ureterovaginal fistula, 136
Urethra, age-related changes in, 76
Urethral bulking agents, for injection,
      102
Urethral diverticulum, diagnostic strate-
      gies for, 168*t*

Urethral prolapse, in pediatric patients, 181
Urinary incontinence
  stress
    pelvic support defects and, 80
    surgery for, 97–102
    surgical management of, information resources, 184
Urinary symptoms, pelvic support defects and, 80
Urinary tract. *See also* Bladder; Ureter(s)
  catheterization, and infection, 135
  disorders, pain caused by, 166t
Urinary tract infection(s)
  microbiology of, 135–136
  postoperative, 135–136
Urinary tract injury(ies)
  in laparoscopy, 125
  surgical, 125, 136
    incidence of, 124
    risk factors for, 124
Urogynecology procedures, antibiotic prophylaxis for, 141, 142t
Uterine artery embolization, for leiomyomas, 106
Uterine bleeding, abnormal, diagnostic hysteroscopy for, 3–4
Uterine cancer, magnetic resonance imaging of, 23, 23f
Uterine perforation, 5–6, 161
Uterine prolapse, surgical repair, 90–92
Uterine septa, hysteroscopic resection of, 4
Uterine suspension procedures, 90–92, 92f
Uterus, septate *versus* bicornuate, ultrasound differentiation of, 19

V
Vacuum aspiration, for nonviable first-trimester pregnancy, 110–111
Vagina
  age-related changes in, 76
  foreign bodies in, in pediatric patients, 181
  pediatric, magnetic resonance imaging of, 22
Vaginal atrophy, in older women, 27
Vaginal bulge, pelvic support defects and, 80
Vaginal ecosystem, 67
Vaginal flora, 67, 140–141
Vaginal lubricants, 76
Vaginal septa, magnetic resonance imaging of, 22
Vaginal splinting, pelvic support defects and, 80
Vaginal support, 78, 79f, 80b
Vaginitis, diagnostic flow chart for, 68f
Vaginoscopy, in prepubertal girl, 178
Valacyclovir, for herpes simplex virus infection, 75t
Valerian, potential perioperative effects of, 41t

Vascular access, obesity and, 46
Vasectomy, 154–155
Vasovagal syncope, intraoperative, 161
Vena cava, injury, in laparoscopy, 13
Vena cava filter, indications for, 135
Venlafaxine, and breast pain, 171b
Venography, in diagnosis of deep vein thrombosis, 134
Venous thromboembolism, 133–135
  causes of, 133
  prevention of, 44, 45t
    combined approach (dual prophylaxis), 46
    for obese patient, 138
    options for, 45–46
  risk, preoperative evaluation for, 133–134
  risk classification for, 44, 45t, 47, 48b, 133–134
  risk factors for, 44, 44b
Veress needle
  with expanding polymeric sleeve, 12
  intraabdominal placement of
    complications of, 9
    for laparoscopy, 9–10
  small bowel puncture by, 128
Verneuil disease. *See* Hidradenitis suppurativa
Vesicopsoas hitch, 127f
Vestibulectomy, for vulvar pain, 65
Vestibulodynia, 63
Viral infection(s), vulvovaginitis caused by, 67, 69b
Virginal ulcers, in pediatric patient, 180
Visceral pain
  etiologic possibilities, 165
  management of, 169
Vitamin B$_6$ deficiency, and venous thromboembolism, 45
Vitamin B$_{12}$ deficiency, 45
  treatment of, 47
  and venous thromboembolism, 45
Vitamin K, and anticoagulation reversal for emergent surgery, 47
Vulva
  benign disorders of, 55–66, 183
  contact dermatitis, 55–56, 56b, 71
  dermatitis of, 55–56, 55f
  dermatoses of, 57–60
  hidradenitis suppurativa of, 61–62, 61f
  lichen planus of, 59–60, 59f
  lichen simplex chronicus of, 55, 57
  psoriasis of, 58–59, 58f
  skin care guidelines for, for prevention and control of vulvar symptoms, 55, 56b
Vulvar cancer
  Human papillomavirus (HPV) and, 60
  lichen sclerosus and, 57–58
Vulvar hygiene, for prevention and control of vulvar symptoms, 55, 56b

Vulvar intraepithelial neoplasia
  epidemiology, 61
  human papillomavirus and, 60
  human papillomavirus-related, 61
  multifocal, 61
  treatment of, 61
  unifocal, 61
Vulvar pain, 55, 63–65. *See also* Vulvodynia
  chronic, diagnostic algorithm for, 64, 65f
  incidence of, 63
  precipitating factors, 63
Vulvar pruritus, 55
Vulvar vestibulitis, 63
Vulvodynia, 55, 63–65
  definition of, 63
  diagnosis of, 63–64
  generalized, 63
  incidence of, 63
  localized, 63
  management of, 63–65, 169
Vulvovaginitis
  candidal, 67, 69–72, 69b
    chronic, recurrent, 71
    clinical features of, 70t
    complicated, 71
    diagnosis of, 71
    and evaluation of sexual partners, 71
    and treatment of sexual partners, 71
    pathogenesis of, 69–71
    prevalence of, 69
    treatment of, 71–72, 72t
  causes, 67, 69b
  diagnostic flow chart for, 68f
  epidemiology, 67
  examination of patient with, 67
  infectious, 67, 69b
  information resources, 184
  noninfectious, 67, 69b
  pediatric, 179–180
  psychologic considerations in, 67
  psychosexual considerations in, 67
  trichomonad. *See* Trichomoniasis

W
Warfarin
  maintenance therapy with, 135
  perioperative management with, 47
Wart(s), genital. *See* Human papillomavirus
White blood cell count, in surgical patient, 41–42
Wickham striae, of lichen planus, 59, 59f
Wound contamination, and surgical site infection, 140

Y
Yeast infection(s). *See* Candidiasis